THOMPSON'S RHEUMATOLOGY POCKET REFERENCE

TABLE OF CONTENTS

Differential Disease	
Adult ...	
Ankyl...	
Antiph...	
Syndro...	
Bacter...	
Behcet...	
Calcium...	
Deposit...	
Churg S... (CSS) 23	
Complex Regional Pain Syndrome (CRPS) 26	
Cutaneous Vasculitis 29	
Diffuse Idiopathic Skeletal Hyperostosis (DISH) 32	
Erythema Nodosum (EN) 34	
Fibromyalgia (FM) 36	
Gonococcal Arthritis 39	
Gout 41	
Inflammatory Myositis 45	
Juvenile Idiopathic Arthritis - Oligoarticular 48	
Juvenile Idiopathic Arthritis - Polyarticular 52	
Juvenile Idiopathic Arthritis - Systemic 57	
Lyme Disease 62	
Microscopic Polyangiitis (MPA) 64	
Mixed Connective Tissue Disease (MCTD) 67	
Neuropathic Arthropathy 70	
Osteoarthritis (OA) 72	
Osteoporosis (OP) 75	
Polymyalgia Rheumatica (PMR) & Giant Cell Arteritis (GCA) 80	

Paget's Disease 83	
Polyarteritis Nodosa (PAN) 85	
... . 88	
... (RP) 91	
... . 94	
... (RP) 97	
... . 99	
... . 103	
Sjogren's Syndrome (SS) 108	
... Lupus Erythematosus (SLE) 111	
Systemic Sclerosis (SSc) 123	
Takayasu Arteritis (TA) 127	
Viral Arthritis 130	
Wegener's Granulomatosis (WG) 134	
Analgesics 138	
Biologics 149	
Corticosteroids 155	
Coxibs 161	
Disease Modifying Anti-Rheumatic Drugs (DMARDs) 163	
Gastroprotection 187	
Medications for Treatment of Gout & Hyperuricemia 190	
Non-Steroidal Anti-Inflammatory Drugs (NSAIDs) 195	
Osteoporosis & Metabolic Bone Disease 211	
Pulmonary Hypertension 224	
Salivary Stimulants 228	
Viscosupplementation 230	
The Rheumatology Laboratory 232	
Classification Criteria of the Rheumatic Diseases 239	
Index 251	

ANDY THOMPSON, MD

Reviewers: John M Esdaile MD, MPH; W Maksymowych MD; Janet E Pope MD MPH; Ed Keystone MD; Dafna Gladman MD; JD Adachi MD; Kenneth T Calamia MD; Kam Shojania MD; Barry Koehler MD; John Watterson MD; Graham Reid MB; Andy Chalmers MD; Alice Klinkhoff MD; Michael C Nimmo MD; Simon Huang MD; Ken Blocka MD; Carter Thorne MD; John Kelsall MD; Howard Stein MD; John P Wade MD; Marlene J Thompson BScPT

Thank-you: Steve and Beth Green (Tarascon) for all of your advice. Dr. Mike Crouzat for his inspiration and help with the cover art work.

✠ DEDICATION ✞

To my wife Marlene & son Callum, for your love, understanding, patience, & support

IMPORTANT - READ THIS!

The information in *Thompson's Rheumatology Pocket Reference* is compiled from sources believed to be reliable. Exhaustive efforts have been put forth to make the book as accurate as possible. ***However, the accuracy and completeness of this work cannot be guaranteed.*** Despite our best efforts this book may contain typographical errors and omissions. *Thompson's Rheumatology Pocket Reference* is intended as a quick and convenient reminder of information you have already learned elsewhere. The contents are to be used as a guide only, and health care professionals should use sound clinical judgement and individualize therapy to each specific patient care situation. This book is sold without warranties of any kind, expressed or implied, and the publisher, reviewers, and author disclaim any liability, loss or damage caused by the contents.

THOMPSON'S RHEUMATOLOGY POCKET REFERENCE, 3RD EDITION, 2006
ISBN 0-9739676-0-9 / 978-0-9739676-0-9 51495

Comments/Suggestions: andy.thompson@rogers.com

DIFFERENTIAL DIAGNOSES

INFECTIOUS ARTHRITIS
(a) Viral: HIV, hepatitis B/C, Parvo B19, EBV, Rubella; *(b) Bacterial:* Gonococcal; Non-Gonococcal (Gram positive (75-80%), Gram negative (20-25%)); Rickettsia; Mycoplasma; *(c) Rheumatic Fever; (d) Bowel Bacterial Overgrowth; (e) SAPHO; (f) Mycobacterium:* Tuberculosis; *(g) Fungal:* Coccidioidomycosis; Sporotrichosis; Blastomycosis; Cryptococcus; Histoplasmosis; *(h) Spirochetes:* Borrelia Burgdorferi (Lyme); Treponema Pallidum (Syphilis)

CRYSTALLINE ARTHROPATHIES
(a) Monosodium Urate Deposition (Gout); (b) Calcium Pyrophosphate Deposition (CPPD); (c) Basic Calcium Phosphate Deposition

RHEUMATOID ARTHRITIS & VARIANTS
(a) Rheumatoid Arthritis; (b) Juvenile Inflammatory Arthritis; (c) Adult Still's Disease

SERONEGATIVE ARTHRITIDES
(a) Psoriatic Arthritis; (b) Ankylosing Spondylitis; (c) Reactive Arthritis; (d) Enteropathic Arthritis; (e) Undifferentiated Spondyloarthropathy

CONNECTIVE TISSUE DISEASES
(a) Systemic Lupus Erythematosus; (b) Sjogren's Syndrome; (c) Inflammatory Myopathies; (d) Systemic Sclerosis; (e) Overlap Syndromes; (f) Mixed Connective Tissue Disease; (g) Undifferentiated CTD; (h) Relapsing Polychondritis; (i) Behcet's Disease. *Vasculities: (a) Large Vessel:* Takayasu Arteritis; Giant-Cell Arteritis; *(b) Medium Vessel:* Polyarteritis Nodosa; Kawasaki's Disease; Isolated CNS vasculitis; *(c) Small Vessel:* Hypersensitivity Vasculitis (drugs, infection); ANCA associated (WG, CSS, MPA) vasculitis; Cryoglobulinemic vasculitis; Henoch Schonlein Purpura; Vasculitis secondary to CTD; Malignancy assoc vasculitis; Vasculitis mimics - Sepsis

DEGENERATIVE ARTHRITIDES
(a) Primary Osteoarthritis; (b) Secondary Osteoarthritis: Hereditary -Type II collagen defect; Mechanical - Post traumatic; Metabolic - Hemochromatosis, CPPD; Neurovascular

ARTHRITIS ASSOCIATED WITH SYSTEMIC DISEASE
(a) Sarcoidosis; (b) Metabolic: Hemochromatosis; Wilson's; Amyloidosis; Lipids; *(c) Endocrine:* Diabetes; Acromegaly; Thyroid; Parathyroid; *(d) Hematologic:* Hemophilia; Sickle Cell; Thalassemia; Leukemia; Myeloma; *(e) Malignancy:* Carcinomatous polyarthritis, metastatic disease; Myositis; Hypertrophic; osteoarthropathy

NEOPLASMS
(a) Pigmented Villo Nodular Synovitis (PVNS); (b) Synovial Chondromatosis; (c) Synovioma

NEUROVASCULAR
(a) Avascular Necrosis (AVN); (b) Neuropathic Arthritis

SOFT-TISSUE RHEUMATISM
(a) Fibromyalgia (FM)

ARTHRITIS ASSOCIATED WITH TRAUMA (BURNS, FROSTBITE ETC)

Acute Monoarthritis: (a) Infection; (b) Crystals; (c) RA & Variant - Monoarticular onset; (d) Seronegative - Monoarticular onset; (e) CTD - Monoarticular onset; (f) Systemic Disease - Sarcoidosis; (g) Osteoarthritis; (h) Neoplasm; (i) Avascular Necrosis, Neuropathic Joint; (j) Traumatic

Chronic Monoarthritis: (a) Infection - atypical mycobacterium; (b) Crystals; (c) RA & variants; (d) Seronegatives; (e) Connective Tissue Diseases; (f) Systemic Disease; (g) Osteoarthritis; (h) Neoplasms; (i) Neurovascular; (j) Traumatic - resulting instability

Acute Oligoarthritis: (a) Infection (gonococcal); (b) Crystals; (c) RA & Variants - ASD, JIA; (d) Seronegatives; (e) Connective Tissue Diseases; (f) Systemic Disease - Sarcoidosis

Chronic Oligoarthritis: (a) Seronegatives; (b) Connective Tissue Diseases; (c) Systemic Disease; (d) Osteoarthritis; (e) Neurovascular

Acute Polyarthritis: (a) Infection (gonococcal & viral); (b) Crystals - rarely; (c) RA & Variants; (d) Seronegatives (reactive); (e) Connective Tissue Diseases; (f) Systemic Disease

Chronic Polyarthritis: (a) Infection - unusual; (b) Crystals - can mimic RA; (c) RA & Variants; (d) Seronegatives; (e) Connective Tissue Diseases; (f) Systemic Disease; (g) Osteoarthritis

Dactylitis: (a) Infection - Tuberculosis; (b) Crystals - Gout; (c) Seronegatives - Psoriatic & Reactive; (d) Systemic Disease (sarcoidosis)

Polyarthritis & Fever: (a) Infection; (b) Crystals; (c) RA & Variants (ASD, Systemic JIA)); (d) Connective Tissue Diseases (SLE, DM/PM, TA, KD, PAN, WG, CSS, MPA, CRYO, Hypersensitivity); (e) Familial Mediterranean Fever; (f) Systemic Disease; (g) Neoplasms

Polyarthritis & Raynaud's: (a) RA & Variants; (b) Connective Tissue Diseases (SSc, SLE, PM/DM, SS, Vasculitis - cryoglobulinemia)

Polyarthritis & Skin Rash: (a) Infection; (b) RA & Variants (ASD, Systemic JIA); (c) Seronegatives; (d) Connective Tissue Diseases (SLE, DM, SS, Behcet's, CSS, MPA, WG, Hypersensitivity, cryoglobulins); (e) Systemic Disease (sarcoidosis)

Polyarthritis & Nodules: (a) Infection; (b) Crystals (gout); (c) RA & Variants; (d) Seronegatives; (e) Connective Tissue Diseases (SLE, SSc (calcific), Behcet's, PAN, SVV); (f) Systemic Disease (lipids); (g) Osteoarthritis; (h) Neoplasms

Polyarthritis & Lung Involvement: (a) Infection; (b) RA & Variants; (c) Seronegatives (AS); (d) Connective Tissue Diseases (SLE, SSc, SS, PM/DM, SVV (WG, CSS, MPA, Hypersensitivity)); (e) Systemic Disease (Sarcoidosis)

Polyarthritis & Cardiac Involvement: (a) Infection (SBE, Rheumatic fever); (b) RA & Variants; (c) Seronegatives (AS); (d) Connective Tissue Diseases (SLE, aCL/LA, SSc, DM/PM, KD, PAN, WG, CSS, MPA, HSV); (e) Systemic Disease (Hemochromatosis)

Polyarthritis & Renal Involvement: (a) Infection (SBE); (b) Crystals (Gout); (c) Connective Tissue Diseases (SLE, SSc, Vasculitis (WG, MPA, CSS, Hypersensitivity, Cryos); (d) Systemic Disease (Amyloidosis)

Polyarthritis & GI Involvement: (a) Infection (Whipple's); (b) Seronegatives (IBD, ReA); (c) Connective Tissue Diseases (SSc, Behcet's, Vasculitis); (d) Systemic Disease (Amyloidosis, Celiac Disease, Collagenous and Microscopic Colitis); (e) Intestinal Bypass Arthritis; (f) Whipple's Disease

Polyarthritis & Hepatic Involvement: (a) Infection (Hep B & C); (b) Seronegatives (IBD); (c) Connective Tissue Diseases (SLE, SSc, SS, Vasculitis); (d) Systemic Disease (Hemochromatosis, Amyloidosis)

Polyarthritis & Ocular Inflammation: (a) Infection; (b) Seronegatives (AS, ReA, IBD); (c) Connective Tissue Diseases (SLE, SS, Behcet's, Relapsing Polychondritis, WG); (d) Systemic Disease (Sarcoidosis)

Low Back Pain: (1) MECHANICAL: Lumbar Strain or Sprain; Discogenic / Herniated Disc; Zygoapophyseal (Facet) arthropathy; Spinal Stenosis; Spondylolisthesis; Traumatic Fracture; Congenital Abnormality; Spondylolysis; **(2) NON-MECHANICAL:** (a) Malignancy: Metastases; Myeloma; Lymphoma & Leukemia; Spinal Cord Tumors; Retroperitoneal Tumors; Primary Vertebral Tumors; (b) Infection: Osteomyelitis; Septic Disciitis; Paraspinal Abscess; Epidural Abscess; **(3) INFLAMMATORY:** Ankylosing Spondylitis; Psoriatic Arthritis; Reactive Arthritis; IBD; Paget's; **(4) VISCERAL:** (a) Pelvic Disease: Prostatitis; Endometriosis; Chronic PID; (b) Renal Disease: Nephrolithiasis; Pyelonephritis; Perinephric Abscess; Aortic Aneurysm; (c) Gastrointestinal Disease: Pancreatitis; Cholecystitis; Penetrating Ulcer

Proximal Muscle Weakness: (1) INFLAMMATORY MYOSITIS: Polymyositis; Dermatomyositis; Inclusion Body Myositis; Overlap Syndromes; Juvenile Dermatomyositis; **(2) DRUGS & TOXINS:** Alcohol; Corticosteroids; Illicit Drugs - Cocaine, Heroin; Colchicine - myoneuropathy; Statins; Anti-malarials; Zidovudine; Amiodarone; **(3) INFECTION:** (a) Viral: Influenza; Parainfluenza; Cocksackie; HIV; CMV, EBV, Adenovirus; (b) Bacterial; (c) Fungal; (d) Parasitic; **(4) MALIGNANCY; (5) ENDOCRINE:** Hypothyroidism; Cushing's Syndrome; **(6) ELECTROLYTE:** Hypokalemia; Hypophosphatemia; Hypocalcemia; Hyper/Hyponatremia; **(7) METABOLIC:** carbohydrate; Lipid

Polymyalgia: (a) Polymyalgia Rheumatica; (b) Seronegative RA; (c) Hypothyroidism; (d) Bacterial Endocarditis; (e) Polymyositis; (f) Amyloidosis; (g) Malignancy; (h) Fibromyalgia

Fibromyalgia: (1) RHEUMATIC DISORDERS: Fibromyalgia; Autoimmune disorders (RA, SLE, Sjogren's, SSc); Seronegative spondyloarthropathies; Inflammatory and metabolic myopathies; Polymyalgia rheumatica; **(2) ENDOCRINOPATHIES:** Hypothyroidism; Addison's disease; Cushing's syndrome; Hyperparathyroidism; **(3) NEUROLOGIC DISORDERS:** Entrapment neuropathies; Cervical spine disease (radiculopathy); Autoimmune disorders (Myasthenia gravis, Multiple sclerosis); **(4) INFECTION:** Parvovirus B19; Hepatitis C; Lyme Disease; **(5) SLEEP DISORDERS:** Obstructive sleep apnea; **(6) MEDICATIONS:** Lipid lowering drugs; antiviral medications; Tapering of corticosteroids; **(7) MALIGNANCY**

Extra-Articular Calcification: (a) Calcium pyrophosphate deposition; (b) Hydroxyapatite deposition; (c) Systemic sclerosis; (d) Juvenile dermatomyositis; (e) Hyperparathyroidism; (f) Myositis ossificans

ADULT STILL'S DISEASE (ASD)

DEFINITION & PATHOPHYSIOLOGY

Definition: Adult Still's Disease (ASD) is a variant of systemic juvenile inflammatory arthritis which occurs in adults and is characterized by an inflammatory seronegative polyarthritis with prominent systemic features

Pathophysiology: The principle hypothesis is ASD results from an infectious agent

PRESENTATION

Identifying Data: Typically a young patient aged 16-35; Male: Female ratio is equal; Prevalence about 0.01% in the population

Onset: Initial features are typically non-specific, including myalgias, arthralgias, malaise, weight-loss, and sore throat. *(a) High Spiking Fever:* Patients develop the dramatic onset of a sudden high-spiking fever to 39 degrees C or higher: The fever occurs once daily (quotidian) or twice daily (double quotidian) but returns to normal; The peak is usually in the late afternoon or early evening; About 20% of patients will have fever spike that does not return to normal; *(b) Rash:* Patients develop the characteristic evanescent salmon-colored rash which is macular or maculopapular: The rash may only be present with the fever spike; The rash may be elicited with heat or by the Koebner phenomenon. Therefore, it can typically be found in areas of mechanical pressure - belt line or beneath the breasts. *(c) Arthritis:* Arthritis is present in all patients: Initially the arthritis may be oligoarticular but can progress into potentially destructive polyarticular disease; The knees and wrists are most commonly affected

Progression: Self-limited (20%) pattern with complete resolution of symptoms, usually within one year; Intermittent (30%) pattern with one or more disease flares surrounding periods of complete remission. Relapses tend to be less severe and of shorter duration; Progressive (50%) pattern with active disease usually due to persistent inflammatory arthritis

Constitutional Features: Prominent fatigue, weight loss, arthralgias, and myalgias

Functional Status: With treatment, functional status is usually quite good with 90% achieving an ACR category 1 functional status

RHEUMATOLOGIC REVIEW OF SYSTEMS

Mucocutaneous Involvement: Pharyngitis: Non-suppurative

Lymphatic Involvement: Lymphadenopathy

Cardiac Involvement: Pericarditis

Respiratory Involvement: Pleuritis; Pneumonitis

Gastrointestinal Involvement: Hepatomegaly; Splenomegaly

RISK FACTORS

No known risk factors

FAMILY HISTORY

Familial cases are exceedingly rare

RED FLAGS

Rule out infection

DIFFERENTIAL DIAGNOSIS

(a) Adult Still's Disease; (b) Rheumatic Fever (c) Connective Tissue Diseases: SLE; Dermatomyositis; MCTD; Vasculitis; (d) Sarcoidosis; (e) Infection; (f) Malignancy

PHYSICAL EXAMINATION

Vitals: Pulse: Elevated if acutely ill and febrile; BP: Low if volume depleted; RR: Normal to elevated; Temperature: Quotidian or diquotidian fever pattern

Cutaneous: Macular evanescent salmon colored rash found commonly on the trunk or in areas under mechanical stress (belt line, underneath the breasts)

Head & Neck: l ymphadenopathy; Erythematous pharynx - pharyngitis
Respiratory: Pleural friction rub due to underlying pleuritis; Reduced breath sounds due to small pleural effusions; Axillary adenopathy
Cardiovascular: Pericardial friction rub
Gastrointestinal: Enlarged liver and/or spleen
Musculoskeletal: Inflammatory arthritis
Neurologic: No specific findings

INVESTIGATIONS

CBC: Normochromic normocytic anemia (occasionally profound); leukocytosis in 90% (80% of cases it is greater than 15,000); reactive thrombocytosis
ESR: Universally elevated
Hypoalbuminemia: Seen in about 50%
Liver Function Tests: Elevation of AST and LDH seen in 75% of patients
Ferritin: Very high elevations of ferritin can be seen in up to 70% of patients. Levels > 3000 should lead to suspicion of ASD.
Rheumatoid Factor: Usually negative
ANA: Usually negative
Radiology: Early in the disease course soft-tissue swelling, effusions, and periarticular osteopenia; Erosive narrowing of the CMC joints and intercarpal joints of the wrist which may become ankylosed

MANAGEMENT

General: Education about the disease; Vocational counseling; Arthritis self management programs
Physical Therapy: Joint protection; Active and passive ROM; Strengthening; Wt loss
Occupational Therapy: Splints & braces; Assistive devices; Ambulatory devices - Canes; Orthotics
NSAIDs: In some cases (25%) NSAIDs or high dose ASA is all that is required to control symptoms adequately. These patients tend to have a good prognosis. Main concern with NSAIDs is hepatotoxicity and frequent monitoring of LFTs is mandatory
Corticosteroids: Indications for corticosteroids include: (a) Poor response to NSAIDs; (b) NSAID toxicity (rising LFTs on NSAIDs); (c) Debilitating joint symptoms; (d) Internal organ involvement (pericarditis with tamponade, myocarditis, pneumonitis); Usual dose of prednisone is 0.5 - 1 mg/kg/day with 30% of patients requiring at least 60 mg of prednisone daily
Disease Modifying Agents: Inflammatory arthritis is the most common cause for chronicity in ASD. Failure to reduce prednisone to an acceptable level prompts the introduction of DMARDs. Methotrexate, sulfasalazine, IM gold, and hydroxychloroquine have all been used; however, no controlled studies have been published. Azathioprine, cyclophosphamide, and cyclosporine have been introduced in more resistant cases
Biologics: Etanercept and infliximab have been used in refractory cases with excellent results. Anakinra has been used in cases refractory to etanercept & infliximab.

PROGNOSIS

Risk Stratification for Poor Progression: (a) Development of polyarthritis early in the disease course; (b) Involvement of root joints (shoulders and hips); (c) The need for more than 2 years of systemic therapy
Prognosis: The median time to enter remission with therapy is 10 months and 2 1/2 years to discontinuation of all therapy; 5 year survival is 90-95%

ANKYLOSING SPONDYLITIS (AS)

DEFINITION & PATHOPHYSIOLOGY

Definition: A chronic inflammatory disease of the axial skeleton resulting in back pain and progressive stiffness and may be associated with characteristic extra-spinal lesions; See the Rome and New York Criteria for the diagnosis of AS (page *239*)

Pathophysiology: The current theory involves AS developing after exposure to a foreign antigen in a genetically susceptible individual (HLAB27 positive)

PRESENTATION

Identifying Data: Typical patient is a young male or young adult (20's or 30's - average age 26); Male: female ratio of about 3:1; Prevalence within the population depends on HLA-B27 positivity (0.1-1%)

Onset: (a) Spine: Insidious onset of low back/alternating buttock pain: Noticeable morning stiffness > 60 minutes; Improves with activity, however, may worsen with too much activity as the day progresses; Worse with overnight rest and sleep is impaired due to pain and stiffness - a definite contributor to fatigue; Thoracic spinal involvement may result in stiffness in the upper back between the scapulae; Cervical involvement may result in neck pain. *(b) Peripheral joint involvement:* A minority of patients may present with associated inflammation of the hips; Other patients may have an associated oligoarthritis that particularly affects the ankles, hips, and knees; *(c) Enthesitis:* Entheseal involvement may be confused with true joint involvement. For example, shoulder involvement is primarily an enthesopathy of the supraspinatus. True joint involvement of the upper limbs is unusual; however, entheseal involvement of the upper limbs is common (up to 15% of patients may have an associated shoulder enthesopathy).

Progression: Pain & stiffness; May be fluctuant and flare on and off over a period of months; Each flare can last days to months; Continued inflammation may result in persistent pain, however, once spinal ankylosis occurs, the pain may improve

Constitutional Features: Fatigue may be prominent due to sleep difficulties

Functional Status: Reduced functional status with difficulties in ADLs; Difficulty at work - Employment affected in 30% of males; Loss of libido; Depression

RHEUMATOLOGIC REVIEW OF SYSTEMS

Musculoskeletal Involvement: Entheseal Involvement: Greater trochanter, plantar fascia, Achilles tendon, pelvis, costochondral junction, patella, rotator cuff insertions (supraspinatus), and elbow; Osteoporosis of the spine

Ocular Involvement: Acute anterior uveitis in 40%. Unilateral and recurrent.

Neurologic Involvement: Cord or root lesions following spinal fracture; Cervical spine subluxation; Cauda equina syndrome due to arachnoiditis

Cardiac Involvement: Aortitis with dilatation of the aortic ring and regurgitation (rare)

Respiratory Involvement: Rigidity of the chest wall with reduced chest expansion; Progressive upper lobe fibrosis in 0.5%

Gastrointestinal Involvement: Subclinical changes in small or large bowel in 60%

Renal Involvement: IgA nephropathy and amyloidosis

RISK FACTORS

(a) HLA-B27 positivity in > 90% of patients with AS vs. 3-7% of the general population; *(b) Family history* is the biggest risk factor: A first degree relative with AS increases the risk to 5-20%; If the child is HLAB27 negative the risk is lower 5% and if the child is HLAB27 positive it increases to 20%

FAMILY HISTORY

Family history is a major risk factor for developing AS (see above)

RED FLAGS

(a) New onset acute back pain or change in chronic back pain; (b) Continuous pain not relieved or worsens with supine position; (c) Constant pain that does not change with activity; (d) Severe night pain that wakes from sleep; (e) Fever, chills, or weight loss; (f) Bladder/bowel dysfunction; (g) Saddle anesthesia; (h) Loss of muscle bulk or weakness; (i) Difficulty walking; (j) Sensory abnormalities; (k) Past history of cancer or osteoporosis; (l) History of major or minor trauma

DIFFERENTIAL DIAGNOSIS

(a) Ank. Spond.; (b) Psoriatic, reactive, and enteropathic arthritides; (c) Mechanical LBP; (d) DISH; (e) Paget's; (f) Infection; (g) Malignancy; (h) Fibromyalgia

PHYSICAL EXAMINATION

Vitals: P: Normal; BP: Normal; RR: Elevated if respiratory involvement; T: Normal

Cutaneous: No specific findings

Head & Neck: Uveitis

Respiratory: Adventitious sounds (crackles) at the apices suggesting apical fibrosis.

Cardiovascular: Murmur of aortic regurgitation - aortitis.

Gastrointestinal: No specific findings

Musculoskeletal: Oligoarticular inflammatory arthritis predominantly affecting the lower extremity; Entheseal pain with shoulder pain (rotator cuff tendonitis), lateral hip pain (greater trochanter), heel pain (Achilles tendonitis), costochondral junction pain, and plantar fascial pain

Neurologic: Cord or root signs if spinal cord or roots are compromised.

EXAMINATION OF THE INFLAMMATORY SPINE

Gait: Trendelenburg gait if associated hip pathology. With severe hip or knee flexion deformities, a patient may need to walk on the toes on that side as the foot won't touch the floor - Rare

Inspection: Flattening of the lumbar lordosis with spinal disease. If the lumbar lordosis is increased, think of hip involvement as associated hip flexion contractures may lead to an increased lumbar lordosis to keep the patient upright. Increased thoracic kyphosis resulting in a stooped posture with a forward set head position and difficulty in looking upwards.

Flexion: Observe the rhythm with flexion (smooth), the extent, and pain (i.e. smooth, full, pain-free flexion of the lumbar spine); Observe as the patient extends to neutral (comes up) from the flexed position – Can see two common abnormalities: (a) Hands placed on the thighs to help walk themselves back up (more commonly seen in mechanical back pain); (b) Reversed spinal rhythm - Patient flexes the knees to bring the hips underneath the body, followed by hip extension bringing the back to a vertical position, finally they simply stand up

Extension: Put patient's thighs against the examination table so they don't cheat and ask them to extend. Again looking for smooth, full, pain-free ROM. (Patient's with inflammatory back disease typically lose their ability to extend)

Lateral Flexion: Ask the patient to stand against the wall with their buttocks and shoulder blades touching the wall and make a mark on the thigh at the position of the tip of the middle finger. Ask the patient to laterally flex (slide down the wall) and make a mark at the tip of the middle finger (maximum lateral flexion). Measure the distance between the two marks (Patient's with inflammatory back disease typically lose lateral flexion early in the disease process).

Rotation: In the sitting position, ask the patient to cross their arms in front of them and rotate to the left and right and compare the ranges of rotation (at least 45 degrees – up to 90 degrees). Rotation is often lost in inflammatory spinal diseases.

Hip Involvement: Loss of internal rotation is a sensitive measure of change for hip involvement. It is a poor prognosticator to have root joints involved.

Occiput to wall distance: Distance from the patient's occiput to wall (normal 0 cm)

Chest Expansion: Tape measure is placed at the level of the xiphisternum. Deep inhalation then deep exhalation followed by a deep inspiration. Measure the distance the tape moves from full expiration to full inspiration. Normal is dependent on age and sex. This measure is more useful for following patients over time.

Measure the fingertip to floor distance: In full flexion

Lateral flexion - See above

Modified Schober test: Mark at S2 (PSIS) with the patient in standing; Place marks 10 cm up and 5 cm down from the original mark at S2; Ask the patient to fully flex and measure the distance between the upper an lower mark; The gap should increase from 15 cm to a minimum of 20 cm with full flexion

Modified modified Schober test: Make a mark at S2 (PSIS) with the patient in standing; Ask the patient to fully flex. While in full flexion, place marks at 10 cm, 20 cm, and 30 cm up from the original mark at S2; In the prone position, ask the patient to do a "sloppy pushup" – hands to the side and do a pushup keeping the pelvis on the table; In full extension measure the compression of the three 10 cm segments (normal from top to bottom should be 2-3 cm, 3-4 cm, and 4-5 cm)

SI Compression Testing: These tests are included for historical purpose only. They are better predictors of mechanical back pain. (a) Cross armed test pushing on either side of the iliac crests; (b) Flex the hip and exert pressure down through the femur; (c) FABER test (Flexion – Abduction, External Rotation); (d) Gainslands Test

Trendelenburg Test: Place hands on both iliac crests; Ask the patient to lift the left leg off the ground and stand on the right leg. The left iliac crest should come up slightly. If the left iliac crest remains or falls then the test is positive. Positive test is due to weak hip abductors on the right side. Switch legs and test the other side.

Thomas Test: To look for hip flexion contractures

INVESTIGATIONS

CBC: Mild normochromic, normocytic anemia

ESR/CRP: Mild elevations

ALP: May be slightly elevated

Immunoglobulins: Mild elevation in IgA

HLA-B27: Occurs in 95% of patients with AS compared to 6% of general population.

Sacroiliac Joints: Sacroiliitis is usually bilateral and the most frequent and earliest radiographic manifestation of AS. (a) Grade 1 – Pseudowidening of the sacroiliac Joints due to erosions of subchondral bone with loss of definition of joint margins, superficial erosions, and surrounding osteopenia. (b) Grade 2 - Bony sclerosis at one or both joint margins (c) Grade 3 - Sclerosis and erosions at both joint margins (d) Grade 4 - Bony fusion and loss of sclerosis

Differential Diagnosis of Sacroiliitis Includes: Ank. Spond; Other seronegative arthropathies; Septic sacroiliitis; Osteitis condensans ilii; Degenerative SI joints;

Symphysis Pubis: Osteitis pubis: Sclerosis & bony irreg. at the symphysis pubis;

Enthesitis: Bony erosions or "whiskering" along the margins of the ischial tuberosities, iliac crests, or the proximal trochanters are indicative of enthesitis

Spine: Spinal involvement is usually present when sacroiliitis is documented or follows shortly thereafter; Most common sites of origin are the thoracolumbar and lumbosacral regions; **Alignment:** Flattening of the normal lumbar lordosis; Dorsal thoracic kyphosis; **Bones:** Squaring of vertebrae with shiny corners; Inflammation at the discovertebral interface (osteitis and erosions); Calcification of the anterior longitudinal ligament fills in the normal concave anterior contour; Ossification of spinal ligaments; Formation of Syndesmophytes - Originate and insert at the upper and lower margins of adjacent vertebral bodies. They are gracile ossifications of the fibers of the annulus fibrosus of the intervertebral disc and are usually bilateral in AS. When many syndesmophytes are present the spine takes on the appearance of the classic bamboo spine. (Syndesmophytes in ReA and PsA tend to be asymmetric and have non-marginal origins and insertions). Generalized Osteopenia - Probably due to immobility and local cytokine release; Zygoapophyseal Joints - Go through a similar process of inflammation and subsequent bony fusion

Complications: (a) Spinal fracture with minimal trauma which can result in a pseudoarthrosis; (b) Spondylodiscitis: A sterile, circumscribed, destructive process involving one vertebral body and adjacent intervertebral disc which may mimic infection; (c) Accelerated segment degeneration; (d) Atlanto-axial instability and subluxation; (e) Dorsal kyphosis; (f) Cauda-Equina syndrome

Peripheral Joints: Can develop an erosive inflammatory arthritis, however, hip and knee involvement is usually non-erosive

Aspiration & Pathology: Subchondral edema is the earliest pathologic finding; Inflammation has a predilection for sites rich in fibrocartilage

MANAGEMENT
General: Education

Physiotherapy: Regular exercise may slow the progression of spinal stiffness and restriction: It is imperative that patients work with a physiotherapist and understand the role of stretching and exercise to minimize the long-term impact of their condition

NSAIDs & Analgesics: May dramatically reduce pain and spinal stiffness; Long-acting NSAIDs taken at night may reduce night discomfort and morning stiffness

Corticosteroids: Local corticosteroid injections may be of value for enthesteal pain and peripheral synovitis; Local corticosteroid injection into the sacroiliac joints may be of benefit; Brief courses of oral or parenteral steroids may be helpful in overcoming severe spinal or peripheral inflammatory disease

DMARDs: Sulfasalazine may be useful in peripheral synovitis but not as effective in spinal involvement; No controlled trials to support the use of Methotrexate

Biologics: Etanercept - Gorman et al, NEJM 2002 - 50% achieving an ASAS50 and >20% achieving an ASAS70; Infliximab - Braun et al, Lancet 2002 - 50% of patients achieved a 50% improvement in BASDAI, better patient global health, reduced CRP, and more spinal mobility. OR 60% patients approved to ASAS 40. Patients with high CRP tended to be better responders; Adalimumab: No published trials.

Bisphosphonates: Improve osteoporosis associated with AS; Pamidronate may also improve inflammatory symptoms of AS

PROGNOSIS
Risk Stratification for Poor Progression: Traditional poor prognosticators include. (a) Hip Involvement; (b) High ESR, (c) Poor efficacy of NSAIDs; (d) Limitation of ROM of Lumbar Spine; (e) Dactylitis; (f) Oligoarthritis; (g) Onset < 16 years of age; If no poor prognosticators then mild disease course is likely. The presence of hip involvement or 3 other factors virtually excludes mild disease and makes the likelihood of severe disease much more but does not completely estimate risk.

Prognosis: Most patients with mild disease are able to continue with a reasonable level of functional activity and full time employment; Disease activity fluctuates over decades with very few individuals entering long term remission (1%); AS does not affect overall mortality; Physiotherapy is extremely important for keeping mobility and reducing contractures

ANTIPHOSPHOLIPID ANTIBODY SYNDROME (APLAS)

DEFINITION & PATHOPHYSIOLOGY

Definition: An autoimmune disease characterized by recurrent arterial or venous thrombosis or recurrent pregnancy losses with the persistent presence of a lupus anticoagulant or anticardiolipin antibodies; See the Criteria for APLAS (page 239).

Pathophysiology: ß2-glycoprotein-1 is thought to be a natural in-vivo anticoagulant because of its ability to bind to negatively charged phospholipids and thereby inhibit contact activation of the intrinsic coagulation pathway. Antiphospholipid antibodies are predominantly targeted towards ß2-glycoprotein-1. Other phospholipid binding proteins described are prothrombin, protein C, protein S, and annexin V. The antigenic specificities of the lupus anticoagulant include prothrombin and ß2-glycoprotein-1. Pathogenic mechanisms of antiphospholipid antibodies include: Inhibition of activated protein C; Inhibition of the antithrombin III pathways; Inhibition of fibrinolysis; Upregulation of tissue factor activity; Interference with the role of ß2-glycoprotein-1. Antiphospholipid antibodies bind to ß2-glycoprotein-1 on the endothelial surface resulting in endothelial cell activation. Inhibit the binding of annexin V to procoagulant surfaces

PRESENTATION

Identifying Data: Typical patient is a young female of reproductive age

Onset: (a) Laboratory Detection: Detection of a lupus anticoagulant or antiphospholipid antibodies in an otherwise asymptomatic patient. ***(b) Thrombosis:*** Most common clinical manifestation is thrombosis. Venous thrombosis occurs in up to 55% of patients and arterial thrombosis in up to 50%. Arterial sites of occlusion include the coronary vessels, eye, kidney, and peripheral arteries. ***(c) Pregnancy Loss:*** Risk of pregnancy loss is greatest from the 10th week of gestation. Criteria for pregnancy loss: (a) 3 or more unexplained spontaneous pregnancy losses prior to 10 weeks with maternal anatomic or hormonal abnormalities and paternal and maternal chromosome abnormalities excluded; (b) 1 or more unexplained deaths of a morphologically normal fetus after 10 weeks; (c) 1 or more premature births of a normal fetus prior to 34 weeks. ***(d) Catastrophic Antiphospholipid Antibody Syndrome:*** Multiorgan involvement of rapid onset associated with high mortality (thrombotic storm). Mortality as high as 50%; Precipitants: Infection, surgery, withdrawal of anticoagulation, drugs (OCP), and malignancy

Progression: Involves recurrent thrombotic events or recurrent fetal losses; The risk of recurrent thromboses, without treatment, is estimated to be 0.15-0.19 thrombotic events per patient year after the initial event – about 30% per year; Risk of thrombosis in patients with pregnancy loss only is unknown; Risk of thrombosis in asymptomatic patients with serologic evidence of LA or aCL is unknown.

Constitutional Features: Fatigue may be a prominent feature

Functional Status: Reduced functional status with difficulties in ADLs due to fatigue and sequelae of thrombosis; Higher incidence of depression

RHEUMATOLOGIC REVIEW OF SYSTEMS

Associated Conditions: Systemic Lupus Erythematosus: 12-30% have anticardiolipin antibodies and 15-34% have a lupus anticoagulant. 50% of those with aCL or LA have a history of thrombosis (6-15%)

Musculoskeletal Involvement: Avascular necrosis

Mucocutaneous Involvement: Livedo reticularis; Digital gangrene; Raynaud's

Hematologic Involvement: Thrombocytopenia: Typically mild and rarely associated with bleeding (100-150); Hemolytic anemia: Rare

Neurologic Involvement: Stroke; Seizure; Migraine headaches; Chorea; Memory loss & Dementia; Multiple sclerosis-like syndromes; Transverse myelopathy

Cardiac Involvement: Valvular vegetations

Respiratory Involvement: Pulmonary embolism

Gastrointestinal Involvement: Budd-Chiari synd. venous thrombosis in the liver

Renal Involvement: Renal artery or vein thrombosis

RISK FACTORS

Risk Factors for Thrombosis: (a) Previous history of thrombosis - Recurrent episodes tend to mimic the original vascular event (venous following venous and arterial following arterial); (b) Presence of a lupus anticoagulant; (c) High titer anticardiolipin antibodies; (d) Pregnancy; (e) Surgery

FAMILY HISTORY

May be an associated family history of blood clotting

RED FLAGS

Anti-phospholipid antibodies can be caused by HIV, medications, and malignancies

DIFFERENTIAL DIAGNOSIS

Differential Diagnosis of Anti-Phospholipid Antibody Production

Primary antiphospholipid antibody syndrome; Secondary APLAS: (a) Systemic lupus erythematosus; (b) Medications: Chlorpromazine; Phenytoin; Hydralazine; Procainamide; Quinidine; (c) Infections: HIV; (d) Neoplasm: Lymphoma

Other Causes of Thrombosis: (a) Factor V Leiden (activated protein-C resistance); (b) Protein C/S deficiency; (c) Antithrombin III deficiency; (d) Dysfibrinoginemia; (e) Hyper-homocysteinemia; (f) Nephrotic syndrome; (g) Meds – oral contraceptives

PHYSICAL EXAMINATION

Vitals: P: Normal; BP: Elevations in BP as may be an indicator of thrombosis (renal); RR: Elevated RR may indicate pulmonary embolism, cardiac valve involvement

Cutaneous: Raynaud's phenomenon; Digital infarcts and gangrene secondary to Raynaud's phenomenon; Livedo reticularis; See SLE *(111)*

Head & Neck: See SLE *(111)*

Respiratory: Pulmonary embolism - Pleural effusion, pleural rub, diminished breath sounds, hemoptysis, and elevated RR; See SLE *(111)*

Cardiovascular: Murmurs assoc. with valvular vegetations; See SLE *(111)*

Gastrointestinal: No specific findings; See SLE *(111)*

Musculoskeletal: Arthralgias; Myalgias; Associated fibromyalgia

Neurologic: Choreaform movements; Upper motor neuron signs related to CVA & transverse myelitis; Lower motor neuron signs related to assoc. multiple sclerosis

INVESTIGATIONS

CBC: Coomb's positive hemolytic anemia, thrombocytopenia (usually mild 100-150)

Persistent Lupus Anticoagulant: (2 positive measurements 6 weeks apart) Presence of a lupus anticoagulant seems to be associated with a higher thrombotic risk. A lupus anticoagulant is defined by the following: Elevated PTT: (a) PTT NOT corrected with mixing study; (b) PTT partially or completely corrects with addition of excess phospholipid; Confirmatory Test - Positive dRVVT or KCT - Confirmation by another phospholipid dependent assay such as the dilute Russell Viper Venom Test (dRVVT) or Kaolin Clotting Time (KCT)

Persistent Anti-Cardiolipin Antibodies: (IgG or IgM) by ELISA (2 positive measurements 6 weeks apart); Higher levels are associated with a higher thrombotic risk and IgG seems to be more thrombogenic than IgM or IgA

False positive VDRL

MANAGEMENT

General: Education

Patient with positive aPL but no clinical events: Treat conservatively with 81 mg ASA per day

Patient with positive aPL and one or more thrombotic events: Long-term anticoagulation with warfarin 3-4 mg/day aiming for a target INR of 3-3.5

Patient with positive aPL and recurrent fetal loss: ASA 81 mg as soon as conception is planned; Heparin 10,000 units BID as soon as a live intrauterine pregnancy is documented (7 weeks) – monitor platelet count weekly for the first 3 weeks of heparin (HIT); Continue heparin to term, stop in labor. Heparin is restarted in the post-partum period for 6 weeks.

Catastrophic APLAS: IV anticoagulation with heparin and IV corticosteroids; Consider plasmapheresis or IVIG

PROGNOSIS

In general, initial arterial thrombotic events are followed by arterial events and venous events are followed by venous events

BACTERIAL ARTHRITIS

DEFINITION & PATHOPHYSIOLOGY
Definition: An inflammatory arthritis secondary to bacterial invasion of a joint
Pathophysiology: Bacteria usually enter a joint through hematogenous spread from a remote extra-articular site of infection (70%). Other ways bacteria can enter a joint include: (a) Direct innoculation (penetrating trauma or iatrogenic infection from arthrocentesis or surgery; (b) Spread from a contiguous site (osteomyelitis); (c) Lymphatic spread. Bacteria enter the joint and deposit in the synovial membrane resulting in an intense inflammatory reaction

PRESENTATION
Identifying Data: Male: female ratio is equal; More common in older individuals
Onset: Patient may have a prodromal infective focus (UTI, respiratory, or skin); Fevers and chills may accompany the infection; The actual joint infection is characterized by an acute and very intense inflammatory response associated with considerable pain, swelling, redness, warmth, and loss of function; A monoarticular presentation is most common (80%) and tends to involve larger peripheral joints such as the knees (50%), hips, ankles, shoulders, wrists, & elbows; An oligoarticular/ polyarticular septic arthritis is less common (20%) and is typically seen in the setting of overwhelming sepsis
Progression: The arthritis can progress quite rapidly. Without rapid detection and appropriate treatment this progression can quickly lead to fulminant joint damage.
Constitutional Features: Fever, chills, night sweats, fatigue, anorexia, and wt. loss
Functional Status: Typically impaired in the setting of acute bacterial arthritis

RHEUMATOLOGIC REVIEW OF SYSTEMS
Associated Conditions: Patient may have associated sepsis

RISK FACTORS
(a) Host Factors: Age > 80 years; Comorbid illness; Immunosuppression; (b) Joint Abnormalities: Presence of a prosthetic joint; Recent joint surgery; Underlying arthritis (RA etc.); (c) Recent Infection: Recent skin infection; (d) Direct Penetrating Trauma

FAMILY HISTORY
No association

RED FLAGS
Aspirate the joint - *"To inject is human, to aspirate divine"* - Dr. Barry Koehler

DIFFERENTIAL DIAGNOSIS
(a) Bacterial arthritis (non-gonococcal); (b) Gonococcal arthritis; (c) Lyme arthritis; (d) Crystalline arthritis (gout/pseudogout); (e) Rheumatoid arthritis with a pseudoseptic joint; (f) Reactive arthritis; (g) Acute traumatic arthritis; (h) Tumor

PHYSICAL EXAMINATION
Vitals: Pulse: May be elevated; BP: May be elevated or low with sepsis, RR: May be elevated; Temperature: May be elevated
Cutaneous: Examine for a predisposing skin infection; Erythema overlying
Head & Neck: No specific findings
Respiratory: No specific findings
Cardiovascular: Murmurs (MR, AR) secondary to associated endocarditis
Gastrointestinal: No specific findings
Musculoskeletal: Intensely painful, erythematous, swollen, warm joint. Patients are typically very resistant to examination and movement of the joint.
Neurologic: No specific findings

INVESTIGATIONS
CBC: Leukocytosis (predominantly PMNs)

ESR/CRP: Elevated

Blood Cultures: Positive in up to 75% but usually less (50%)

Initial Radiographic Findings: Done initially to look for contiguous osteomyelitis; Usually normal with soft-tissue swelling at the time of initial diagnosis

Later Radiographic Findings: The hallmark of septic arthritis is aggressively rapid changing features (lysis, fragmentation) mixed with slower processes (sclerosis and periosteal bone reaction); ***Soft-Tissue:*** Edema; calcification may develop secondary to necrosis; ***Alignment:*** May be normal early on and proceed to joint deformity; ***Bones: Septic Arthritis:*** Normal; Periarticular osteopenia; Marginal erosions with destruction; Poorly defined bony destruction with "fuzzy" osseous margins; ***Contiguous Osteomyelitis:*** Periosteal reaction; Mixed lytic and sclerotic reaction; Sequestration (bone fragmentation); ***Joints:*** Joint space loss with erosions and bony ankylosis

Scintigraphy: Tc99 Pyrophosphate bone scan; Indium-111 labeled WBC scan - Useful in prosthetic joint infections and looking for osteomyelitis

Synovial Fluid: Cell Count: Ranges from 30 - 150 x 10^9 cells/L (30,000 - 150,000 cells/mm3), 85 - 90% are PMNs; Crystals: Co-existent crystals may exist; Gram Stain: Positive in 50-80% of cases with gram positive organisms easier to detect than gram negative ones; Culture: Positive in up to 95% of cases

Organisms: Gram positive cocci (80%): (a) Staphylococcus (60+%): Staphylococcus aureus (60%) - Commonest pathogen overall, it can affect any patient; Staphylococcus epidermidis - Common in prosthetic joints; (b) Streptococcus (20%): Streptococcus pneumoniae; Streptococcus pyogenes (group a); Streptococcus agalactiae (group b); Streptococcus viridans; (c) Enterococcus

Organisms: Gram negative (15%): Immune compromised (diabetics, alcoholics, malignancies, elderly, neonates, and IV drug abusers: Haemophilus influenzae; E. Coli; Pseudomonas aeruginosa; Serratia Marcescens

Organisms Anaerobes: Immune compromised: Clostridium perferingens; Bacteroides fragilis

MANAGEMENT

General: Rest, ice, & elevation; Physiotherapy for gentle range of motion

Analgesia: Acetaminophen; Narcotic analgesics; NSAIDS & COXIBs

Anti-Microbial Therapy (Antibiotics): Initial broad spectrum coverage: ***Gram positive organisms:*** Cefazolin; Vancomycin; Clindamycin; ***Gram negative organisms:*** Third generation cephalosporin (Cefotaxime, Ceftriaxone, or Ceftazidime); Aminoglycoside (Gentamicin); ***Anaerobes:*** Clindamycin, Cefoxitin, Penicillin, Vancomycin; ***Duration of Treatment:*** 4-6 weeks of IV antibiotics (2 weeks has been used for uncomplicated infections)

Surgical: Daily joint aspiration when amenable; Surgical drainage is indicated in: (a) Septic arthritis of the hip or shoulder or other difficult joints to drain; (b) Infected prosthetic joints; (c) Extra-articular extension (osteomyelitis); (d) Long-standing infection (adhesions created); (e) Underlying joint disease (rheumatoid arthritis)

PROGNOSIS

Risk Stratification for Poor Progression: (a) Polyarticular disease; (b) Delayed diagnosis; (c) Older individuals; (d) Prosthetic joint; (e) Concurrent immunosuppression; (f) Pre-existing joint disease (rheumatoid arthritis)

Prognosis: (a) Mortality: 10% in monarticular infections to 30% in polyarticular; Rheumatoid arthritis up to 20% mortality in monoarticular infections and up to 60% in polyarticular; ***(b) Morbidity:*** Poor outcome in up to 30% of cases with severe functional decline requiring prosthetic joint replacement, amputation, or arthrodesis

BEHCET'S DISEASE (BD)

DEFINITION & PATHOPHYSIOLOGY

Definition: Behcet's disease is a chronic inflammatory vascular disorder (vasculitis) characterized by recurrent mucocutaneous lesions (oral and genital ulceration), ocular inflammation, and potential involvement of other sites. Classification criteria for Behcet's (page 240).

Pathophysiology: The current theory is an environmental stimulus triggers the disease in patients who are genetically susceptible (HLA B51 positivity)

PRESENTATION

Identifying Data: Predominantly a disease of young adults with the mean age of onset between the ages of 25-30; Males and females are roughly affected equally, however, in western countries it is more common in females; The prevalence is highest in countries of the Eastern Mediterranean, the Middle East, and the Eastern Asian rim; In Turkey the prevalence is 3 per 1000 and in the Asian rim it is 0.15 per 1000

Onset: Aphthous oral ulceration (97-100% of patients): The most common initial manifestation of the disease (25-75%); The keratinized mucosa of the hard palate and dorsum of the tongue is rarely involved; These ulcers are painful, round or oval, with an erythematous rim. They may be quite persistent in some individuals.

Progression: (a) Genital ulceration: Occurs in 80-100% of patients and occur on the penis or scrotum and in the vagina or on the vulva; These lesions may heal with scarring; Vaginal ulceration may result in painless discharge; ***(b) Skin Lesions:*** Consist of erythema nodosum, pseudofolliculitis, papulopustular lesions, or acneiform nodules; ***(c) Positive pathergy test*** (hyperirritability of the skin): Insert a 20-gauge needle perpendicularly into the skin to a depth of about 5mm. 24-48 hours later an erythematous papule or pustule > 2 mm in diameter confers a positive test. Pathergy is less common in North American and Northern European patients ***(d) Ocular Lesions:*** Hypopyon-uveitis in 1/3 of patients; Panuveitis (posterior and anterior uveitis and retinal vasculitis) is the primary cause of vision loss; Typically follows the mucocutaneous symptoms, affects both eyes, and relapses in a chronic course

Constitutional Features: May include fatigue, anorexia, and weight loss. Fever may be due to large vessel disease or to infection.

Functional Status: May experience considerable functional impairment with active disease

RHEUMATOLOGIC REVIEW OF SYSTEMS

Associated Conditions: Amyloidosis; MAGIC Syndrome - Mouth And Genital ulceration with Inflamed Cartilage

Musculoskeletal Involvement: Monoarthritis or oligoarthritis of the knees, ankles, wrists, and/or hands; Episodic in nature and does not necessarily correlate with other disease activity; Synovial biopsies reveal neutrophilic infiltration

Vascular Involvement: Aortic aneurysms from vasculitis of the vasa vasorum; Pulmonary artery vasculitis presenting with hemoptysis due to pulmonary artery-bronchial fistula; Superficial thrombophlebitis; Vena cava occlusion (high risk of mortality); Budd-Chiari syndrome, Cerebral venous thrombosis

Neurologic Involvement: Aseptic meningitis; Parenchymal CNS lesions (stroke like); Peripheral neuropathy - unusual

Cardiac Involvement: Uncommon

Gastrointestinal Involvement: Much more common in Japanese patients; Abdominal pain due to ulcerative lesions involving the terminal ileum and cecum (but any area can be involved) which have a tendency to bleed or perforate

Renal Involvement: Unusual

Genitourinary Involvement: Epididymitis

RISK FACTORS
HLA-B51 positivity

FAMILY HISTORY
Familial Behcet's disease is uncommon but does occur

RED FLAGS
Rule out other causes of aphthous stomatitis (HIV, medications, IBD, other CTD)
Evidence of vascular involvement is a major source of morbidity and mortality

DIFFERENTIAL DIAGNOSIS
Differential Diagnosis for Recurrent Aphthous Ulceration: (a) Behcet's disease / MAGIC syndrome; (b) Inflammatory bowel disease; (c) Systemic lupus erythematosus; (d) Celiac disease; (e) Medications - NSAIDs; (f) Infections - HIV, fungal; (g) Contact stomatitis; (h) Vitamin deficiencies - Iron, folic acid, vitamin B1, B2, B6, B12; (i) Hematologic disorders - Cyclic neutropenia, benign familial neutropenia; (j) Sweet's syndrome

PHYSICAL EXAMINATION
Vitals: Pulse: May be elevated if acutely unwell; BP: Variable; RR: Variable; Temperature: May have an associated fever (if present consider large vessel vasculitis or infection)

Cutaneous: Superficial thrombophlebitis; Erythema nodosum, pseudofolliculitis, papulopustular lesions, or acneiform lesions; Varices (collateral veins)

Head & Neck: Ocular involvement - Reduced vision, hypopyon, retinal vasculitis; Oral ulceration

Respiratory: SOB due to pulmonary arterial involvement (unusual)

Cardiovascular: Murmurs due to pulmonary arterial involvement (unusual)

Gastrointestinal: Abdominal tenderness and evidence of bleeding; Enlarged liver; Genital ulceration

Musculoskeletal: Inflammatory arthritis - usually mono or oligoarthritis

Neurologic: Meningeal irritation; Upper motor neuron signs as a result of CVA

INVESTIGATIONS
CBC: Microcytic normochromic anemia and thrombocytosis (reactive)

ESR/CRP: May be elevated

Creatinine: May be mildly elevated

HLA-B51: More common in Behcet's disease (along the Silk Route)

Radiology: Non-erosive arthritis

Biopsy: Vasculitis may be seen on biopsy, but is often non-specific; Lymphocytic infiltration with liquefaction-degeneration at the dermal-epidermal border explains the ulcer formation and necrosis; The cellular infiltration may be perivascular or with findings typical of a leukocytoclastic vasculitis: Endothelial cell swelling; Nuclear dust from leukocytoclasia; Extravasation of RBC; Fibrinoid necrosis of the vessel wall; Mixed cellular infiltrate; Neutrophilic infiltrates in acute lesions and on pathergy testing

MANAGEMENT
General: Education; Vocational counseling; Arthritis self management programs

Physical Therapy: Joint protection; Active and passive ROM; Strengthening; Weight loss

Occupational Therapy: Splints, braces, and orthotics; Assistive devices; Ambulatory devices

Mucocutaneous lesions: (a) Topical or intralesional corticosteroids; (b) Oral colchicine 0.6 mg PO OD-TID; (c) Oral corticosteroids (best avoided for aphthosis if at all possible); (d) Thalidomide 200 mg/day and dapsone 100-200 mg/day have also been shown to be effective; (e) Methotrexate has been tried in refractory cases

Ocular disease: (a) Corticosteroids - Do not appear to prevent blindness in serious ocular disease; (b) Immunosuppressants (azathioprine, cyclosporine, chlorambucil, cyclophosphamide); (c) Interferon alpha and infliximab have been tried in resistant cases. No controlled studies.

Musculoskeletal: (a) NSAIDs; (b) Colchicine; (c) Other immunosuppressants

Systemic disease (CNS, gastrointestinal, CVS, & vascular): (a) Low dose ASA if vascular disease (arterial): Vascular disease may require treatment with corticosteroids and immunosuppressants as inflammation is likely the cause of thrombosis. Thrombosis may continue in the face of warfarin therapy alone; (b) Oral corticosteroids: May have a role in the treatment of inflammation but have variable results on mucocutaneous and CNS disease; (c) Immunosuppressants: Azathioprine (2.5 mg/kg/day); Chlorambucil; Cyclosporine; Cyclophosphamide; (d) Biologics: Etanercept: May be useful for aphthosis; Infliximab: Anecdotal evidence suggests it may be effective

Surgery: Repair of arterial aneurysms

PROGNOSIS

Risk Stratification for Poor Progression: (a) Younger patients; (b) Male patients; (c) Patients from the Middle or Far East

Prognosis: A variable course filled with exacerbations and remissions. Over time the disease may become less severe.

CALCIUM PYROPHOSPHATE DEPOSITION DISEASE (CPPD)

DEFINITION & PATHOPHYSIOLOGY

Definition: Calcium pyrophosphate is a salt which is deposited in cartilage and appears as chondrocalcinosis on radiographs. Alternatively, the crystalline form can be released into the joint resulting in an acute inflammatory arthritis known as pseudogout.

Pathophysiology: An inflammatory response to CPPD crystals shed from cartilaginous structures into the synovial cavity

PRESENTATION

Identifying Data: Most patients with primary pseudogout are older (>55-60)

Onset: CPPD can present in one of 5 ways: *(a) Asymptomatic Chondrocalcinosis:* Characteristic sites of CPPD deposition are: Lateral and medial menisci in the knee, acetabular labrum in the hip, fibrocartilaginous symphysis pubis, triangular discs of the distal radio-ulnar joint, annulus fibrosus of the intervertebral discs, and articular capsule or synovial calcification of large joints; *(b) Acute Pseudogout (25%):* An acute inflammatory arthritis with rapid onset of pain, swelling, erythema, and warmth. Occasionally accompanied by systemic features such as malaise and fever. The attacks mimic acute gout but tend to be less intense and take longer to reach peak and lasts for several days to two weeks. It tends to present as a monoarthritis with the knees most commonly affected, however, almost all joints have been reported. *(c) Pseudo Osteoarthritis (50%):* Overlap with the distribution of primary OA, however, the distribution of joint degeneration with CPPD is distinct. It can result in severe degeneration in joints not typically affected by OA, including changes in the MCPs, wrists, elbows, shoulders, and knees. In the knees, CPPD is more likely to affect the lateral compartment and isolated patello-femoral degeneration is also a common presentation. X-rays show chondrocalcinosis and extensive osteophyte formation. *(d) Pseudo Rheumatoid Arthritis (5%):* May present clinically identical to rheumatoid arthritis, however, it is non-erosive and radiographic changes are more typical of osteoarthritis. *(e) Pseudo Neuropathic Joint:* CPPD crystal deposition in association with severe joint destruction resembling a neuropathic joint. Neurologic function in this setting is normal.

Constitutional Features: Fever and malaise may accompany attacks of acute pseudogout

Functional Status: Reduced functional status resulting in difficulties with ADLs

RHEUMATOLOGIC REVIEW OF SYSTEMS

Associated Conditions: Associated with secondary causes of CPPD (see Risk Factors)

RISK FACTORS

(a) Hemochromatosis; (b) Hyperparathyroidism; (c) Hypophosphatasia; (d) Hypomagnesemia; (e) Hypothyroidism; (f) Amyloidosis; (g) Post-traumatic pseudogout (acute illness, surgery, trauma); (h) Aging; (i) Familial/hereditary forms

FAMILY HISTORY

There are reported familial/hereditary forms of CPPD

RED FLAGS

Think about septic arthritis in the setting of acute pseudogout; Concomitant gout; Acute pseudogout is frequently precipitated by an urgent medical illness

DIFFERENTIAL DIAGNOSIS

Differential Diagnosis of Acute Pseudogout: (a) CPPD deposition; (b) Acute gout; (c) Infectious arthritis: Bacterial, Non-gonococcal, Gonococcal, Viral; (d) Reactive arthritis; (e) Trauma

Differential Diagnosis of Extra-Articular Calcification: (a) Calcium pyrophosphate deposition; (b) Hydroxyapatite deposition; (c) Systemic sclerosis; (d) Juvenile dermatomyositis; (e) Hyperparathyroidism; (f) Myositis ossificans

PHYSICAL EXAMINATION

Vitals: Pulse: Normal; BP: Normal; RR: Normal; Temperature: May be elevated in pseudogout

Cutaneous: Bronzing of the skin suggestive of hemochromatosis

Head & Neck: Acute neck pain with calcification surrounding the odontoid process (crowded dens syndrome); Thyroid enlargement

Respiratory: No specific findings

Cardiovascular: Normal unless concomitant hemochromatosis or hypothyroidism

Gastrointestinal: Normal unless associated hemochromatosis, hyperparathyroidism, or hypothyroidism

Musculoskeletal: OA changes in the DIPs, PIPs, MCPs, and wrists; Pseudo-rheumatoid changes; Carpal tunnel syndrome; Acute inflammatory arthritis with pain, swelling, erythema, and warmth

Neurologic: Features associated with hypothyroidism, hyperparathyroidism, and amyloidosis

INVESTIGATIONS

CBC: Leukocytosis with a left shift

ESR: Elevated

Screening Investigations: Serum calcium and albumin, magnesium, & phosphate; Ferritin and transferrin saturation; Alkaline phosphatase; TSH

Radiology: Radiographic features divided into Articular & Periarticular Calcification and Pyrophosphate Arthropathy as follows:

Articular and Periarticular Calcification: Associated with calcification of articular and periarticular structures; These deposits can be located in cartilage, synovium, capsule, tendons, bursae, ligaments, soft-tissues, and vessels; Chondrocalcinosis (cartilage calcification) – Found most often in fibrocartilage such as: Knees – menisci; Symphysis pubis; Wrist – Triangular fibrocartilaginous complex (TFCC); Intervertebral disc – Annulus fibrosus; Hip – Acetabular labrum; Shoulder – Glenoid labrum; Hyaline cartilage calcification may also occur and is more common in the wrist, knee, elbow, and hip

Pyrophosphate Arthropathy: Found most commonly in the knee, wrist, and metacarpophalangeal joints; It is similar to degenerative joint diseases with loss of articular space, subchondral sclerosis, subchondral cysts. However, it differs in the following ways: ***(a) Unusual articular distribution*** – Seen in unusual places for degenerative disease – wrist, elbow, shoulders; ***(b) Unusual intra-articular distribution*** – Isolated or significant involvement of the radiocarpal or trapezioscaphoid articulations of the wrist, patellofemoral compartment of the knee, and the talocalcaneal articulation of the midfoot; ***(c) Prominent sub-chondral cyst formation*** – Very numerous and large cysts; ***(d) Destructive bone changes*** – Severe and progressive. May be associated with extensive and rapid subchondral bone collapse and fragmentation and the appearance of single or multiple intra-articular osseous bodies. These features resemble those of a neuroarthropathy. This destructive arthropathy may be evident in the hips, knees, shoulders, elbows, wrists, symphysis pubis, ankles, metacarpophalangeal and mid-tarsal joints; (e) *Variable osteophyte formation* – large irregular bony excrescences may be noted about involved articulations

Synovial Fluid: Cloudy/opaque; Prominent leukocytosis consisting of PMNs; Rhomboid shaped crystals seen under polarized light microscopy. They are weakly positively birefringent which means they appear blue when viewed under polarized light with the long axis of the crystal parallel to the direction of slow vibration of light in the first order red compensator. Remember ABC (Alignment Blue Calcium).

MANAGEMENT

General: Rest, ice, elevation & joint immobilization; Physical therapy for gentle range of motion

Acute Pseudogout

Intra-articular corticosteroids: (a) Small Joint: 5-10 mg Depo-medrol, 10 mg Triamcinolone Acetonide, 10 mg Triamcinolone Hexacetonide; (b) Medium Joint: 20-40 mg Depo-medrol, 20 mg Triamcinolone Acetonide, 20 mg Triamcinolone Hexacetonide; (c) Large Joint: 40-80 mg Depo-medrol, 30 mg Triamcinolone Acetonide, 40 mg Triamcinolone Hexacetonide

Analgesics & NSAIDs: For symptomatic relief

Systemic Corticosteroids: Used of severe polyarticular attacks unresponsive to NSAIDs and injection. Prednisone 30 mg PO to start tapering by 5 mg every other day until finished (12 days) - Anecdotal evidence only

Colchicine: 0.6 mg PO BID - TID (rarely used)

PROGNOSIS

Varies depending on associated diseases and presentation

CHURG-STRAUSS SYNDROME (CSS)

DEFINITION & PATHOPHYSIOLOGY

Definition: Churg-Strauss syndrome is otherwise known as allergic granulomatosis and angiitis. It is a granulomatous inflammatory disease of small and medium sized blood vessels associated with extravascular granulomas and hypereosinophilia. See the Classification Criteria for Churg Strauss syndrome (page *240*)

Pathophysiology: The initiating factor(s) responsible for the development of vasculitis is/are unknown; Endothelial cells are quickly activated and upregulate adhesion molecules, cytokines, growth factors, and receptors recruiting and activating components of the innate and adaptive immune systems; PMNs express antigens (MPO, PR3) on their surface and are activated through ANCA binding to these antigens. Activated PMNs release MPO, PR3, & reactive oxygen species upregulating the immune response, which may result in damage to endothelial cells

PRESENTATION

Identifying Data: Male=Female; Any age (Average age of onset 40 - 50 years)

Onset: Onset typically follows the following stages: *(a) First Phase (Prodromal):* The prodromal phase consists of allergic rhinitis, nasal polyposis, and asthma. It may have been present for many years, however, asthma can sometimes occur concomitantly with the vasculitis (20%). *(b) Second Phase (Eosinophilic):* Onset of peripheral blood & tissue eosinophilia manifests as Loffler's syndrome, chronic eosinophilic pneumonia, or eosinophilic gastroenteritis. *(c) Third Phase (Vasculitic):* Onset of systemic vasculitis which occurs a mean of 3 years after the onset of asthma. Treatment of asthma with corticosteroids may suppress the vasculitic component which may become apparent as the steroid dose is reduced.

Progression: May be indolent or progressive. Inflammation in organs may result in permanent damage and/or deformity with new organs becoming involved over time.

Constitutional Features: Fatigue, fevers, anorexia, weight loss, night sweats

Functional Status: May be significantly impaired with active vasculitis

RHEUMATOLOGIC REVIEW OF SYSTEMS

Musculoskeletal Involvement: Arthralgia, myalgia, & arthritis present during the vasculitic phase; Muscle weakness

Mucocutaneous Involvement: Palpable purpura (LCV); Subcutaneous nodules (up to 30%); Splinter hemorrhages; Livedo reticularis and skin infarction

Neurologic Involvement: Peripheral neuropathy - Usually mononeuritis multiplex, but mononeuropathy & distal sensory neuropathy are also seen; Central Nervous System - Optic neuritis (rare) & cranial neuropathies

Cardiac Involvement: Accounts for 50% of deaths due to CSS. A granulomatous infiltration of the myocardium and coronary vessel vasculitis are the cause of: Congestive heart failure; Pericardial effusion; Restrictive pericarditis

Respiratory Involvement: *(a) Asthma:* Occurs in > 95% of patients; Typically becomes worse with the onset of vasculitis; Severity of asthma often necessitates the use of systemic corticosteroids; *(b) Pulmonary Infiltrates:* Occur in 30-70% of patients, typically in the eosinophilic phase; Transient and patchy infiltrates with an alveolar pattern are most common, however a diffuse interstitial pattern can be seen; *(c) Pleural effusions:* Up to 30%

Gastrointestinal Involvement: Eosinophilic gastroenteritis - Abdominal pain, diarrhea, & bleeding thought secondary to: Mesenteric vasculitis; Bowel wall infiltration with eosinophils

Renal Involvement: Characterized by a focal segmental glomerulonephritis with necrotizing features, including crescents; Rare (5%)

RISK FACTORS
History of asthma; Leukotriene receptor antagonists have been associated with CSS and improve asthma and subsequent reduction in prednisone may unmask CSS.

FAMILY HISTORY
No known association

RED FLAGS
Must always rule out sepsis as it can present as multi-organ failure and can mimic vasculitis; Refractory vasculitis is an infection until proven otherwise

DIFFERENTIAL DIAGNOSIS
Hypereosinophilia: (a) Churg-Strauss syndrome; (b) Infection: Helminthic infections: Strongyloides stercoralis, Hookworm, & Toxocara canis; Fungal Infections: Allergic bronchopulmonary aspergillosis & Coccidioidomycosis; HIV; (c) Hematologic abnormalities: Hypereosinophilic syndrome; Systemic mastocytosis; Eosinophilic leukemia; Lymphoma; (d) Allergic disorders; (e) Adrenal insufficiency
Small Vessel Vasculitis: See Page 3

PHYSICAL EXAMINATION
Vitals: P: Normal to elevated; BP: Low if very ill, elevated if hypertensive with renal disease; RR: Frequently elevated with accompanying asthma; Temp: Fever
Cutaneous: Splinter hemorrhages & nail-fold infarcts; Palpable purpura; Subcutaneous nodules; Livedo reticularis
Head & Neck: Cranial nerve palsies; Optic neuritis
Respiratory: Reduced breath sounds and diffuse wheezes with asthmatic component; Adventitious sounds, pleural friction rubs (with effusion)
Cardiovascular: CHF with renal failure, flow murmurs with anemia, pericardial friction rub with pericarditis
Gastrointestinal: Abdominal tenderness with GI involvement
Musculoskeletal: Arthralgia & myalgias; Inflammatory arthritis
Neurologic: Peripheral neuropathy (mononeuritis multiplex)

INVESTIGATIONS
CBC: Normochromic, normocytic anemia, leukocytosis, and thrombocytosis; Eosinophilia - Can range from 1.5 - 29 x 109/L
Albumin: Low
Complement: Normal or elevated C3, C4
ESR/CRP: Elevated
Creatinine: May be elevated (85%)
Urinalysis: Microscopic hematuria & proteinuria if renal involvement
ANCA: p-ANCA in 70% (myeloperoxidase); c-ANCA rare but has been reported (proteinase-3)
Chest Radiographs: Transient and patchy opacities which are not distributed in a lobar or segmental manner (scattered); Diffuse interstitial pattern; Widespread opacities with pulmonary hemorrhage; Pleural effusion
Aspiration & Pathology: Open lung biopsy is considered the "gold standard". Transbronchial biopsies are not useful. Pathologic findings include: (a) Eosinophilic infiltration; (b) Small necrotizing granulomas - Usually perivascular and extravascular, composed of a central eosinophil surrounded by macrophages and giant cells - "Churg-Strauss granuloma"; (c) Necrotizing vasculitis of small blood vessels; (d) Lung necrosis

MANAGEMENT
General: Education, Vocational counseling, Arthritis self management programs
Physical Therapy: Joint protection, Active & passive ROM, Strengthening, Wt loss

Occupational Therapy: Splints & braces, Assistive devices, Ambulatory devices

Supportive: Supportive care with ventilatory support for pulmonary/cardiac involvement; Respirology consult

High-Dose Corticosteroids: Patients with Churg-Strauss syndrome typically respond well to corticosteroids; Pulsed methylprednisolone 1 gram IV over 60 minutes daily for 3-5 days; After 3 days give prednisone 1 mg/kg PO OD - This can be given in 3-4 divided daily doses for 7-10 days consolidating to a single morning dose by 2-3 weeks; With clinical improvement and normalization of ESR the prednisone can be slowly tapered. *Example Tapering Regimens:* Taper to 50% original dose by decreasing by 2.5 mg q10days; Maintain dose for 3 weeks; Taper to 20 mg by decreasing 2.5 mg qweekly; Taper to 10 mg by decreasing 1 mg q2weeks; Maintain at 10 mg for 3 weeks; Taper to 0 by decreasing by 1 mg qmonthly **OR** Taper by 5 mg on alternate days qweekly gradually converting the treatment regimen to alt. daily prednisone; Tapered by 2.5-5 mg qweekly until it is discontinued

Cyclophosphamide: Cyclophosphamide is typically used as a second line treatment in patients who have failed corticosteroids. Indications for cyclophosphamide are as follows: (a) Factor Five (b) Score of one or greater; (c) Failure of Corticosteroids

Pulsed IV Cyclophosphamide: Initial pulses may vary from 0.25 to 2.5 grams at intervals of 1 week to 1 month. In Europe, mini-pulses given more frequently are routinely used. Example orders see page 166.

Oral Cyclophosphamide: More effective (less relapoco) and used second line when IV falls; Given as 1-2 mg/kg/day orally for a maximum of one year. Use cyclophosphamide as the induction agent aiming to stop it at 3-6 months and continue with one of the maintenance agents. The initial NIH regimen states to continue cyclophosphamide one year after remission then taper by 25 mg every 2-3 months, however, they do state that the "necessary duration of treatment is open to question and our views have changed over the years".

European Union Vasculitis Study Group used the CYCAZAREM: regimen in patients with WG. **Induction:** Oral Cyclophosphamide 2 mg/kg/day for 3 months; **Remission:** Oral Cyclophosphamide 1.5 mg/kg/day plus azathioprine 2 mg/kg/day for 6 months. **Maintenance:** Azathioprine 1.5 mg/kg/day

Methotrexate: Has been used for maintenance of remission in patients with Wegener's Granulomatosis (not CSS). Oral cyclophosphamide was used to initiate disease remission and weekly methotrexate was substituted given 1-2 days after the last dose of CYC.

Mycophenolate Mofetil: Under investigation as a maintenance agent

IVIG: Benefit in 1991 study in CSS *(J Allergy & Clin Immunol 1991;88:823)*

Plasmapheresis/Plasma Exchange: Uncertain benefit & undeniable risks *(J Rheum 1991)*

Interferon-alpha: Refractory to steroids and cyclophosphamide. (A Int Med 1988)

PROGNOSIS

Risk Stratification for Poor Progression: Five Factor Score (FFS) (total of 5 points): (a) Proteinuria > 1 gram/day (1 point); (b) Renal insufficiency with creatinine > 140 umol/L (1 point); (c) Cardiomyopathy (1 point); (d) Gastrointestinal tract involvement (1 point); (e) CNS involvement (1 point); 5 year mortality as follows: FFS = 0 (12%), FFS = 1 (26%), FFS > 1 (46%)

Prognosis: The major cause of mortality, which accounts for 50% of deaths, is cardiac involvement with myocardial infarction and congestive heart failure; Other causes of mortality include renal failure, cerebral hemorrhage, gastrointestinal tract perforation and hemorrhage, status asthmaticus, and respiratory failure

COMPLEX REGIONAL PAIN SYNDROME (CRPS)

DEFINITION & PATHOPHYSIOLOGY

Definition: Complex regional pain syndrome (previously known as Reflex Sympathetic Dystrophy (RSD)) consists of extremity pain, swelling, vasomotor instability, and stiffness, often leading to disability. It frequently follows a traumatic event or is associated with a disease or a drug. The characteristic features are: (a) Diffuse, non-dermatomal pain which may include allodynia (a normally non-noxious stimuli causing pain) and hyperalgesia (prolonged pain). The pain is out of keeping with the inciting event. (b) Edema: Swelling; (c) Abnormal blood flow: Color changes; (d) Autonomic dysfunction: Fluctuations in temperature (cool/warm) and moisture (sweaty/dry). *Type 1 CRPS:* Develops after a noxious event (no definable nerve lesion); *Type 2 CRPS:* Develops after a nerve injury

Pathophysiology: The pathogenesis is unclear; The current theory involves the gate control theory of pain: Normally, discharge from myelinated A fibers prevents signals from noxious unmyelinated C fibers from reaching the brain, thus acting as a closed gate. If enough C fibers fire at a rapid rate the stimulus will break through the gate and result in the perception of pain. In CRPS, the afferent nerves are damaged resulting in: (a) Damaged A fibers which can no longer act as a gate; (b) Damaged C fibers which become overly sensitive and fire spontaneously. The increased signals from the noxious C fibers are transmitted to the brain resulting in constant pain. With pain, the sympathetic nervous system is stimulated, releasing chemicals which serve only to stimulate the damaged C fibers resulting in a runaway cycle of increasing pain

PRESENTATION

Identifying Data: More common in women (2-3:1) and in older age groups (40-60)

Onset: The initial stage is known as the *acute phase* (3-6 months). It can occur early after an inciting event or take months to occur. It is characterized by: (a) A burning or chronic aching pain in an extremity which is very sensitive to movement and temperature fluctuations; (b) Localized swelling of the extremity; (c) Color and temperature fluctuations; (d) Immobilization of the extremity to reduce symptoms

Progression: The second stage is known as the *dystrophic phase* (3-12 months) and is characterized by: (a) Continued pain; (b) Immobilization of the extremity now results in stiffness and muscle wasting; (c) The edema continues and becomes brawny and the nails become brittle; The extremity feels cold; The third stage is known as the *atrophic stage* and is characterized by: (a) Continued pain which may begin to diminish; (b) Prolonged immobilization results in continued stiffness with reduced range of motion and development of contractures; (c) Continued atrophy of the muscles; (d) The skin is now tethered and glossy due to subcutaneous tissue atrophy; (e) The nails become brittle; (f) The extremity may spasm or a tremor may be present. The pain may involve the extremity on the opposite side in about 25% of cases which is typically not as severe as the original lesion.

Constitutional Features: Anorexia and weight loss due to chronic pain

Functional Status: The psychological impact of chronic pain may result in: Loss of employment; Depression; Social withdrawal and family problems

RHEUMATOLOGIC REVIEW OF SYSTEMS

Associated Conditions: Associated fibromyalgia

RISK FACTORS

CRPS is more common with the following associated diseases: (a) Diabetes mellitus; (b) Alcohol abuse; (c) Smoking; (d) Hyperthyroidism, (e) Hyperparathyroidism; (f) Multiple sclerosis; (g) Hyperlipidemia

Inciting events associated with CRPS include: (a) Trauma to the affected extremity (physical, thermal, or chemical); (b) Neurologic disorders (CVA, Tumor); (c) Immobilization (casting); (d) Acute medical illness (MI), Surgery; (e) Medications (barbiturates, cyclosporine); (f) Malignancy; (g) Emotional disturbances (stress); (h) Pregnancy

FAMILY HISTORY
No known associated family history

RED FLAGS
Exclude other causes of pain including fracture, infection, inflammatory arthritis, and nerve injury

DIFFERENTIAL DIAGNOSIS
(a) Arterial insufficiency or thromboembolism; (b) Arthritis - crystalline, inflammatory, infectious; (c) Infection - osteomyelitis; (d) Erythromelalgia - Associated with thrombocytosis; (e) Nerve injury (cervical spine, thoracic outlet, brachial plexus, carpal tunnel, peripheral neuropathy, vasculitis); (f) Vasculitis; (g) Fracture; (h) Raynaud's phenomenon

PHYSICAL EXAMINATION
Vitals: Pulse: Normal; BP: Normal; RR: Normal; Temperature: Normal
Cutaneous: Atrophy of the subcutaneous fat; Brawny edema of the overlying skin; May be edematous or atrophied with brittle nails; Fluctuating temperature and abnormal sweating
Head & Neck: No specific findings
Respiratory: No specific findings
Cardiovascular: No specific findings
Gastrointestinal: No specific findings
Musculoskeletal: Exquisitely sensitive extremity worse with movement or touch; Contractures and associated muscle wasting (e.g. claw hand); Elbow is not usually involved; Shoulder may be exquisitely painful and swollen with reduced range of motion; Cervical spine disease
Neurologic: Hyperesthesia and dysesthesia of the affected limb; Muscular wasting

INVESTIGATIONS
CBC, ESR/CRP, and chemistries: Usually normal
Plain Radiographs: (a) Patchy periarticular osteoporosis (mottled appearance) known as Sudek's atrophy; (b) Subperiosteal cortical bone resorption results in a ragged appearance of the outer margins of the bone. Endosteal resorption results in thinning of the cortices. Intracortical bone resorption results in striation within the cortex; (c) Juxta-articular erosions like those seen in RA commonest in the MCP and MTP joints with preservation of the joint space; (d) Destruction of joints may occasionally occur
Bone Scan: (a) Very early lesions: Bone scans typically show reduced flow phase; (b) Stage 1 (6 weeks after onset): Increased flow phase with early, increased, and prolonged juxta-articular pooling; (b) Stage 2: Normal flow phase and early, normal, but prolonged juxta-articular pooling; (c) Stage 3: May be normal
Synovial biopsy: Edema, hyperplasia and hypertrophy of synoviocytes, neovascular proliferation, fibrosis in the deep layers, and lymphocyte infiltration (occasionally)

MANAGEMENT
Education: Understanding the disease process; Stress management; Smoking cessation
Physical & Occupational Therapy: Can begin once the pain is better controlled; Early treatment consists of mobilization, edema control, and isometric

strengthening; Later treatment consists of stress loading, isotonic strengthening, range of motion, postural normalization, and aerobic conditioning; Vocational rehabilitation

Psychotherapy: Consists of imagery, self-hypnosis, biofeedback, relaxation techniques, behavioral modification, and psychometric testing

Pain Control: Prior to physical or occupational therapy, pain control must be attempted; Pain control is best achieved when approached from multiple levels including topical agents, systemic agents, local nerve blocks, and others.

Topical Agents: (a) Capsaicin; (b) Topical NSAIDs

Systemic Agents: (a) Acetaminophen: Usually of little value; ***(b) NSAIDs:*** May be useful in early disease; ***(c) Narcotics; (d) Corticosteroids:*** Can give good relief and pain reduction in some patients. They seem to work better in "warm" disease of the upper extremity. The recommended 28 course of prednisone is as follows: 15 mg qid x 4 days; 10 mg qid x 4 days; 10 mg tid x 4 days; 10 mg bid x 4 days; 15 mg qd x 4 days; 10 mg qd x 4 days; 5 mg qd x 4 days; Stop; ***(e) Calcitonin:*** Subcutaneous or intranasal seems to be effective in up to 60% of patients given over a 20 day period. It is usually effective within the first few days; ***(f) Bisphosphonates:*** Benefit seen with intravenous pamidronate and oral alendronate; ***(g) Beta-Blockers:*** Good results have been seen with pindolol and propranolol. They should not be given to those patients with cold-onset CRPS.; ***(h) Alpha-Blockers:*** Prazosin with varied success; ***(i) Chronic Pain medications:*** Gabapentin - Starting with doses of 300 mg qd x 1 day, 300 mg bid x 1 day, then 300 mg tid. Anecdotal experience has reported very good results.; Amitriptyline may improve sleep and decrease pain.; Carbamazepine

Regional Nerve Blocks: (a) Stellate ganglion block: Abandon if does not work first or second attempts; ***(b) Bier blocks:*** Regional intravenous perfusion with ketorolac or methylprednisolone; ***(c) Surgical sympathectomy:*** Potential therapy for patients who receive excellent but temporary relief from sympathetic blockade.

PROGNOSIS

Risk Stratification for Poor Progression: (a) Longer disease duration; (b) Low skin temperature (cool extremity); (c) Lack of edema

Prognosis: Difficult to predict; Some patients experience reduced symptoms or apparent recovery; Some patients continue to experience significant disability

CUTANEOUS VASCULITIS

DEFINITION & PATHOPHYSIOLOGY

Definition: Cutaneous vasculitis (leukocytoclastic vasculitis) is defined as a polymorphonuclear inflammatory infiltration of the walls of small to medium sized blood vessels that supply the skin; Cutaneous vasculitis may represent an underlying systemic disorder which may or may not have recognizable abnormalities in other organ systems; Cutaneous vasculitis can be the result of a hypersensitivity reaction to a foreign antigen (e.g. medications, viral illness)

Pathophysiology: Cutaneous vasculitis is believed to result from the deposition of circulating immune complexes (usually IgG or IgM) between endothelial cells in the vessel wall. Immune complexes can result in complement activation resulting in: Direct attack by the MAC; Release of chemotactic factors attracting PMNs which release lysozomal enzymes; Initial inflammatory infiltrate is polymorphonuclear with the mononuclear cells coming later to clear destroyed tissue.

PRESENTATION

Identifying Data: Men & women equally; Affects any age; Caucasians

Onset: If the cutaneous vasculitis is secondary to a hypersensitivity reaction the lesions typically appear 7 to 21 days following the initial exposure; *(a) Purpuric Lesions:* The most frequent typical onset is usually a non-palpable purpuric rash (flat erythematous lesions which do no blanche) which is found most frequently on dependent surfaces (legs and buttocks), in areas of trauma, or under tight fitting clothing. The lesions vary in size from small 1 mm lesions to ones which are several centimeters. The lesions may coalesce. *(b) Urticarial Lesions:* The second most common presentation with raised erythematous urticaria which typically last for 6-72 hours; *(c) Other skin lesions:* including livedo reticularis, bullous lesions, nodules, ulceration, erythematous plaques, and erythema multiforme like lesions; Patients usually only have one type of skin lesion

Progression: (a) Purpuric Lesions: These are dynamic and tend to become palpable with time. The lesions tend to last about a week but not usually longer than 4 weeks. With healing the skin may hyperpigment. In more persistent lesions nodules, vesicles and bullae may form. The lesions occasionally ulcerate and become necrotic. *(b) Systemic manifestations:* May also be present including arthralgias and myalgias. Up to 50% of patients may develop systemic involvement including the following: Arthralgias, myalgias, myositis, arthritis; Renal involvement with proteinuria, hematuria, hypertension, and renal insufficiency; Gastrointestinal involvement with pain, ulceration, and hemorrhage; Pulmonary involvement with infiltrates, pleuritis, and nodular lesions; Neurologic involvement; Cardiac involvement with pericarditis or myocarditis

Constitutional Features: General malaise, fatigue, loss of appetite, mild weight loss, and fevers may be associated.

Functional Status: Significant reduction in functional status may be observed during periods of active disease.

RHEUMATOLOGIC REVIEW OF SYSTEMS

Musculoskeletal Involvement: Myalgias and arthralgias; Arthritis; Myositis

Mucocutaneous Involvement: Palpable purpura; Urticarial lesions; Livedo reticularis; Nodular lesions; Vesicles and bullae

Ear, Nose, & Throat Involvement: Chronic sinusitis & hematochezia if associated with Wegener's

Lymphatic Involvement: Lymphadenopathy

Hematologic Involvement: If a systemic inflammatory or malignant disease

Ocular Involvement: If the cutaneous vasculitis is associated with a systemic disease process then ocular involvement may be seen.

Neurologic Involvement: Peripheral neuropathy - mononeuritis multiplex

Psychiatric Involvement: If associated with a systemic disorder such as SLE

Cardiac Involvement: Pericarditis, myocarditis; Ask about infectious risk and risks of subacute bacterial endocarditis

Respiratory Involvement: Pulmonary infiltrates; Pleuritic chest pain; Cough & hemoptysis if assoc. with Wegener's; History of asthma if assoc. with Churg Strauss

Gastrointestinal Involvement: Abdominal pain and colic; Ulceration, perforation, or hemorrhage; Pancreatitis; Ask about risk factors for hepatitis B & C infection

Renal Involvement: Proteinuria, hematuria, hypertension, azotemia

RISK FACTORS

Recent infection such as URTI (strep) & viral hepatitis; History of drug exposure

FAMILY HISTORY

No associated family history

RED FLAGS

Systemic involvement including pulmonary, cardiac, neurologic, and gastrointestinal involvement should raise suspicion for an underlying disease process

DIFFERENTIAL DIAGNOSIS

Differential Diagnosis of Diseases Associated with Cutaneous Vasculitis: (a) Idiopathic (45-55%); (b) Medication (10-15%): Penicillins; Cephalosporins; Sulfonamides; Phenytoin; Allopurinol; (c) Infection (15-20%): Hep B & C; HIV; Subacute bacterial endocarditis; (d) Collagen Vascular Disease (15-20%): Wegener's granulomatosis, Churg-Strauss syndrome, polyarteritis nodosa; Cryoglobulinemia secondary to hepatitis C; Rheumatoid arthritis, SLE, Sjogren's syndrome, dermatomyositis; Henoch-Schonlein Purpura; (e) Malignancy (<5%)

Differential Diagnosis of Small Vessel Vasculitis: See page (3)

PHYSICAL EXAMINATION

Vitals: P: Usually normal, may be elevated with systemic involvement; BP: Usually normal, may be elevated with renal involvement; RR: Usually normal, may be elevated with cardiorespiratory involvement; Temp: May have a low-grade fever

Cutaneous: Palpable purpuric lesions on dependant areas which may be small and discrete or larger and coalescent; Non-blanchable & non-tender; Hyperpigmentation in areas of healed lesions; Ulceration and necrosis can sometimes be seen with the lesions; Urticarial lesions; Other rashes include: Livedo reticularis, nodular lesions, bullous lesions and vesicles, erythema multiforme lesions, and erythematous plaques

Head & Neck: Normal unless associated with an underlying systemic disease

Respiratory: Usually normal, however, look for adventitious sounds, pleural effusions, and pleural rubs which may represent pulmonary involvement

Cardiovascular: Usually normal

Gastrointestinal: Usually normal

Musculoskeletal: True inflammatory arthritis is uncommon in isolated cutaneous vasculitis. Arthralgia and myalgia are more common. If associated with an underlying systemic disease may see evidence of inflammatory arthritis or myositis

Neurologic: Usually normal, however, with systemic involvement can have neurologic involvement including both CNS and PNS

INVESTIGATIONS

CBC: Examine for evidence of an underlying inflammatory/malignant process

ESR/CRP: Evidence of inflammatory disease

Creatinine & Urinalysis: Renal involvement with hematuria, proteinuria, and elevated creatinine

AST, ALT, ALP, Albumin: Look for evidence of viral hepatitis

Hepatitis B & C Serology

HIV Serology: When clinically indicated

Rheumatoid Factor, ANA, ENA, ds-DNA: Evidence of collagen vascular disease

Cryoglobulins

ANCA: If appropriate

Immunoglobulins: Elevated IgA may suggest Henoch Schonlein purpura

Also consider: Complement studies (C3, C4, CH50), blood cultures, anticardiolipin antibodies when indicated

Chest X-Ray: To examine for evidence of pulmonary involvement

Skin Biopsy of a Lesion typically shows a Leukocytoclastic Vasculitis with the following characteristics: Small blood vessels (usually post-capillary venules) are infiltrated by a polymorphonuclear cellular infiltrate. This infiltration is transmural. With time, fibrinoid necrosis of the blood vessel wall occurs and fragments of leukocytes (leukocytoclasis) are seen; With healing the predominant infiltrate is lymphocytic; Immunofluorescence may show immune complex deposition. IgA and C3 deposition is seen in HSP.

MANAGEMENT

General: Stop any suspected medications; Anecdotal evidence for trial of elimination diets to remove possible causes such as foods, food additives, or other supplements. Treatment of underlying conditions such as resection of tumors, antiviral agents for viral hepatitis and HIV may be beneficial in resolving an associated cutaneous vasculitis

NSAIDs: NSAIDs can be useful for some cases but findings have not been universal

Anti-histamines: Patients with burning or itching from urticarial lesions may benefit from antihistamines using H1 antagonists combined with H2 antagonists

Corticosteroids: If given in high enough doses, corticosteroids are almost always effective for controlling cutaneous lesions; Corticosteroids are indicated in extensive skin involvement, severe skin involvement with bullae, vesicles, or ulceration, and systemic involvement; Doses used typically begin at 40-60 mg of prednisone per day with tapering after disease control has been established

Colchicine: Colchicine 0.6 mg PO BID may be beneficial for chronic or recurrent isolated cutaneous vasculitis. The response occurs within a few days and a lack of response after 14 days should prompt discontinuation.

Dapsone: Dapsone 50-100 mg PO OD for chronic or recurrent cutaneous lesions

IVIG: Used successfully to treat resistant urticarial vasculitis (2 g/kg IV over 2-4 days)

Immunosuppressants: Hydroxychloroquine may be useful for urticarial vasculitis; Azathioprine and Methotrexate may be useful as steroid sparing agents in patients with chronic recalcitrant cutaneous vasculitis; Cyclophosphamide is usually reserved for cases where severe systemic involvement is associated

PROGNOSIS

Risk Stratification for Poor Progression: (a) Extensive or severe skin involvement; (b) Persistent or frequently recurrent eruptions; (c) Need for persistent corticosteroids; (d) Associated systemic disease

Prognosis: The prognosis of cutaneous hypersensitivity vasculitis associated with drugs or infection is excellent. Up to 60% of patients require no treatment with 25% using NSAIDs alone and 15% requiring corticosteroids. The prognosis is worse for patients with cutaneous vasculitis associated with an underlying systemic disease.

DIFFUSE IDIOPATHIC SKELETAL HYPEROSTOSIS (DISH)

DEFINITION & PATHOPHYSIOLOGY

Definition: A non-inflammatory disease characterized by calcification and ossification of spinal ligaments and peripheral entheses. It is not an arthropathy and there is no abnormality of articular cartilage, adjacent bone margins, or synovium.

Diagnostic Criteria: The presence of flowing calcification or ossification along the anterolateral aspects of at least 4 contiguous vertebral levels. Relative preservation of the intervertebral disc height in the involved vertebral segment without the extensive changes of primary degenerative disc disease. The absence of apophyseal joint ankylosis or sacroiliac joint erosions, sclerosis, or widespread intra-articular bony ankylosis

Pathophysiology: The etiology of DISH is unknown

PRESENTATION

Identifying Data: Typical patient is an older male (rarely diagnosed < 40); Male: female ratio of about 2:1; Prevalence about 3-4% in the general population (>40) and 7-10% (for those >70)

Onset: DISH is often found incidentally on routine radiographs. Otherwise it presents as intermittent pain and/or stiffness in the cervical spine (40-80%), thoracic spine, lumbar spine, or extremities (shoulder, elbow, & knee). Morning stiffness is present in 80% along with gelling phenomenon. Dysphagia may be present due to prominent cervical osteophytes

Progression: Slowly progressive with many patients having disease for years (10) prior to diagnosis. Spinal stenosis may occur in patients with a long standing history.

Constitutional Features: Fatigue may be associated with poor sleep and weight loss due to dysphagia

Functional Status: Reduced functional status with difficulties with ADLs versus healthy controls.

RHEUMATOLOGIC REVIEW OF SYSTEMS

Musculoskeletal Involvement: Enthesitis including Plantar fascia, Achilles tendon, pelvis, costochondral junction, patella, rotator cuff insertions; Recurrent shoulder tendonitis; Recurrent lateral or medial epicondylitis

Neurologic Involvement: Cord or root lesions following spinal fracture; Cervical spine subluxation (atlanto-axial); Spinal stenosis

Respiratory Involvement: Rigidity of the chest wall with reduced chest expansion; Stridor, nocturnal dyspnea, and vocal cord paralysis

Gastrointestinal Involvement: Dysphagia due to prominent cervical osteophytes

RISK FACTORS

Gender – Male; Age – More common in older individuals; Obesity; Diabetes

FAMILY HISTORY

May be a genetic component as there is a particularly high prevalence of DISH in the Pima Indians in Arizona, USA.

RED FLAGS

(a) New onset acute back pain or change in chronic back pain; (b) Continuous pain not relieved or worsens with supine position; (c) Constant pain that does not change with activity; (d) Severe night pain that wakes from sleep; (e) Fever, chills, or weight loss; (f) Bladder / bowel dysfunction; (g) Saddle anesthesia; (h) Loss of muscle bulk or weakness; (i) Difficulty walking; (j) Sensory abnormalities; (k) Past history of cancer; (l) Osteoporosis; (m) History of major or minor trauma

DIFFERENTIAL DIAGNOSIS
(a) DISH; (b) Ankylosing spondylitis; (c) Spondylitis deformans; (d) Other seronegative spondyloarthropathies – Psoriatic, reactive, enteropathic; (e) Acromegaly; (f) Hypoparathyroidism; (g) Fluorosis; (h) Ochronosis; (i) Retinoids; (j) Trauma

PHYSICAL EXAMINATION
Vitals: Pulse: Usually normal; BP: Usually normal; RR: Usually normal
Cutaneous: No specific findings
Head & Neck: No specific findings
Respiratory: Reduced chest expansion; Stridor, dysphonia due to vocal cord paralysis
Cardiovascular: No specific findings
Gastrointestinal: No specific findings
Musculoskeletal: Peripheral osteoarthritis; Rotator cuff tendonitis, subacromial bursitis; Enthesitis: Patellar tendonitis, Achilles tendonitis, plantar fasciitis, medial and lateral epicondylitis; Pain and reduced range of motion in the cervical, thoracic, or lumbar spine
Neurologic: Lower motor neuron lesions secondary to spinal cord compromise (stenosis, vertebral instability)

INVESTIGATIONS
Bloodwork & Urinalysis: No consistent lab abnormalities associated with DISH
Thoracic Spine: Calcification and ossification of the anterior longitudinal ligament which is separated from the vertebral bodies by a thin radiolucent line. Most evident in the mid-thoracic level but can be seen in cervical and lumbar levels. Osteophytes arise a few millimeters from the margins of the vertebral bodies best seen on the lateral projection. More prominent on the right side. Lack of associated disc degeneration or zygoapophyseal joint involvement
Cervical Spine: Bony outgrowths at the inferior margin of the vertebral bodies and extend inferiorly around the disc. Most common in the lower cervical spine
Lumbar Spine: Same as cervical spine but the outgrowths tend to grow up
Pelvis and Hips: Bony proliferation (whiskering) of the iliac crests, greater trochanter, & ischial tuberosity. Para-articular osteophytes
Knees: Patellar osteophytes at the insertion of the patellar tendon on the tibial tuberosity
Ankles and Feet: Osteophytes on the posterior and plantar surfaces of the calcaneus, dorsal surface of the talus, dorsal and medial tarsal navicular, lateral and plantar aspects of the cuboid, and the base of the 5th metatarsal

MANAGEMENT
General: Education
Physiotherapy: Regular exercise for spinal stiffness and restriction; Swimming; Orthotics
Analgesics: Acetaminophen may be useful for mild pain
NSAIDs: May reduce pain and spinal stiffness; Long-Acting NSAIDs taken at night may reduce night discomfort and morning stiffness
Corticosteroids: Local corticosteroid injections may be of value for entheseal pain and peripheral synovitis

PROGNOSIS
Variable, depending on degree and location of involvement

ERYTHEMA NODOSUM (EN)

DEFINITION & PATHOPHYSIOLOGY

Definition: Painful, erythematous, subcutaneous nodules typically found in the pretibial area

Pathophysiology: Erythema nodosum is thought to be a delayed hypersensitivity reaction stimulated by a number of different antigenic stimuli (infection, malignancy, drugs, immune disorders)

PRESENTATION

Identifying Data: Occurs more commonly in younger patients (20-30 years of age); Male:Female ratio is 1:4

Onset: Erythema nodosum usually presents systemically with a flu-like illness which may include a fever, myalgias, arthralgias, and malaise. The rash occurs simultaneously or shortly afterwards and is characterized by: Painful and tender red or violet subcutaneous nodules; The lesions typically become firm and painful over the initial week; Range in size from 1-6 cm in diameter; Typically form on the shins but may also occur on the forearms, thighs, and trunk. Actually, any skin surface may be involved. Bilateral.

Progression: Individual lesions usually last for 2-3 weeks, however, new lesions may develop prolonging the course of the illness; During the second week the color of the lesions changes from red to a bluish color and finally to a yellowish hue resembling a bruise; The lesions resolve without scarring as the overlying skin desquamates

Constitutional Features: Fatigue, arthralgias, myalgias, and general malaise

Functional Status: Erythema nodosum is usually a self-limited process. The functional status is dependant upon the associated disease.

RHEUMATOLOGIC REVIEW OF SYSTEMS

Musculoskeletal Involvement: Arthritis/Arthralgia - Predominantly affects the ankles, knees, and wrists

Mucocutaneous Involvement: Pharyngitis with streptococcal infection if associated; Oral or ocular complaints if associated with Behcet's

Respiratory Involvement: Hilar adenopathy if associated with sarcoidosis; Dyspnea or cough if associated with infection

Gastrointestinal Involvement: May occur if associated with infection, inflammatory bowel disease, or Behcet's disease

RISK FACTORS

No known risk factors

RED FLAGS

Rule out infection and malignancy

FAMILY HISTORY

Not applicable

DIFFERENTIAL DIAGNOSIS

Differential Diagnosis of Erythema Nodosum: (a) Erythema Nodosum; (b) Nodular Vasculitis (erythema induratum): Looks like EN but is atypical in that it occurs on the posterior legs, tends to recur, may ulcerate, and heal with scarring; Most commonly associated with tuberculosis; (c) Weber-Christian Disease: Relapsing febrile nodular vasculitis; More commonly found on the thighs and trunk; (d) Cutaneous Vasculitis; (e) Infection; (f) Superficial Thrombophlebitis

Diseases Associated with Erythema Nodosum: (a) Idiopathic - In up to 50% of cases no discernible cause can be found; (b) Infection: Bacterial: Streptococcal; Myobacterium tuberculosis; Mycoplasma pneumoniae; Yersinia enterocolitica;

Salmonella; Campylobacter; Leprosy. Fungal: Coccidioidomycosis (San Joaquin Valley Fever); Histoplasmosis; Blastomycosis; (c) Drugs: Sulfonamides; Oral contraceptive pills; (d) Sarcoidosis; (e) Inflammatory Bowel Disease; (f) Behcet's Disease; (g) Hodgkin's Lymphoma; (h) Pregnancy

PHYSICAL EXAMINATION

Vitals: Pulse: Elevated if acutely ill and febrile; BP: Low if volume depleted; RR: Usually normal to elevated if associated infection; Temperature: May be febrile

Cutaneous: Bilateral, raised, erythematous, tender nodules most often found on the shins; May have associated peripheral edema

Head & Neck: Lymphadenopathy; Pharyngeal erythema

Respiratory: Usually normal, however, EN may be secondary to an associated respiratory tract infection

Cardiovascular: No specific findings

Gastrointestinal: Tenderness if EN associated with IBD or infection

Musculoskeletal: Inflammatory arthritis most commonly affecting the wrists, knees, and ankles

Neurologic: No specific findings

INVESTIGATIONS

CBC: Look for evidence of infection, malignancy, or autoimmune disease

ESR: Often elevated

ASOT Titer: Streptococcal Infection (normal values do not exclude this)

PPD Skin Test: Tuberculosis

Beta-HCG: If associated with pregnancy

Possible Culture Sites: Pharynx; Stool; Blood

Chest X-ray: To look for evidence of sarcoidosis (hilar adenopathy) and tuberculosis

Biopsy: A deep incisional biopsy is required to sample the subcutaneous fat. A punch biopsy is inadequate. The pathology is that of a septal panniculitis with the following features: (a) Early lesions show widening of the septae due to edema; (b) Infiltration by lymphocytes, histiocytes, and multinucleated giant cells; (c) Fibrosis of the septae; (d) Vasculitis is not present

MANAGEMENT

General: Discontinue any offending medications; Treat any underlying illness if associated

Education: Erythema nodosum is usually a self-limited disease typically requiring symptomatic control with rest and NSAIDs in most cases; Rest, elevate the legs, and compression stockings may provide symptomatic relief

NSAIDs: The first choice for treatment and in most cases all that is required

Corticosteroids: Effective in self-limited disease, although, rarely required; Used in recurrent or refractory disease; Usual dose of prednisone is 10-20 mg/day

Colchicine: May be used in refractory cases

Potassium Iodide: Usual dose is 300 mg 3 times daily for 3-4 weeks

PROGNOSIS

Risk Stratification for Poor Progression: Chronic erythema nodosum

Prognosis: Usually a self-limited process lasting 3-8 weeks; Recurrences may occur in some patients; Patients treated early in the disease course respond more favorably than those with chronic EN

FIBROMYALGIA (FM)

DEFINITION & PATHOPHYSIOLOGY

Definition: Fibromyalgia is a non-inflammatory disorder consisting of chronic widespread pain and fatigue with specific tender points on physical examination.

Pathophysiology: The etiology of fibromyalgia is unknown, however, current theories emphasize abnormal amplified pain perception within the CNS. The mechanism of amplified pain perception is not fully understood but the following abnormalities have been observed: (a) Disturbance of normal sleep patterns; (b) Abnormalities of the descending analgesic pathways; (c) Reduced serotonin within the brain; (d) Decreased blood flow to areas such as the thalamus and caudate nucleus; (e) Autonomic instability (orthostatic hypotension, resting tachycardia); (f) Dysfunction within the hypothalamic-pituitary axis; (g) Elevated levels of substance P within the spinal fluid

PRESENTATION

Identifying Data: Female: male = 10:1; Can occur at any age but is more frequent between the ages of 35-55; May occur in up to 0.5% of men and 5% of women

Onset: Fibromyalgia may be triggered by preceding physical or emotional stress such as a medical illness or physical trauma. It has the following characteristics: *(a) Diffuse widespread pain:* May initially begin with localized pain (typically in the neck or back) eventually becoming diffuse; The diffuse pain affects both upper and lower halves of the body, both right and left sides, and usually involves the axial skeleton; The pain is distributed in a non-dermatomal fashion and described as a chronic aching sensation which may be associated with paresthesias and dysesthesias; The pain is frequently attributed to muscle or bones; The pain may be quite fluctuant aggravated by stress, lack of sleep, physical exertion, or changes in weather; *(b) Morning stiffness and soft-tissue swelling:* Morning stiffness may be prominent lasting > 60 minutes; Subjective feeling of soft-tissue swelling, however, no joint swelling exists on physical examination; *(c) Fatigue:* May be the principal complaint; Associated with non-restorative sleep

Progression: The pain and fatigue typically progress resulting in significant functional impairment

Constitutional Features: Fatigue

Functional Status: Functional status may be significantly impaired due to chronic pain and fatigue; Social functioning may decline; Depression and mood disorders are more common which also affect functioning

RHEUMATOLOGIC REVIEW OF SYSTEMS

Associated Conditions: Mood disorder; Visual disturbances; TMJ syndrome; Non-cardiac chest pain; Non-ulcer; dyspepsia; Irritable bowel syndrome; Chronic pelvic pain; Interstitial cystitis; Primary dysmenorrhea; Chronic fatigue syndrome; *Sleep Disorder:* Stage IV sleep (delta wave) is disrupted and significantly reduced by frequent bursts of alpha waves which produces a non-restorative sleep pattern; Bruxism; Restless legs syndrome; Obstructive sleep apnea

Mucocutaneous Involvement: Sicca features occur in 15% of patients; Raynaud's phenomenon is more common than found in the general population

Neurologic & Psychiatric Involvement: Migraine & tension headaches; Cognitive difficulties with memory problems; Depression - Up to 1/3 may suffer a serious depression; Anxiety

RISK FACTORS

Female sex; Inflammatory arthritis (RA, SLE)

FAMILY HISTORY
More common in family members with fibromyalgia
RED FLAGS
Rule out organic causes of chronic pain and fatigue
DIFFERENTIAL DIAGNOSIS
(a) Rheumatic Disorders: Fibromyalgia; Autoimmune disorders (RA, SLE, Sjogren's, SSc); Seronegative spondyloarthropathies; Inflammatory and metabolic myopathies; Polymyalgia rheumatica; *(b) Endocrinopathies:* Hypothyroidism; Addison's disease; Cushing's syndrome; Hyperparathyroidism; *(c) Neurologic disorders:* Entrapment neuropathies; Cervical spine disease (radiculopathy); Autoimmune disorders (myasthenia gravis, multiple sclerosis); *(d) Infections:* Parvovirus B19; Hepatitis C; Lyme disease; *(e) Sleep disorders:* Obstructive sleep apnea; *(f) Medications:* Lipid lowering drugs; Antiviral medications; Tapering of corticosteroids; *(g) Malignancy*
PHYSICAL EXAMINATION
Vitals: Pulse: Normal, may have a resting tachycardia; BP: Normal; RR: Normal; Temp: Normal
Cutaneous: No specific findings
Head & Neck: Xerostomia and xerophthalmia
Respiratory: No specific findings

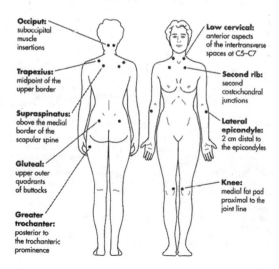

Occiput: suboccipital muscle insertions

Trapezius: midpoint of the upper border

Supraspinatus: above the medial border of the scapular spine

Gluteal: upper outer quadrants of buttocks

Greater trochanter: posterior to the trochanteric prominence

Low cervical: anterior aspects of the intertransverse spaces at C5–C7

Second rib: second costochondral junctions

Lateral epicondyle: 2 cm distal to the epicondyles

Knee: medial fat pad proximal to the joint line

Cardiovascular: No specific findings

Gastrointestinal: Diffuse tenderness

Musculoskeletal: Raynaud's phenomenon; 11 out of 18 fibromyalgia tender points

Neurologic: No specific findings

Fibromyalgia Tender Points: (a) Occiput: Bilateral, at the suboccipital muscle insertions; *(b) Low cervical:* Bilateral, at the anterior aspects of the intertransverse spaces at C5-C7; *(c) Trapezius:* Bilateral, at the midpoint of the upper border; *(d) Supraspinatus:* Bilateral, at origins, above the scapular spine near the medial border; *(e) Second rib:* Bilateral, at the second costochondral junctions, just lateral to the junctions on upper surfaces; *(f) Lateral epicondyle:* Bilateral, 2 cm distal to the epicondyles; *(g) Gluteal:* Bilateral, in upper outer quadrants of buttocks in anterior fold of muscle; *(h) Greater trochanter:* Bilateral, posterior to the trochanteric prominence; *(i) Knee:* Bilateral, at the medial fat pad proximal to the joint line

Control Tender Points: Mid forehead; Thumbnail; Volar surface of mid forearm; Anterior mid thigh

INVESTIGATIONS

Bloodwork & Urinalysis: All hematology panels, chemistries, serology should be normal

Screening Investigations: CBC; Electrolytes including Ca, Mg, PO4; Creatinine; Liver enzymes - AST, ALT, ALP, LDH, albumin; CK; TSH; ESR/CRP; ANA - If symptoms suggestive of SLE; RF - If symptoms suggestive of inflammatory arthritis; Sleep study - If OSA is questioned

MANAGEMENT

Education: Reassurance that fibromyalgia is a real condition; Reassurance that other illnesses have been ruled out

Physical Therapy with Aerobic Exercise: Begin very gradually under the guidance of a physical therapist and explain that their disease may flare initially; Aerobic, non-impact (water aerobics, walking, and biking) exercise is more beneficial than stretching programs; The goals of exercise are to: Improve overall muscle conditioning, aid in the restoration of sleep, and increase endogenous endorphins within the CNS; Core muscle strengthening has been shown to be of benefit

Cognitive Behavioral therapy: Relaxation training, activity pacing, visual imagery techniques, problem solving, and goal setting

Sleep Hygiene: No stressful activities at least one hour prior to bed (TV, work, exercise); Avoid caffeine; Go to bed at the same time each evening; Use the bedroom only for sleep, keep it dark, cool (65 degrees), and quiet; If not asleep after 30 minutes - get out of bed and leave the room; Try not to take worries to bed

Analgesia: Acetaminophen & NSAIDs may be of benefit; Corticosteroids are of no benefit

CNS Active Medications: Tricyclic anti-depressants (Amitriptyline and Cylcobenzaprine); Selective serotonin reuptake inhibitors (SSRIs); Gabapentin

Complementary therapies: Trigger point injections; Acupuncture; Myofascial release; Chiropractic therapy

PROGNOSIS

Risk Stratification for Poor Progression: (a) Older patients; (b) Female sex; (c) Persistent pain; (d) Long duration of symptoms

Prognosis: The majority of patients experience symptoms despite specific treatment; Half of patients may experience some improvement and 25% of patients experience substantial improvement

GONOCOCCAL ARTHRITIS

DEFINITION & PATHOPHYSIOLOGY

Definition: Gonococcal infection is due to hematologic dissemination of Neisseria Gonococcus as a result of sexual transmission of the organism

Pathophysiology: Neisseria gonorrhea infects mucosal surfaces including the urethra, cervix, pharynx, and rectum. The organism disseminates hematologically via defects in mucosal surfaces. Gonococcal arthritis is a result of the hematologic dissemination of the organism. The migratory polyarthritis may be immunologically driven as organisms are often absent from the affected joints.

PRESENTATION

Identifying Data: Young women more commonly than men (3-4:1); More prevalent in developing countries and is on the decline in North America and Europe

Onset: (a) Bacteremic Form: Begins with fever & chills accompanied by an intense asymmetric polyarthralgia which may be migratory or may be additive; *(b) Suppurative Form:* Arthritis (usually monoarticular) is the major feature

Progression: Bacteremic Form: The arthralgia takes a few days to peak and may resolve spontaneously; Skin lesions are non-pruritic and seen as tiny pustules on an erythematous base. The skin lesions spare the face and scalp. Tenosynovitis may accompany the presentation in up to 66% of patients involving the dorsum of the hands, wrists, and ankles. Tenosynovial involvement does not necessarily mean underlying joint involvement. An actual inflammatory arthritis occurs in less than 50% of patients and is usually monoarticular.

Constitutional Features: May be accompanied by fever

Functional Status: Reduced functional status with difficulties in ADLs

RHEUMATOLOGIC REVIEW OF SYSTEMS

Musculoskeletal Involvement: Tenosynovitis; Osteomyelitis; Pyomyositis

Mucocutaneous Involvement: Dermatitis

Neurologic Involvement: Meningitis

Cardiac Involvement: Gonococcal endocarditis; Myocarditis, Pericarditis

Gastrointestinal Involvement: Hepatitis

Endocrine Involvement: Waterhouse – Friedrichsen syndrome

RISK FACTORS

(a) Female sex; (b) Pregnancy; (c) Menstruation; (d) Multiple sexual partners; (e) Low socioeconomic class; (f) IV drug use; (g) Complement deficiency; (h) Systemic lupus erythematosus; (i) HIV infection

FAMILY HISTORY

Family history is not a risk factor

RED FLAGS

Aspirate the joint to rule out other causes of septic arthritis

DIFFERENTIAL DIAGNOSIS

(a) Gonococcal arthritis; (b) Other septic arthritis; (c) Crystalline arthritis (gout or CPPD); (d) Seronegative arthritis with a monoarticular onset (ReA, PsA); (e) Trauma with hemarthrosis; (f) RA – Rarely can get a pseudoseptic joint

PHYSICAL EXAMINATION

Vitals: P: Normal to elevated with pain; BP: Normal; RR: Usually normal; T: May have an associated fever

Cutaneous: Dermatitis

Head & Neck: No specific findings

Respiratory: No specific findings

Cardiovascular: Congestive heart failure as a result of myocarditis or pericarditis; Pericardial friction rub - pericarditis; Murmurs secondary to endocarditis

Gastrointestinal: Right upper quadrant tenderness with hepatitis

Musculoskeletal: Tenosynovitis - Over the dorsum of the hands and wrists, over the fingers (dactylitis), over the ankles and feet, and over the toes (dactylitis); Arthralgia & myalgia; Acute septic arthritis if bacteremic form

Neurologic: Meningeal irritation if associated gonococcal meningitis

INVESTIGATIONS

CBC: Leukocytosis and thrombocytosis

ESR: Elevated

Culture Sites: Cervical cultures in women (Positive in 70 – 80%); Urethral cultures in men (Positive in 70 – 80%); Pharyngeal cultures (Positive in 20%); Rectal cultures (Positive in 10%); Blood cultures (Positive in only 5%); Culture the partner

Radiology: Soft tissue fusiform swelling, otherwise usually normal

Aspiration & Pathology: Synovial fluid should be aspirated whenever possible; WBC counts range from 10 – 100 billion cells per liter (10,000 – 100,000 cells/mm3); Gram stain is negative in over 50% of culture positive fluids; Synovial fluid cultures are positive in only 50% of patients.

MANAGEMENT

General: Establish the diagnosis by culture whenever possible; Think about complications of dissemination including endocarditis and meningitis; Test for other sexually transmitted diseases at time of diagnosis and 6 weeks afterwards. These include: (a) Chlamydia; (b) HIV; (c) Syphilis

Test the patient's partner(s); Educate the patient and his or her partner about safe sexual practices: Sexual mode of transmission; Preventing sexually acquired infections;

If the patient has a purulent arthritis the joint must be repeatedly aspirated on a daily basis

Analgesics & NSAIDs: For symptomatic relief

Parenteral (IV or IM) antibiotics: First-line treatment and should be continued for 24-48 hours after improvement or resolution of signs and symptoms. Purulent effusions may require longer IV antibiotic treatment. The first line choice is a ***3rd generation cephalosporin:*** IV Ceftriaxone 1-2 grams q24h; IV Cefotaxime 1 gram q8h; ***If severe penicillin allergy use:*** Spectinomycin 2 grams IM q12h;

Oral (PO) antibiotics: Once the patient has improved they may be changed to oral therapy to complete at least a 7 day course of antibiotics. The choice of oral antibiotics depends upon the sensitivity of the organism: Cefixime 400 mg PO BID; Cefuroxime 500 mg PO BID; Clavulin 500 mg PO q8h; Ciprofloxacin 500 mg PO BID; Amoxicillin 500 mg PO q8h; Treat chlamydial infections with doxycycline 100 mg PO BID for 7 days or azithromycin 1 gram single oral dose

PROGNOSIS

Risk Stratification for Poor Progression: Delay in seeking medical treatment

Prognosis: The prognosis is excellent provided appropriate prompt antibiotic treatment is given early

GOUT

DEFINITION & PATHOPHYSIOLOGY

Definition: Acute gout is an inflammatory arthritis produced by the deposition of uric acid crystals into a joint

Pathophysiology: Hyperuricemia is seen in all patients with gout. Most (90%) are underexcretors. The first attack of gout typically occurs after 15-20 years of asymptomatic hyperuricemia. For some reason urate crystallizes in over saturated joints as a monosodium salt. Precipitation is favored by: The degree of supersaturation; Local temperatures (urate is less soluble at temps <37); Plasma proteins: The binding of albumin to urate increases the solubility and prevents precipitation; Abnormal aggrecans (OA) which reduce solubility and increase crystallization. The urate crystals are deposited in the synovium. These urate crystals are able to initiate and maintain intense attacks of acute inflammation because of their capacity to stimulate the release of numerous inflammatory mediators. Macrophages and synovial cells are induced to release phospholipase A2, cyclooxygenase, lipoxygenase, TNF, IL-1, IL-6, and IL-8. These cytokines then promote endothelial-neutrophil adhesion with the subsequent neutrophilic influx. The ingress of neutrophils appears to be the most important event for developing acute urate crystal-induced synovitis. IL-1, TNF, IL-6, and IL-8 release into the venous circulation appears to be responsible for the systemic manifestations

PRESENTATION

Identifying Data: Men > women (20:1); Onset in men between the ages of 35-50; Onset in women 15-20 years after menopause

Onset: Intense pain, swelling, & erythema of the affected joint with inflammation of contiguous structures such as tenosynovium; Typically begins in the morning; The disease is monoarticular in 80% of cases and the most common joint affected is the 1st MTP. Precipitants include: (a) minimal trauma, (b) acute illness, (c) surgery, (d) excessive alcohol intake, (e) changes in medications (Stopping or starting allopurinol may result in a flare of acute gout)

Progression: The inflammation reaches maximum intensity over a few hours. Untreated, it will usually resolve in 7-10 days; *Chronic Tophaceous Gout:* Clinically apparent tophi may present 10-20 years after an initial attack; Tophi are most commonly found over the dorsal fingers and toes and extensor surfaces of the forearms; Less dramatic, but more persistent joint inflammation which may resemble rheumatoid arthritis

Constitutional Features: May be accompanied by fever

Functional Status: Reduced functional status with difficulties with ADLs

RHEUMATOLOGIC REVIEW OF SYSTEMS

Associated Conditions: Hypertension; Obesity; Hyperlipidemia; Atherosclerosis

Mucocutaneous Involvement: Development of tophi

Renal Involvement: Renal calculi

Endocrine Involvement: Insulin resistance

RISK FACTORS

Uric Acid Overproduction (10%): (a) PRPP synthetase overactivity; (b) HGPRT deficiency; (c) Myeloproliferative & lymphoproliferative disorders; (d) Psoriasis; (e) Hemolytic anemia; (f) Excessive alcohol use

Uric Acid Underexcretion (90%): (a) Family history of gout; (b) Starvation; (c) Dehydration; (d) Acidosis - Ketoacidosis & lactic acidosis; (e) Chronic renal failure; (f) Endocrinopathies; (g) Hypothyroidism; (h) Hyperparathyroidism; (i) Medications

(Thiazide diuretics; Loop diuretics; Low-dose ASA; Cyclosporine; Nicotinic acid; Ethambutol; Pyrazinamide); (j) Obesity

Renal Handling of Uric Acid

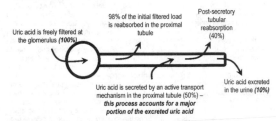

Uric acid is freely filtered at the glomerulus *(100%)*

98% of the initial filtered load is reabsorbed in the proximal tubule

Post-secretory tubular reabsorption (40%)

Uric acid excreted in the urine *(10%)*

Uric acid is secreted by an active transport mechanism in the proximal tubule (50%) – *this process accounts for a major portion of the excreted uric acid*

FAMILY HISTORY
A family history of gout is an independent risk factor for gout

RED FLAGS
Aspirate the joint to rule out septic arthritis

DIFFERENTIAL DIAGNOSIS
(a) Septic arthritis; (b) Crystalline arthritis (CPPD); (c) Seronegative arthritis with a monoarticular onset (ReA, PsA); (d) Trauma with hemarthrosis; (e) RA - Rarely can get a pseudoseptic joint

PHYSICAL EXAMINATION
Vitals: Pulse: Normal to elevated with pain; BP: Patient may have concomitant hypertension; RR: Usually normal; Temperature: May have an associated fever with acute gout

Cutaneous: Tophaceous deposits over the DIPs, PIPs, MCPs, extensor surfaces of the forearms, the olecranon bursa, and the pinnae of the ears

Head & Neck: Tophaceous deposits on the pinnae of the ears

Respiratory: No specific findings

Cardiovascular: Look for signs of hyperlipidemia

Gastrointestinal: No specific findings

Musculoskeletal: Acute inflammatory radiographic arthritis which can resemble a septic joint; Tenosynovitis with edema of the soft tissues around the joint; Inflammatory arthritis which may resemble rheumatoid arthritis

Neurologic: No specific findings

INVESTIGATIONS
CBC: Leukocytosis, reactive thrombocytosis

ESR: Elevated

Uric Acid: Elevated (can fall in the face of an acute attack)

Creatinine: May be elevated

Serum Cholesterol: May be elevated

Radiology: The most common radiographic finding in patients with clinical evidence of gout is a completely normal joint and likely some soft tissue swelling. This is true even for patients whose symptoms have spanned many years; *(a) Soft Tissue:*

Eccentric asymmetric nodular soft tissue prominence accompanies soft tissue deposition of urates. These lesions may not be visible until they reach larger sizes (5-10 mm). Calcification of a tophus is unusual and may reflect a coexisting abnormality of calcium metabolism. Associated peripheral arterial calcification has been described in gout; *(b) Bones:* Bone Density: Extensive loss of bone density is not a feature; Erosions: Bony erosions are common in gout; They are produced by tophaceous deposits and may be intra-articular, para-articular, or located a considerable distance from the joint; The erosions usually start in the marginal areas of the joint and proceed centrally; Erosions are generally round and may be surrounded by a sclerotic border producing a "punched out" effect; Erosions have a typical appearance with overhanging edges which is not pathognomonic but is strongly suggestive of the "gout"; Cyst formation in gout may represent tophaceous deposits within bone; *(c) Cartilage:* A relative preservation of the normal interosseous space in an articulation with extensive erosions is a characteristic feature of gout; This relates to the relative integrity of the cartilage adjacent to areas of extensive cartilaginous and osseous destruction; In later stages, joint space narrowing is frequent and may be uniform; Bony ankylosis of joint spaces is rare and only seen in the interphalangeal joints; *(d) Distribution:* Chronic polyarticular gout tends to be distributed in an asymmetric fashion with a predilection for the lower extremities; Commonly involved areas include the foot and ankle, knees, hands, wrists, and elbows. Involvement of the shoulders, hips, spine, & SI joints has been reported but is rare. *(e) Remember with Gout:* Normal radiographs most common, however, soft tissue swelling can be observed; A preserved joint space in the face of extensive erosions is a clue; Bone density is not usually changed; Erosions are usually marginal (away from the joint surface) and have sclerotic margins and may have overhanging edges; Cyst formation is seen (tophi in bone); Distributed in an asymmetric manner

Aspiration & Pathology: Identification of intracellular monosodium urate crystals in synovial fluid leukocytes is the gold standard; Negatively birefringent needle-shaped crystals on polarized microscopy

MANAGEMENT

General: Rest & elevation; Ice; Physical therapy for gentle range of motion

Pharmacologic Treatment of Acute Gout: See Next Page

Prevention of Future Attacks: Most attacks are usually self-limited and treating each attack is a perfectly reasonable approach; Use hypouricemic agents (Allopurinol) if: (a) Recurrent acute episodes of gout affecting lifestyle; (b) Patients at risk from complications of treatments required for acute attacks; (c) Patient acceptance of the need for LIFELONG medication compliance. Remember gout is a relatively benign disease with a potentially harmful treatment (allopurinol).

Pharmacologic Treatment of Chronic Tophaceous Gout: The goal of therapy is to lower the serum uric acid thereby creating a concentration gradient encouraging uric acid in the tissues to move into the circulation; *(a) Allopurinol:* Most appropriate therapy for patients with chronic tophaceous gout; Should not be initiated during an acute attack of gout; Start at doses of 50-200 mg/day increasing every 1-3 weeks aiming to reduce the serum uric acid level to the lower limit of normal; On initiation of Allopurinol, patients may experience a flare of their gout "mobilization gout" and should be warned; *(b) Probenecid & Sulfinpyrazone:* Increase uric acid excretion by the kidneys; These agents are not as effective in the setting of renal impairment

PROGNOSIS

Risk Stratification for Poor Progression: (a) Early age of onset; (b) Multiple recurrent attacks; (c) High serum uric acid levels; (d) Polyarticular disease

Prognosis: Recurrence rates for acute gout: 60% in the 1st year; 80% by 2 years; 90% by 5 years

ALGORITHM FOR THE TREATMENT OF ACUTE GOUT

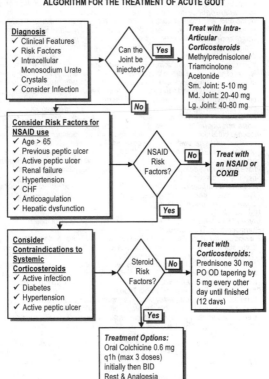

INFLAMMATORY MYOSITIS

(POLYMYOSITIS (PM) & DERMATOMYOSITIS (DM))

DEFINITION & PATHOPHYSIOLOGY

Definition: An inflammatory myopathy characterized by proximal muscle weakness and non-suppurative inflammation

Pathophysiology: Believed to be triggered by environmental factors in genetically susceptible individuals; Virus are thought to be the environmental triggers due to: Seasonal variation of the disease; Chronic myositis is known to develop after infection with picornovirus

PRESENTATION

Identifying Data: Bimodal distribution age 10-15 and ages 45-60; Patients with "malignancy associated" myositis are typically > 50; Male: female ratio of about 1:2; Prevalence rare – at most 0.001% in the population (10 per million)

Onset: Initial symptoms of muscle weakness are insidious occurring over 3 to 6 months involving the shoulder and hip girdles most severely. The weakness is symmetrical and proximal.

Progression: As the disease progresses the muscle weakness slowly worsens with 50% of patients developing neck flexor weakness. The disease can be severe enough to cause people to be bed ridden.

Constitutional Features: Fatigue may be prominent, weight loss due to anorexia and the inflammatory burden, and morning stiffness

Functional Status: Reduced functional status with difficulties in ADLs; Difficulty at work

RHEUMATOLOGIC REVIEW OF SYSTEMS

Associated Conditions: Overlap with SLE and SSc

Musculoskeletal Involvement: Involvement of pharyngeal muscles can result in dysphonia or dysphagia. This should be regarded as very serious with a high risk of aspiration pneumonia. Non-erosive Inflammatory polyarthritis. Arthralgias and myalgias are usually a mild feature unlike polymyalgia rheumatica

Mucocutaneous Involvement: May come up to one year prior to the onset of clinical muscle weakness; Gottren's Papules: Lacy violaceous areas on the dorsal aspect of the interphalangeal joints, elbows, patella, and medial malleoli – these are pathognomonic for dermatomyositis; Heliotrope discolorations of the eyelids with periorbital edema; Macular erythema of the posterior shoulders and neck (Shawl Sign), anterior neck (V-Sign), face, and forehead; Periungal telangiectasia and nailfold capillary changes; Mechanic's hands in Anti-Synthetase Syndrome

Vascular Involvement: Raynaud's Phenomenon - More common with the anti-synthetase syndrome

Cardiac Involvement: Myocardial muscle involvement; Asymptomatic ECG abnormalities are most common; Supraventricular tachycardia; Cardiomyopathy and congestive heart failure

Respiratory Involvement: Interstitial fibrosis (5-10%); Aspiration pneumonia – Significant cause of morbidity and mortality; Respiratory muscle weakness - Poor cough and sputum clearance

Gastrointestinal Involvement: Dysphagia from esophageal dysmotility

RISK FACTORS

HLA-DR3; *HLADR52* in ALL patients with anti-Jo-1; Malignancy: Malignancies are more commonly associated with dermatomyositis than polymyositis; Can occur 2 years prior to onset to 2 years after onset of myositis; Ovarian, gastric, cervical, and lung malignancies seem to be more common

FAMILY HISTORY
No known associated family history

RED FLAGS
Pharyngeal and respiratory muscle involvement confer a worse prognosis; Malignancy (see below); Infection; Think of overlap with SLE and SSc

DIFFERENTIAL DIAGNOSIS
(a) Inflammatory myopathies; *(b) Inflammatory myopathy secondary to malignancy*; *(c) Inclusion body myositis:* Affects older white males (> 50); Affects both proximal and distal muscles; Legs affected > arms; May have an associated neuropathy; CK may be normal in 20-30% of cases; Responds poorly to therapy; *(d) Drug-induced myositis:* Corticosteroids: Does not usually cause an elevation in CK; Less likely to involve the neck flexors; If in doubt look at the MRI for evidence of persistent inflammation; HMG-CoA reductase Inhibitors; Alcohol; AZT; Plaquenil; Colchicine; *(e) Endocrine:* Hypothyroidism; Hyperthyroidism; Cushing's disease; Addison's disease; *(f) Infectious myositis:* Bacterial – Pyomyositis; Viral – HIV; Parasitic – Toxoplasma; *(g) Neuromuscular disorders:* Myasthenia gravis; Eaton Lambert; Amyotrophic lateral sclerosis; *(h) Metabolic myopathies:* Glycogen storage disorders; Lipid metabolic abnormalities; Mitochondrial myopathies

PHYSICAL EXAMINATION
Vitals: Pulse: Normal; BP: Normal; RR: Increased if pulmonary involvement; Temperature: May have an associated fever

Cutaneous: Gottren's papules; Periungal erythema with dilated capillaries with dropout; Raynaud's phenomenon; Mechanic's hands; Rash over the olecranon process; Heliotrope rash with periorbital edema; Erythematous rash on forehead and face; V-sign or shawl sign

Head & Neck: Dysphonia; Salivation due to swallowing difficulty

Respiratory: Crackles secondary to interstitial fibrosis; Reduced chest expansion due to muscle weakness; Cough due to retained secretions or aspiration

Cardiovascular: Tachycardia; Congestive heart failure

Gastrointestinal: No specific findings

Musculoskeletal: Proximal muscle weakness – Needs to be graded (0-5); Inflammatory arthritis affecting the small joints

Neurologic: Atrophy and weakness distally if inclusion body myositis

INVESTIGATIONS
CBC: Anemia with active disease, reactive thrombocytosis

Creatinine Kinase: Usually elevated. A normal CK may be found for the following reasons: Early disease, burnt out disease, or circulating inhibitors of creatinine kinase

AST, ALT, LDH, Aldolase: Elevated as released from muscle

ESR: Normal in 50%

ANA: 80% of cases

Anti-Jo-1 (antibody to histidyl-t-RNA synthetase): 11-20% of cases present with the antisynthetase syndrome characterized by: Relatively acute onset; Mechanic's hands; Raynaud's phenomenon; Inflammatory arthritis; Interstitial lung involvement; Moderate control with a tendency of disease persistence

Anti-Mi-2 (helicase components of histone acetylase complexes): (5-10%) Acute classic dermatomyositis with the "V" and "Shawl" signs with cuticular overgrowth – good prognosis and good response to steroids

Anti-SRP (signal recognition particle): (< 5%) Polymyositis with very acute onset of severe weakness, occurs often in the fall, and has a tendency for cardiac involvement. Poor responder to treatment.

Screening for Malignancy: Full history and physical exam including breast, rectal, and pelvic exams; Bloodwork (CBC, Cr, LFT's, Ca, ESR, urine); Stool for occult blood; Mammogram for all women; CXR; CT-Chest, abdomen, and pelvis; Ca-125

Electromyography (EMG): (a) Increased insertional activity with fibrillations and sharp positive waves; (b) Spontaneous, high-frequency discharges; (c) Polyphasic motor units of low amplitude and short duration

Magnetic Resonance Imaging (MRI): Ask for STIR images which show active inflammation, edema, fibrosis, and calcification of the muscle

Muscle Biopsy: (a) Polymyositis: Muscle fiber necrosis with degenerating and regenerating fibers scattered throughout the fascicle; Increased CD8+ T-Cells invading muscle fibers; Endomysial inflammation; **(b) Dermatomyositis:** Muscle fiber necrosis with degenerating and regenerating fibers in a perifascicular distribution; Perimysial and perivascular inflammation with CD4+ T-Cells; Complement deposition (MAC) in blood vessel walls

MANAGEMENT

General: Education; Avoidance of Sunlight for those with DM; Speech pathology involvement with dysphagia

Physiotherapy: Improve ROM; Improve functional abilities by increasing muscle strength, endurance, and aerobic capacity; Chest physiotherapy and follow-up of respiratory function with daily bedside spirometry

Occupational Therapy: Joint protection; Fatigue management; Assistive devices

Corticosteroids: Start prednisone at 1mg/kg (60 mg) and continue until muscle strength begins to return and enzymes normalize; Once the enzymes have normalized the prednisone can be slowly tapered following the patients muscle strength closely; If at 3 months the patient is not responding or requiring large doses of prednisone a second agent should be introduced (review the initial diagnosis if the patient is not responding to corticosteroids); If the muscles are weak with normal enzymes – think about steroid myopathy; Don't forget the osteoprotective meds (Calcium, Vitamin D, and bisphosphonates)

DMARDs: Methotrexate or Azathioprine may be used first-line in patients with poor prognostic features; No direct head to head comparisons of MTX vs. AZA; Some suggestion that MTX may be better in anti-synthetase syndrome

IVIG: 2 grams once monthly for 3 months – small trial with only 15 treatment resistant patients; Life threatening disease may also be an indication

Cyclosporine: Has been effective in treating a few patients with DM

Hydroxychloroquine & Mycophenolate Mofetil: May be useful in patients with refractory rash

PROGNOSIS

Risk Stratification for Poor Progression: (a) Disease present > 6 months prior to treatment; (b) Severe weakness; (c) Dysphagia; (d) Anti-signal recognition peptide (SRP)

Prognosis: Overall 5-year survival with PM or DM is about 85% with following 5-year survival for these subgroups: anti-Mi-2: 90%; anti-Jo-1: 65%; anti SRP: 30%; Malignancy associated myositis has a worse prognosis

JUVENILE IDIOPATHIC ARTHRITIS - OLIGOARTICULAR

DEFINITION & PATHOPHYSIOLOGY

Definition: Pauciarticular juvenile idiopathic arthritis is a subset of juvenile idiopathic arthritis resulting in inflammation of the synovial membrane in 4 or fewer of the diarthrodial joints

Pathophysiology: The most widely accepted hypothesis is that the disease is triggered by an unknown antigen in a genetically susceptible individual. The initial stages consist of infiltration and clonal expansion of T cells into the synovial membrane. The early inflammatory response results in recruitment of other cells to the synovium which is facilitated by upregulation of adhesion molecules and proliferation of new blood vessels. T-cells activate macrophages to secrete pro-inflammatory cytokines (TNF, IL-1, IFN). Tumor Necrosis Factor has the following actions: Activates neutrophils, macrophages, and synovial fibroblasts; Stimulates other cytokine production (IL-1), IL-6, GM-CSF etc; Upregulates adhesion molecules; Promotes the proliferation of synoviocytes and fibroblasts; Activates and induces differentiation of osteoclasts; Stimulates the release of matrix metalloproteinases (MMPs) resulting in proteolysis and tissue destruction. The natural anti-inflammatory and regulatory mechanisms are overwhelmed resulting in a runaway inflammatory process leading to the destruction of cartilage and bone

PRESENTATION

Identifying Data: Occurs in children < 6 years of age with peak onset between 1 and 3 years of age. Rarely presents after age 10 and children who do present after age 10 are usually diagnosed with an enthesitis related arthritis. Females:males = 4:1

Onset: In 1/3 to 1/2 of children the arthritis begins as a monoarthritis. Usually presents in young girls as a painless limp which begins insidiously. The time of onset of the illness is often difficult to determine as typically there are no complaints of pain. The knee is the most common joint affected followed by the ankle and then small joints of the hands (including the wrists), and the elbows. The joint is often swollen and warm but usually not very painful, tender, or erythematous. Pauciarticular JIA affecting the hip is extremely uncommon and the diagnosis should be questioned under these circumstances.

Progression: The arthritis may not progress and remain confined to the joint(s) at initial presentation. This occurs in up to 1/3 of children. Other children have progression of the disease with the addition of one or two more joints, however, the burden of disease remains oligoarticular. In some children (up to 50%) the disease may progress to a polyarticular form

Constitutional Features: Constitutional features are typically absent with pauciarticular JIA

Functional Status: Alterations in age specific ADLs; Difficulty at school with physical activity; Weakness and difficulty ambulating

RHEUMATOLOGIC REVIEW OF SYSTEMS

Musculoskeletal Involvement: Leg Length Discrepancy: Second most common complication of Pauci-articular JIA

Ocular Involvement: Uveitis or Iridocyclitis: Occurs in 20% of children and 50% of cases are asymptomatic. Presenting symptoms (in 50%) could include pain, redness, headache, photophobia, and altered vision. Bilateral in 2/3 of cases; Activity of uveitis does not parallel that of the arthritis; Typically presents within 5 - 7 years of joint involvement and is present in < 10% of patients prior to the onset of arthritis; Risk factors include: (a) Female sex; (b) Young age of onset; (c) Arthritis present less than four years; (d) Negative rheumatoid factor; (e) Positive ANA

RISK FACTORS
HLA DR5, DR8, DR11, DR13, and DPw2 genetic factors

FAMILY HISTORY
Uncommon to have multiple members of a family affected. Small increased risk to family members of a patient with JRA.

RED FLAGS
Anemia and elevated acute phase reactants are rare and alternate diagnosis should be considered in this situation; Children with significant pain should be evaluated for infectious or neoplastic disease

DIFFERENTIAL DIAGNOSIS
(a) Juvenile idiopathic pauciarticular arthritis; (b) Infectious arthritis: Bacterial; Viral; Lyme disease; Tuberculosis; (c) Psoriatic arthritis; (d) Enthesitis associated arthritis; (e) Neoplastic disease; (f) Connective tissue diseases; (g) Sarcoidosis; (h) Pigmented Villonodular Synovitis

PHYSICAL EXAMINATION
Vitals: Pulse: Normal; BP: Normal; RR: Normal; Temperature - Normal

Cutaneous: No specific findings

Head & Neck: Ocular involvement with uveitis which is usually not apparent without slit lamp examination. In some children the iris may appear irregular due to posterior synechiae although this is a late finding.

Respiratory: No specific findings

Cardiovascular: No specific findings

Gastrointestinal: No specific findings

Musculoskeletal: The involved joints are usually swollen and warm with minimal pain, tenderness, and lack of erythema; Range of motion may appear to be preserved but should be compared to the other side as children have much greater range of motion than adults; Typical joints involved include the knees, ankles, wrists, elbows, and small joints of the hands

Neurologic: No specific findings

INVESTIGATIONS
CBC: Normal hemoglobin, normal WBC, normal platelet count

ESR/CRP: Normal

Rheumatoid Factor: Negative

ANA: Present in 40-85% of patients and associated with chronic anterior uveitis

ENA Panel: Negative

Plain Radiographs: (a) Soft Tissue: Periarticular swelling & evidence of joint effusions; *(b) Alignment:* Damage to joints results in mal-alignment; *(c) Bones:* Periarticular osteopenia, bone destruction, under or overgrowth of long bones, accelerated epiphyseal maturation; *(d) Joints:* Uniform joint space narrowing (cartilage destruction) and erosions

Synovial Fluid: Inflammatory cellular picture 5000 – 15,000 cells/mm3 which are predominantly polymorphonuclear leukocytes.

Synovial Biopsy: (a) Hyperplasia of the synovial lining layer: Becomes 6-10 cells thick (normal 1-3); Cells hypertrophy; Cellular infiltrate: Predominantly CD4 T-cells & macrophages; Also see B-cells, dendritic cells, PMNs, and activated fibroblasts; Synovial neovascularization

MANAGEMENT
Education & Psychological Support: Measures to empower patients and their families to improve compliance and coping skills include disease education, and advice regarding pain self-management. Clinically significant psychologic

dysfunction may occur in children and their parents, especially at the time of diagnosis. Adolescents appear to be particularly vulnerable. Provide adequate psychologic counseling for both patients and their families. Ensure teachers and other caregivers have an accurate understanding of an individual child's disease helping to optimize the school experience for the child

Physiotherapy: Education of the parents and child about the goals of physiotherapy; Regular involvement in age appropriate physical activities is encouraged to improve fitness and help the child fulfill psychological needs. Pain relieving strategies and interventions; Maintenance or increase in joint range of motion; Maintenance or increase in muscular strength; Mobility aids and braces; Serial casting for flexion contractures

Occupational Therapy: Required to adequately assess the functional capacities of the child; Improve efficiency with joint protective measures and energy conservation strategies; Increase independence with the use of assistive devices and techniques; Splints to correct or prevent deformities, correct or prevent contractures, and to aid flexion and extension of involved areas; Shoes, insoles, and lifts for leg length discrepancy

Nutrition: To ensure a balanced diet with adequate caloric content for the child with JIA and to discourage the use of a "special diet" for children with JIA. Dietary management of the over-weight child & weight-gain associated with corticosteroids.

Possible Pharmacologic Strategy: Begin with NSAIDs in appropriate doses and review after a period of approximately 2 months. If the child is improved continue the NSAID for a total of 4-6 months and taper off the NSAID. If the child is not improved after the initial NSAID consider intra-articular corticosteroid injection and/or increase the dose of the NSAID. Follow the child every 2-3 months and if persistent inflammation remains after intra-articular injection and adequate trials of NSAIDs re-consider the diagnosis. If inflammation persists consider using sulfasalazine or methotrexate. Hydroxychloroquine could be considered for very mild disease. With this approach, all patients should be on a DMARD within 6 months of persistent inflammation.

NSAIDs and COXIBs: NSAIDs possess both analgesic and anti-inflammatory properties and are typically the first line of therapy for pauciarticular JIA; Most children respond by 4 weeks and in some it may take up to 12 weeks. Pain usually responds initially, however, a reduction in swelling may take longer. NSAIDs should be used for 3 months before deeming a treatment failure; Common NSAIDs used: (a) Naproxen in doses of 15-20 mg/kg/day divided into two daily doses; (b) Ibuprofen in doses of 35 mg/kg/day divided into four daily doses; (c) Diclofenac 2.0-3.0 mg/kg/day divided into three daily doses. Not approved in children; (d) Piroxicam 0.2-0.3 mg/kg/day given as a single daily dose. Not approved in children.

Intra-Articular Corticosteroids: Intra-articular corticosteroids are typically used when patients have failed NSAID therapy, have had significant NSAID toxicity, or have developed joint deformity, growth disturbance, or muscle wasting. Almost all patients experience rapid resolution of joint symptoms within a few days and some achieve remission for 12 months or more after a single injection. Triamcinolone Hexacetonide has been shown to be superior to both betamethasone (celestone) and methylprednisolone (solumedrol). Triamcinolone Hexacetonide (Aristospan) has not been appropriately compared to Triamcinolone Acetonide (Kenolog). Immobilization of joints after injection is common practice in some clinics, however, some rheumatologists advise normal activity but to avoid high-impact physical activity

DMARDs: Children who fail to respond to appropriate trials of NSAIDs or intra-articular corticosteroids are often treated with a conventional DMARD. Common initial DMARD choices include hydroxychloroquine and methotrexate.

Hydroxychloroquine: Typically takes 2-3 months for therapeutic effect; if no improvement after 6 months it should be discontinued; Administered in doses of 5-6 mg/kg/day. Only comes in 200 mg tablets which makes accurate dosing difficult. Some rheumatologists calculate the total weekly dose and divide the 200 mg tablets accordingly. Ocular monitoring should be done q6months.

Methotrexate: Typically takes 2-3 months for therapeutic effect; If no improvement after three to six months consider changing to parenteral compound or discontinuing; Administered in doses of 0.3-0.6 mg/kg/week up to 1.0 mg/kg/week for resistant disease. Consider parenteral methotrexate in those patients who have a poor response to oral methotrexate, need excess doses of oral methotrexate to control disease, or develop significant GI toxicity. Folic acid 1 mg/day or folinic acid once weekly at 1/2 the total dose of methotrexate can be used for GI intolerance.

Sulfasalazine: Typical therapeutic responses seen within 2-3 months; Initially administered starting 500 mg/day and increasing by 500 mg/day until a maximum dose of 50 mg/kg/day or 2000 mg/day is reached; Enteric coated sulfasalazine may be better tolerated.

Gold: Rarely used due to other available choices; If given started with a 5 mg IM test dose and then gradually increased to 0.75 - 1.0 mg/kg/week (maximum 50 mg/week). Requires weekly monitoring for renal and bone marrow toxicity.

Corticosteroids: Low dose corticosteroids can be highly effective in controlling symptoms in patients with active JIA but are rarely used in the child with pauciarticular JIA; Can be used as bridge therapy until DMARD has taken effect.

Biologics: Etanercept is the only approved anti-TNF agent for use in patients with polyarticular juvenile inflammatory arthritis who have failed methotrexate. However, it has been used clinically in patients with unresponsive pauciarticular disease; Typical dose is 0.4 mg/kg twice weekly.

Management of Uveitis: (1) Ocular Examinations: (a) No prior history of uveitis: At initial visit then every 3 months for 2 years, then every 4-6 months for 7 years then once a year; (b) Prior history of uveitis: Every 3 months with inactive disease. As indicated by response to therapy with active disease. (2) Treatment: Should be supervised by an experienced ophthalmologist; First Line: Glucocorticoid eye drops (dexamethasone or methylprednisolone) with or without a mydriatic to dilate the pupil. Glucocorticoid drips given hourly along with glucocorticoid ointment with unresponsive disease. Second Line: Oral corticosteroids are typically used in children who are unresponsive to topical preparations. Cyclosporine and mycophenolate mofetil have been used in refractory disease.

PROGNOSIS

Risk Stratification for Poor Prognosis: (a) Unremitting course / progression to polyarticular disease; (b) Rheumatoid factor positive; (c) Erosions on radiographs. Uveitis: Onset before or shortly after the diagnosis of arthritis.

Prognosis: A common misconception is that pauciarticular JIA will disappear as the patient enters adulthood. In fact, in some studies, 30-70% of patients continued to have active disease 10 years after onset. Patients whose disease remains pauciarticular tend to have the best prognosis. Those patients who progress to polyarticular involvement tend to have a more guarded outcome (especially if they are RF positive). Uveitis: Permanent visual damage may occur in as many as 15% of patients. Cataracts are a long-term consequence of the disease or its treatment.

JUVENILE IDIOPATHIC ARTHRITIS - POLYARTICULAR

DEFINITION & PATHOPHYSIOLOGY

Definition: Polyarticular juvenile idiopathic arthritis is a subset of juvenile idiopathic arthritis resulting in inflammation of the synovial membrane in 5 or more of the diarthrodial joints during the first six months of the disease. This subset comprises about 30-40% of patients with JIA. Children are excluded from this category if (a) they have psoriasis or there is a history of psoriasis in a first degree relative; (b) the patient is and HLA B27 positive male with arthritis beginning over the age of 6 years; (c) there is a family history of HLA B27 associated disease in a first degree relative; (d) the patient has features of systemic JIA. If there are two positive tests for rheumatoid factor at least 3 months apart, the patient is said to have rheumatoid factor positive polyarthritis. (ILAR Criteria, 2004)

Pathophysiology: The most widely accepted hypothesis is that the disease is triggered by an unknown antigen in a genetically susceptible individual. The initial stages consist of infiltration and clonal expansion of T cells into the synovial membrane. The early inflammatory response results in recruitment of other cells to the synovium which is facilitated by upregulation of adhesion molecules and proliferation of new blood vessels. T-cells activate macrophages to secrete pro-inflammatory cytokines (TNF, IL-1, IFN). Tumor Necrosis Factor has the following actions: Activates neutrophils, macrophages, and synovial fibroblasts; Stimulates other cytokine production (IL-1, IL-6, GM-CSF etc); Upregulates adhesion molecules; Promotes the proliferation of synoviocytes and fibroblasts; Activates and induces differentiation of osteoclasts; Stimulates the release of matrix metalloproteinases (MMPs) resulting in proteolysis and tissue destruction. The natural anti-inflammatory and regulatory mechanisms are overwhelmed resulting in a runaway inflammatory process leading to the destruction of cartilage and bone

PRESENTATION

Identifying Data: Bimodal distribution with the first peak incidence between 2-5 years and the second between 10-14 years; Females:males = 3:1

Onset: The onset is insidious with joint pain and swelling in 5 or more joints during the first 6 months of disease. Can rarely begin with a subacute or an acute presentation but this would not be typical. In general there are two broad groups of children: (a) Younger children who are RF negative who typically have a lower burden of disease which can be asymmetric; (b) Older children who are RF positive who often develop a pattern of arthritis similar to adult onset RA. Dactylitis suggests psoriatic arthritis and enthesitis suggests enthesitis related arthritis rather than polyarthritis. Morning stiffness > 60 minutes & gelling are common.

Progression: As the disease progresses additional joints become involved leading to a symmetric polyarthritis; The arthritis tends to be symmetric with the knees, wrists, elbows, and ankles being the most commonly involved. Small joints of the hands or feet may be affected early or late in the course of the disease

Constitutional Features: Low-grade fevers; A very high or quotidian fever suggests systemic JIA; Significant fatigue resulting in a lack of energy, increased requirement for sleep, or general irritability; Anorexia and wt loss; General growth disturbance

Functional Status: Reduced functional status and difficulties with ADLs; Difficulty at school with physical activity; Weakness and difficulty ambulating

RHEUMATOLOGIC REVIEW OF SYSTEMS

Associated Conditions: Poor nutritional status, delayed growth, delayed sexual maturation all reflecting active disease

Musculoskeletal Involvement: (a) General Growth Abnormalities: Normal linear growth is often slowed during periods of active disease; Steroids may also result in slowing of growth; *(b) Localized Growth Disturbances:* Localized growth disturbances in polyarticular JIA are more likely to occur in the fingers; leg length inequalities are typical of oligoarticular disease with one affected knee; With early active inflammation, shortening or lengthening of affected limbs can occur. If the skeleton is immature (young child) the affected limb tends to grow longer as the development of ossification centers of long bones are accelerated. If the skeleton is more mature (just prior to fusion of the physis) then shortening of the affected limb is more likely due to premature fusion of the epiphyses. Micrognathia is a striking example of localized growth retardation; *(c) Flexion Contractures*; *(d) Osteopathy:* Pts with polyarticular JIA fail to adequately mineralize bone and it is common for them to fail to undergo normal increase in bone mass during puberty.

Mucocutaneous Involvement: Rheumatoid nodules are very uncommon (2-5%). They are almost always associated with a positive RF & generally regarded as a poor prognostic sign; Dark discoloration over the skin of the PIP joints (rare)

Lymphatic Involvement: Asymmetric lymphedema (rare); Lymphadenopathy - uncommon and if prominent suggests systemic JIA

Vascular Involvement: Rheumatoid vasculitis in older onset seropositive disease

Hematological Involvement: Anemia of chronic inflammation; Leukocytosis; Thrombocytosis

Ocular Involvement: Uveitis or Iridocyclitis: Occurs in 5% of children and almost all cases are asymptomatic. Presenting symptoms in (50%) could include pain, redness, headache, photophobia, and altered vision. Bilateral in 2/3 of cases. Activity of uveitis does not parallel the disease; Typically presents within 5 - 7 years of joint involvement and is present in < 10% of patients prior to the onset of arthritis. Risk factors include: (a) Female sex; (b) Young age of onset of arthritis; (c) Arthritis present less than four years; (d) Negative rheumatoid factor; (e) Positive ANA

Gastrointestinal Involvement: NSAID gastritis; Mild to mod. hepatosplenomegaly

Endocrine Involvement: Delay of puberty & Sec. sexual charact. in active disease

RISK FACTORS
No known risk factors; Genetic factors

FAMILY HISTORY
Small increased risk to family members of a patient with JIA

RED FLAGS
Important subset of JIA patients are those who are usually girls in late childhood or adolescence who are RF positive. In these patients the pattern of arthritis is very similar to adult onset rheumatoid arthritis.

DIFFERENTIAL DIAGNOSIS
(a) Polyarthritis related to infection: Viral induced polyarthritis; Reactive arthritis; Lyme disease; (b) Juvenile idiopathic arthritis: Polyarticular; Psoriatic arthritis; Enthesitis-related arthritis (Juvenile ankylosing spondylitis); Enteropathic associated arthritis; (c) Connective tissue disease: Systemic lupus erythematosus; Vasculitis; (d) Arthritis associated with systemic disease: Sarcoidosis; Familial hypertrophic synovitis syndromes; Mucopolysaccharidoses

PHYSICAL EXAMINATION
Vitals: Pulse: Normal; may be elevated in presence of anemia or significantly active disease; BP: Normal; RR: Normal; Temp: Normal to low-grade fever

Cutaneous: Dark discoloration across the PIP joints (very uncommon); Rheumatoid nodules often found below the olecranon (very uncommon)

Head & Neck: Ocular involvement with uveitis which is usually not apparent without slit lamp examination. In some children the pupil may appear irregular due to posterior synechiae although this is a late finding.

Respiratory: No specific findings

Cardiovascular: No specific findings

Gastrointestinal: Mild to moderate hepatomegaly; Splenomegaly: mild enlargement occasionally, splenomegaly with neutropenia (Felty's syndrome) is rare

Musculoskeletal: (a) Joint Involvement: The involved joints are usually swollen and warm with minimal pain, tenderness, and lack of erythema; Range of motion may appear to be preserved but should be compared to the other side as children have much greater range of motion than adults; Muscle atrophy and flexion contractures may develop; Typical joints involved include the knees, ankles, wrists, elbows, small joints of the hands, and cervical spine; TMJ involvement may result in limited or asymmetric oral opening, abnormal mandibular alignment and crepitations; *(b) Bone Involvement:* General short stature due to a general growth disturbance; Localized bone overgrowths in common areas such as the knee or wrist; Micrognathia due to mandibular hypoplasia and loss of condyle

Neurologic: No specific findings

INVESTIGATIONS

CBC: Normal hemoglobin to anemia of chronic inflammation, normal WBC to a mild leukocytosis, normal platelet count to a moderate thrombocytosis

Liver Enzymes: May be slightly elevated

ESR/CRP: Usually elevated in active disease

Rheumatoid Factor: May be positive especially in females between ages 12 & 16.

ANA: Present in 50-70% of RF +ve patients and 25% of patients who are RF -ve.

ENA Panel: Negative

Plain Radiographs: (a) Soft Tissue: Periarticular swelling & evidence of joint effusions; *(b) Alignment:* Damage to joints results in malalignment; *(c) Bones:* Periarticular osteopenia, bone destruction, under or overgrowth of long bones, accelerated epiphyseal maturation; *(d) Joints:* Uniform joint space narrowing (cartilage destruction) and erosions

Synovial Fluid: Inflammatory cellular picture 5000 – 15,000 cells/mm3 which are predominantly polymorphonuclear leukocytes.

Synovial Biopsy: (a) Hyperplasia of the synovial lining layer: Becomes 6-10 cells thick (normal 1-3); Cells hypertrophy; (b) Cellular infiltrate: Predominantly CD4 T-cells & macrophages; Also see B-cells, dendritic cells, PMNs, and activated fibroblasts; (c) Synovial neovascularization

MANAGEMENT

Education & Psychological Support: Measures to empower patients and their families to improve compliance and coping skills include disease education and advice regarding pain self-management. Clinically significant psychologic dysfunction may occur in children and their parents, especially at the time of diagnosis. Adolescents appear to be particularly vulnerable. Provide adequate psychologic counseling for both patients and their families. Ensure teachers and other caregivers have an accurate understanding of an individual child's disease helping to optimize the school experience for the child.

Physiotherapy: Education of the parents and child about the goals of physiotherapy. Regular involvement in age appropriate physical activities is encouraged to improve fitness and help the child fulfill psychosocial needs. Pain relieving strategies and interventions; Maintenance or increase in joint range of motion; Maintenance or increase in muscular strength; Mobility aids and braces; Serial casting for flexion contractures

Occupational Therapy: Required to assess functional capacities of the child. Improve efficiency with joint protective measures & energy conservation strategies; Increase independence with the use of assistive devices and techniques; Splints to correct or prevent deformities, correct or prevent contractures, and to aid flexion and extension of involved areas; Shoes, insoles, and lifts for leg length discrepancy

Nutrition: To ensure a balanced diet with adequate caloric content for the child with JIA and to discourage the use of a "special diet" for children with JIA; Dietary management of the over-weight child and weight-gain assoc. with corticosteroids

Possible Pharmacologic Strategy: The best opportunity to obtain remission is in the first 2 years of the disease. Avoid accepting low-grade inflammation as acceptable until failure to suppress inflammation with a combination of at least two DMARDs. Begin with NSAIDs in adequate doses. Review the child after about 2 months of NSAID treatment, If improvement occurs follow every 3 months with the goal of remission. If the child does not improve or remit with NSAIDs then consider adding a DMARD such as oral methotrexate or sulfasalazine. If remission does not occur after adequate exposure or intolerance to the initial DMARD consider changing to subcutaneous methotrexate or using DMARD combination therapy. If further improvement does not occur other choices include the biologics and cyclosporine.

NSAIDs and COXIBs: NSAIDs possess both analgesic and anti inflammatory properties and are typically the first line of therapy for polyarticular JIA; Most children respond by 4 weeks and in some it may take up to 12 weeks. Pain usually responds initially, however, a reduction in swelling may take longer. NSAIDs should be used for 3 months before considered a treatment failure; Common NSAIDs used: (a) Naproxen in doses of 15-20 mg/kg/day divided into two daily doses; (b) Ibuprofen in doses of 35 mg/kg/day divided into four daily doses; (c) Diclofenac 2.0-3.0 mg/kg/ day divided into three daily doses (Not approved for use in children); (d) Piroxicam 0.2-0.3 mg/kg/day given as a single daily dose (Not approved for use in children); (e) COXIBs (Not approved for use in children)

DMARDs: In children who fail to respond to appropriate trials of NSAIDs the addition of a DMARD (usually methotrexate) is indicated.

Methotrexate: Typically takes 2-3 months for therapeutic effect; If no improvement after three to 6 months consider changing to parenteral compound or discontinuing; Administered in doses of 0.3-0.6 mg/kg/week up to 1.0 mg/kg/week for resistant disease. Consider parenteral methotrexate in those patients who have a poor response to oral methotrexate, need excess doses of oral methotrexate to control disease, or develop significant GI toxicity. Folic acid 1 mg/day or folinic acid once weekly at 1/2 the total dose of methotrexate can be used to minimize GI, bone marrow, or hepatic toxicity

Hydroxychloroquine: Typically takes 2-3 months for therapeutic effect; if no improvement after 6 months it should be discontinued; Doses of 5-6 mg/kg/day. Comes in 200 mg tablets which makes accurate dosing difficult. Rheumatologists may calculate the total weekly dose and divide the 200 mg tablets accordingly. Ocular monitoring (visual fields and color discrimination) should be done q12months

Sulfasalazine: Typical therapeutic responses seen within 2-3 months; Initially administered starting 500 mg/day & increasing by 500 mg/day to a max dose of 50 mg/kg/day or 2000 mg/day; Enteric coated sulfasalazine may be better tolerated

Leflunomide: Has been shown to be effective for the treatment of polyarticular JIA. However, it is typically used in patients who fail other DMARDs due to the lack of evidence and potential toxicity; Doses used in studies have been based on the weight of the child: < 20 kg = 100 mg loading dose for one day then 10 mg every other day; 20 - 40 kg = 100 mg loading dose for 2 days then 10 mg every day; > 40 kg = 100 mg loading dose for 3 days then 20 mg every day

Gold: Rarely used due to other available choices, however, it does remain a viable treatment option in some cases; If given started with a 5 mg IM test dose and then gradually increased to 0.75 - 1.0 mg/kg/week (maximum 50 mg/week). Requires weekly monitoring for renal and bone marrow toxicity.

Cyclosporine & Azathioprine: Have been used in treatment resistant cases

Corticosteroids: Low dose corticosteroids can be highly effective in controlling symptoms in patients with active polyarticular JIA but rarely used in the child with pauciarticular JIA; Bridge therapy until the DMARD has taken effect; Typical doses are 0.25 mg/kg/day of prednisone given in 1 to 3 doses a day; Concern with higher doses of prednisone and incidence of side-effects (growth retardation).

Intra-Articular Corticosteroids: Intra-articular corticosteroids are typically used as adjuvant therapy for specific problematic joints; Almost all patients experience rapid resolution of joint symptoms within a few days and some achieve control for 12 months or more after a single injection; Triamcinolone Hexacetonide has been shown to be superior to both betamethasone (celestone) and methylprednisolone (solumedrol). Triamcinolone Hexacetonide (Aristospan) has not been appropriately compared to Triamcinolone Acetonide (Kenolog); Most rheumatologists advise normal activity but to avoid high-impact physical activity. Immobilization of joints after injection is practice in some clinics, however, some will only immobilize if casting to reduce a flexion deformity.

Biologics: Etanercept is the only approved anti-TNF agent for use in patients with polyarticular juvenile inflammatory arthritis who have failed methotrexate; The typical dose of etanercept is 0.4 mg/kg twice weekly; Although not formally approved, Infliximab has been used successfully in open-labeled trials

Management of Uveitis: (a) Ocular Examinations: (a) No prior history of uveitis: At initial visit then every 4-6 months for 5 years, then once a year; (b) Prior history of uveitis: Every 3 months with inactive disease. As indicated by response to therapy with active disease. (b) Treatment: Should be supervised by an experienced ophthalmologist; (a) First Line: Glucocorticoid eye drops (dexamethasone or methylprednisolone) with or without a mydriatic to dilate the pupil. Glucocorticoid drips given hourly along with glucocorticoid ointment with unresponsive disease. (b) Second Line: Oral or high dose intravenous corticosteroids are typically used in children who are unresponsive to topical preparations. Cyclosporine, methotrexate, and mycophenolate mofetil have been used in refractory disease.

PROGNOSIS

Risk Stratification for Poor Prognosis: (a) Older age at onset; (b) Early involvement of small joints of the hands and feet; (c) RF positive; (d) Rheumatoid nodules; (e) Erosions on radiographs; (f) Poorer functional class; *Uveitis:* Onset before or shortly after the diagnosis of arthritis

Prognosis: Guarded prognosis for all patients with polyarticular JIA as the disease can be persistent into adulthood in the majority. Younger patients who are ANA seropositive tend to have a more favorable outcome. Adolescents with RF positive disease likely represent adult onset RA and are at significant risk for persistent disease and may be treated more aggressively. *Uveitis:* Permanent visual damage may occur in as many as 15% of patients. Cataracts are a long-term consequence of the disease or its treatment.

JUVENILE IDIOPATHIC ARTHRITIS - SYSTEMIC

DEFINITION & PATHOPHYSIOLOGY

Definition: Systemic onset juvenile idiopathic arthritis is a subset of juvenile idiopathic arthritis resulting in inflammation of the joints, fever, and an accompanying rash. This subset comprises about 10-20% of patients with JIA.

Pathophysiology: The most widely accepted hypothesis is that the disease is triggered by an unknown antigen in a genetically susceptible individual. The initial stages consist of infiltration and clonal expansion of T cells into the synovial membrane. The early inflammatory response results in recruitment of other cells to the synovium which is facilitated by upregulation of adhesion molecules and proliferation of new blood vessels. T-cells activate macrophages to secrete pro-inflammatory cytokines (TNF, IL-1, IFN). Tumor Necrosis Factor has the following actions: Activates neutrophils, macrophages, and anemia. Stimulates other cytokine production (IL-1), IL-6, GM-CSF etc; Upregulates adhesion molecules; Promotes the proliferation of synoviocytes and fibroblasts; Activates and induces differentiation of osteoclasts; Stimulates the release of matrix metalloproteinases (MMPs) resulting in proteolysis and tissue destruction. The natural anti-inflammatory and regulatory mechanisms are overwhelmed resulting in a runaway inflammatory process leading to the destruction of cartilage and bone

PRESENTATION

Identifying Data: Can affect any age, Affects males and females equally

Onset: The initial presentation is usually high-spiking fevers. The child may also have an associated rash, leukocytosis, and anemia. Many children may be thought to initially have an infection or leukemia. *(a) High Spiking Fevers:* The fevers are typically dramatic in onset reaching temperatures of 39 degrees C or higher. The fever occurs once daily (quotidian) or twice daily (double quotidian) but returns to normal; The child appears very unwell during the fever but seem to improve when their temperature returns to normal; The peak is usually in the late afternoon or early evening; A small number of children will have fever spike that does not return to normal but this is rare and the diagnosis should be questioned in this circumstance. *(b) Rash:* Children develop the characteristic evanescent salmon-colored rash which is macular or maculopapular. The rash may only be present with the fever spike; The rash is typically found in the axillae or around the waist but can occur anywhere; The rash may be elicited with heat or by the Koebner phenomenon. Therefore, it can typically be found in areas of mechanical pressure - belt line. *(c) Arthritis.* Sig. arthralgia but true arthritis may not be evident on initial presentation.

Progression: With time a true inflammatory arthritis develops, however, this may occur weeks to months after the initial onset of the disease. The systemic symptoms (fever, rash, pericarditis) tend to resolve during the initial months to years of disease but may occur with exacerbations of arthritis.

Constitutional Features: Fatigue resulting in a lack of energy, an increased requirement for sleep, or irritability; Anorexia & wt loss; General growth disturbance

Functional Status: Reduced functional status and difficulties with ADLs; Difficulty at school with physical activity; Weakness and difficulty ambulating

RHEUMATOLOGIC REVIEW OF SYSTEMS

Associated Conditions: Amyloidosis; Poor nutritional status; *Macrophage Activation Syndrome (MAS):* A rare, potentially fatal complication that is most common in boys. May be triggered by viral infections, medication changes, or spontaneously. Characterized by rapid development of fever, hepatosplenomegaly, neurologic symptoms (encephalopathy), purpura and mucosal bleeding, rash, and lymphadenopathy. Laboratory abnormalities include leukopenia, anemia, thrombocytopenia, and elevated liver enzymes. Prolongation of PT and aPTT with hypofibrinogenemia induced by a consumptive coagulopathy and DIC. Due to hypofibrinogenemia the ESR may be paradoxically low

Musculoskeletal Involvement: (a) General Growth Abnormalities: Normal linear growth is often slowed during periods of active disease; Steroids may also result in slowing of growth; *(b) Localized Growth Disturbances:* With early active inflammation, shortening or lengthening of affected limbs can occur. If the skeleton is immature (young child) then the affected limb tends to grow longer as the development of ossification centers of long bones are accelerated. If the skeleton is more mature (just prior to fusion of the physis) then shortening of the affected limb is more likely due to premature fusion of the epiphyses. Micrognathia is a striking example of localized growth retardation; *(c) Flexion Contractures; (d) Osteopenia:* Patients with systemic onset JIA fail to adequately mineralize bone and it is common for them to fail to undergo normal increase in bone mass during puberty.

Mucocutaneous Involvement: Characteristic evanescent salmon-colored rash which is macular or maculopapular as described above; Rheumatoid nodules development is rare (5%)

Lymphatic Involvement: Significant symmetric lymphadenopathy in cervical, axillary, and inguinal regions

Hematologic Involvement: Anemia secondary to chronic inflammation; Leukocytosis; Thrombocytosis

Ocular Involvement: Uveitis or Iridocyclitis: Rare in children with systemic-onset JIA

Cardiac Involvement: Pericarditis and pericardial effusions which can occur any time during the course of the disease but tend to come with a systemic exacerbation

Respiratory Involvement: Pleural effusions with a systemic exacerbation; Interstitial pulmonary disease - rare

Gastrointestinal Involvement: Gastritis secondary to NSAID use; Splenomegaly which may be quite prominent and is generally most prominent in the early years; Hepatomegaly with mild abnormalities in liver function

Endocrine Involvement: Puberty and the appearance of secondary sexual characteristics may be delayed in children with active disease

RISK FACTORS
Unknown; Genetic factors

FAMILY HISTORY
Uncommon to have multiple members of a family affected.

RED FLAGS
Development of the macrophage activation syndrome or DIC triggered by viral infections or the initiation of new medications; Thrombocytopenia is rare and should consider bone marrow problem or MAS if present; RF and ANA are typically negative and should consider an alternate diagnosis if they are positive

DIFFERENTIAL DIAGNOSIS
(a) Infection: Viral induced polyarthritis (e.g. infectious mononucleosis); Reactive arthritis; Rheumatic fever; Endocarditis; Malaria; (b) Connective tissue disease: SLE; Vasculitis; Juvenile dermatomyositis; (c) Malignancy: Leukemia; Lymphoma; Solid Tumor; (d) Inflammatory bowel disease; (e) Castelman's disease; (f) Familial Mediterranean fever; (g) Hyper IgD syndrome and other periodic fever syndromes

PHYSICAL EXAMINATION
Vitals: P: Normal; Elevated in presence of anemia or sig. active disease; BP: Normal; RR: Elevated in sig. active disease; T: Quotidian or diquotidian high-spiking fevers

Cutaneous: Characteristic evanescent salmon colored rash

Head & Neck. Ocular involvement with uveitis which is usually not apparent without slit lamp examination although this is rare; Cervical lymphadenopathy

Respiratory: Dullness at bases or reduced breath sounds at bases with overlying bronchial breath sounds due to the presence of a pleural effusion; Axillary adenopathy; Adventitious sounds due to the presence of interstitial disease

Cardiovascular: Pericarditis with a pericardial friction rub; Pericardial effusion with diminished heart sounds, tachycardia, cardiomegaly, and a pericardial friction rub; Cardiac tamponade (rare) with venous distension, hepatomegaly, peripheral edema, and pulsus paradoxus

Gastrointestinal: Hepatosplenomegaly; Splenomegaly; Inguinal adenopathy

Musculoskeletal: (a) Joint Involvement: Initially, signs of true synovitis (swelling, warmth) may not be observed; With time, the involved joints are usually swollen and warm with minimal pain, tenderness, and lack of erythema; Range of motion may appear to be preserved but should be compared to the other side as children have much greater range of motion than adults; Muscle atrophy and flexion contractures may develop; Typical joints involved include the knees, ankles, wrists, elbows, and small joints of the hands; TMJ involvement may result in limited oral opening, abnormal mandibular alignment and crepitations; *(b) Bone Involvement:* Short stature due to a general growth disturbance; Localized bone overgrowth in common areas such as the knee or wrist; Micrognathia due to mandibular hypoplasia

Neurologic: Encephalopathy with MAS.

INVESTIGATIONS

CBC: Anemia is common and profound due to decreased RBC synthesis and poor absorption of oral iron; Leukocytosis is profound with levels commonly being 20-30,000 WBC/mm3 which may exceed 60-80,000 WBC/mm3; Thrombocytosis

Liver Enzymes: May be slightly elevated

Albumin: Usually low

ESR/CRP: Elevated with active disease

Rheumatoid Factor: Usually negative

ANA: Usually negative

Urinalysis: Should be normal (Occasionally see low grade proteinuria)

Plain Radiographs: (a) Soft Tissue: Periarticular swelling & joint effusions; *(b) Alignment:* Malalignment due to damage; *(c) Bones:* Periarticular osteopenia, bone destruction, under/overgrowth of long bones, accel. epiphyseal maturation; *(d) Joints:* Uniform joint space narrowing (cartilage destruction) & erosions

Synovial Fluid: Inflammatory cellular picture 5000 – 15,000 cells/mm3 which are predominantly polymorphonuclear leukocytes.

Synovial Biopsy: (a) Hyperplasia of the synovial lining layer: 6-10 cells thick (normal 1-3); Cells hypertrophy; (b) Cellular infiltrate: CD4 T-cells & macrophages; Also see B-cells, dendritic cells, PMNs, & act. fibroblasts; (c) Synovial neovascularization

MANAGEMENT

Education & Psychological Support: Measures to empower patients and their families to improve compliance and coping skills include disease education, and advice regarding pain self-management. Clinically significant psychologic dysfunction may occur in children and their parents, especially at the time of diagnosis. Adolescents appear to be particularly vulnerable. Provide adequate psychologic counseling for both patients and their families. Ensure teachers and other caregivers have an accurate understanding of an individual child's disease helping to optimize the school experience for the child

Physiotherapy: Education of the parents and child about the goals of physiotherapy. Regular involvement in age appropriate physical activities is encouraged to improve fitness and help the child fulfill psychological needs. Pain relieving strategies and interventions; Mobility aids and braces; Exercise to improve ROM, muscle strength, aerobic conditioning, and core stability training; Weight loss; Manual therapy (manipulation) when appropriate; Serial casting for flexion contractures

Occupational Therapy: Splints; Shoes, insoles, and lifts for leg length discrepancy; Joint protection & energy conservation; Assistive devices; Lifestyle management

Nutrition: To ensure a balanced diet with adequate caloric content for the child with JIA and to discourage the use of a "special diet" for children with JIA; Dietary management of the over-weight child and weight-gain assoc. with corticosteroids

Pharmacologic Approach: The initial pharmacologic approach to the child with systemic onset JIA typically consists of starting NSAIDs and then considering the addition of oral or IV pulse corticosteroids depending on the severity of illness. The child should be reviewed very frequently.

NSAIDs and COXIBs: Possess both analgesic and anti-inflammatory properties and are one of the first lines of therapy for systemic JIA; Common NSAIDs used: (a) Naproxen in doses of 15-20 mg/kg/day divided into two daily doses; (b) Ibuprofen in doses of 20-40 mg/kg/day divided into four daily doses; (c) Indomethacin 2-4 mg/kg/day divided into three daily doses; (d) Diclofenac 3-5 mg/kg/day divided into three daily doses (Not approved in children); (e) Piroxicam 0.2-0.6 mg/kg/day given as a single daily dose (Not approved in children); (f) Coxibs (Not approved in children)

Corticosteroids: Corticosteroids can be highly effective in controlling symptoms in patients with active systemic JIA. Typical starting doses of oral prednisone are 2 mg/kg/day of prednisone and pulse IV methylprednisolone 10-30 mg/kg/day for 1-3 days may be required if severe systemic symptoms (especially cardiac involvement). The concern with higher doses of corticosteroids centers around the higher incidence of side-effects, particularly growth retardation. If the systemic features are resolving then the steroids can be tapered. If the child remains in remission for about 6 months, treatment can be discontinued. If the child remains unwell with corticosteroids and NSAIDs or the child flares with tapering the corticosteroids then DMARDs are usually initiated.

DMARDs: Failures to respond to appropriate trials of NSAIDs/corticosteroids are treated with conventional DMARDs. Common initial DMARD choice is methotrexate.

Methotrexate: First line DMARD in the treatment of systemic onset JIA; Takes 2-3 months for therapeutic effect; If no improvement after 3-6 months consider changing to parenteral compound or discontinuing; Administered in doses of 0.3-0.6 mg/kg/week up to 1.0 mg/kg/week; Consider parenteral methotrexate in those patients who have a poor response to oral methotrexate, need excess doses of oral methotrexate to control disease, or develop significant GI toxicity; Folic acid 1 mg/day or folinic acid once weekly at 1/2 the total dose of methotrexate can be used for GI intolerance

Hydroxychloroquine: Usually not used alone for the treatment of systemic onset JIA; Takes 2-3 months for therapeutic effect; if no improvement after 6 months it should be discontinued; Administered in doses of 5-6 mg/kg/day. Only comes in 200 mg tablets which makes accurate dosing difficult; Some rheumatologists calculate the total weekly dose and divide the 200 mg tablets accordingly; Ocular monitoring for visual fields and color discrimination should be done q12months

Sulfasalazine: Some evidence that sulfasalazine used in the acute phases of systemic JIA may be associated with the development of macrophage activation syndrome 57. Sulfasalazine may be useful in select cases, but it is not typically used during the acute systemic phases this disease; Typical therapeutic responses seen within 2-3 months; Initially administered starting 500 mg/day and increasing by 500 mg/day until a maximum dose of 50 mg/kg/day or 2000 mg/day is reached; Enteric coated sulfasalazine may be better tolerated

Leflunomide: Has been shown to be effective for the treatment of polyarticular JIA but there is little evidence for its use in systemic onset JIA

Gold: Some evidence that gold used in the acute phases of systemic JIA may be associated with the development of macrophage activation syndrome; Gold is usually avoided in patients with systemic onset JIA

Cyclosporine: Has been used successfully in treatment resistant cases resulting in a dramatic improvement. However, other children do not receive any benefit. This discrepancy is unclear. Useful for treatment of MAS/DIC.

Cyclophosphamide, Chlorambucil, & Azathioprine: Used with varying degrees of success and appear to be effective for only subsets of children with JIA

Thalidomide: Has been used successfully in recalcitrant systemic onset JIA; Often limited by neuropathy and sedative effects

IVIG: Limited use due to limited benefits, high cost, and potential toxicity

Biologics: Etanercept: Efficacious in 50-60% of children in open clinical trials; The typical dose of etanercept is 0.4 mg/kg twice weekly; *Infliximab:* Efficacious in 60% of children in open clinical trials; *Anakinra:* May have increased efficacy in systemic onset JIA with up to 70% of children responding to therapy

Intra-Articular Corticosteroids: Intra-articular corticosteroids are typically used as adjuvant therapy for specific problematic joints; Triamcinolone Hexacetonide has been shown to be superior to both betamethasone (celestone) and methylprednisolone (solumedrol). Triamcinolone Hexacetonide (Aristospan) has not been appropriately compared to Triamcinolone Acetonide (Kenolog). Immobilization of joints after injection is common practice in some clinics, however, some rheumatologists advise normal activity but avoid high-impact physical activity

Management of Uveitis: (a) Ocular Examinations: No prior history of uveitis: At initial visit then once a year; Prior history of uveitis: Every 3 months with inactive disease. As indicated by response to therapy with active disease. *(b) Treatment:* Should be supervised by an experienced ophthalmologist; First Line: Glucocorticoid eye drops (dexamethasone or methylprednisolone) with or without a mydriatic to dilate the pupil. Glucocorticoid drips given hourly along with glucocorticoid ointment with unresponsive disease. Second Line: Oral corticosteroids are typically used in children who are unresponsive to topical preparations. Cyclosporine and mycophenolate mofetil have been used in refractory disease.

PROGNOSIS

Risk Stratification for Poor Prognosis: Fever, thrombocytosis, or corticosteroid therapy lasting > 6 months; Evolution to a polyarthritis

Prognosis: Typically, children experience an initial 4-6 month period of active disease (spiking fevers & rash) with varying degrees of arthralgia/arthritis before the disease becomes quiescent. Arthritis will resolve completely in about 50% of children. Some will have oligoarticular disease for a period of time prior to resolution. Some children may have relapses even after years of remission. The other 50% of children will continue to show progression of the disease: (a) The fever and rash may resolve as the arthritis progresses. However, some children have persistent systemic symptoms along with progression of the arthritis. (b) The arthritis may eventually evolve into a chronic polyarthritis. This disease is indistinguishable from polyarticular JIA 57. 25% of patients will have erosive arthritis.

LYME DISEASE

DEFINITION & PATHOPHYSIOLOGY

Definition: Lyme disease is a multi-system inflammatory disorder that occurs in stages. It is caused by the tick-borne spirochete Borrelia burgdorferi.

Pathophysiology: It is unknown how Borrelia burgdorferi escapes the inoculation site and disseminates to cause Lyme disease. Borrelia burgdorferi has been cultured from erythema migrans lesions, synovial fluid, and spinal fluids. The tick takes about 24 hours to attach from initial exposure. Once the tick has attached it may take up to 38 hours for the bug to be spread. Therefore the best way to prevent disease to wash thoroughly with a washcloth to remove the ticks before the organism can be spread. Ticks like warm, moist areas and thus tend to attach in the groins, behind the knees, in the axilla, or along the beltline.

PRESENTATION

Identifying Data: The disease is most prevalent from May to November in endemic areas; 90% of cases are found in the U.S. states of New York, New Jersey, Connecticut, Massachusetts, Minnesota, Wisconsin, Pennsylvania, and Rhode Island; Can affect any age and any sex

Onset: The first stage of early localized disease is characterized by: The development of the erythema migrans rash which occurs in 90% of infected individuals. The rash typically starts 7-10 days after the initial bite (up to 30 days) at the site of the tick bite (groins, popliteal area, axilla, & belt-line) as a red macule or papule; The rash will expand over a few days to form a large annular lesion with or without central clearing (classic bull's eye lesion is rare); Patients may complain of mild constitutional features including low-grade fevers, malaise, headache, myalgias, and arthralgias

Progression: The second stage of early disseminated disease occurs within days and up to 9 months of the tick bite. This is due to spirochetemia and is associated with multiple erythema migrans lesions; The main systems affected are the neurologic and cardiac: Cardiac disease is manifest as conduction defects (AV block), myo or pancarditis, and mild cardiomyopathy; Neurologic disease can include a seventh nerve palsy (Bell's), meningitis, headache, cranial neuropathies, and radiculoneuropathies. The third and final stage of late disease occurs months to years after a tick bite and is due to spirochetemic seeding. The main systems affected are the musculoskeletal and neurologic; Lyme arthritis is characterized by recurrent episodic mono or oligoarticular attacks predominantly involving the knees. Attacks become more persistent and chronic with time and are characterized by large effusions with more stiffness than pain. The synovitis may persist for years and resolve spontaneously. The arthritis is accompanied by fatigue. Neurologic involvement in late disease is called tertiary neuroborreliosis characterized by cognitive dysfunction

Constitutional Features: Fevers, fatigue, headaches, myalgias, & arthralgias

Functional Status: May be significantly impaired with arthritis or a fibromyalgia

RHEUMATOLOGIC REVIEW OF SYSTEMS

Associated Conditions: Fibromyalgia; Chronic headaches; Chronic fatigue

Ocular Involvement: Ocular inflammation

Gastrointestinal Involvement: Mild hepatitis in early disease; Splenitis

RISK FACTORS

Exposure to ticks in endemic areas

FAMILY HISTORY

Family members may also contract disease if exposed

RED FLAGS
Rule out other causes of skin rashes

DIFFERENTIAL DIAGNOSIS
Differential Diagnosis of Polyarthritis & Rash: (a) Infectious arthritis; (b) Adult onset Still's disease; (c) Systemic onset juvenile rheumatoid arthritis; (d) Inflammatory bowel disease; (e) Psoriatic arthritis; (f) Connective tissue diseases (SLE, myositis, Sjogren's, MCTD); (g) Vasculitis; (h) Sarcoidosis

PHYSICAL EXAMINATION
Vitals: Pulse: Usually normal to slightly elevated; BP: Usually normal; RR: usually normal; Temperature – Mild elevation
Cutaneous: Erythema migrans
Head & Neck: Cranial nerve palsies; Ocular inflammation
Respiratory: No specific findings
Cardiovascular: Irregular rhythms due to conduction disturbances; Friction rub with pancarditis
Gastrointestinal: Abdominal tenderness
Musculoskeletal: Inflammatory mono or oligoarthritis most often affecting the knees
Neurologic: Cognitive dysfunction

INVESTIGATIONS
ELISA testing for antibodies (IgM and IgG) to Borrelia burgdorferi: IgM is only useful in early disease and IgG in late disease; Positive titers only reflect prior exposure and say nothing about the activity of the disease; Most patients with later manifestations (arthritis & neurologic disease) are strongly seropositive
Western Blot: To confirm ELISA; Can have false positive rates up to 5%
Lyme urinary antigen testing: Usually not helpful
Radiology: Arthritis associated with Lyme disease is typically non-erosive, however, erosions, cysts, deformities, and osteopenia have been reported
Aspiration & Pathology: Can test synovial and spinal fluids for antibodies

MANAGEMENT
General: Education about the disease; Arthritis self management programs
Physical Therapy: Joint protection; Active & passive ROM; Strengthening; Wt. loss
Occupational Therapy: Splints & braces; Assistive devices; Ambulatory devices - Canes; Orthotics
Oral Antibiotics: Doxycycline 100 mg PO BID; Amoxicillin 500 mg PO TID
Intravenous Antibiotics: Ceftriaxone 2 grams IV q24h; Cefotaxime 2 grams IV q8h
How to Treat: (a) Patients presenting with symptoms of erythema migrans, mild carditis (First degree AV block with PR < 0.3 seconds), or isolated Bell's palsy (early localized disease or early disseminated disease) can be treated with 3-4 weeks of oral antibiotics; (b) Patients presenting with arthritis alone can be treated with 4-6 weeks of oral antibiotics; (c) Patients presenting with other neurologic manifestations or more severe carditis can be treated with 2-4 weeks of intravenous antibiotics; (d) Patients presenting with refractory arthritis or tertiary neuroborreliosis should be treated with 4 weeks of Intravenous antibiotics

PROGNOSIS
Risk Stratification for Poor Progression: Responds well to antibiotic treatment
Prognosis: Responds very well to antibiotic treatment (over 90%) with relapses responding equally well. Re-infection has been documented in patients who do not mount initial antibody responses and with different strains of Borrelia burgdorferi although this is rare. Some patients develop post-Lyme disease syndromes including fibromyalgia, arthralgia, fatigue, headache, and memory difficulties.

MICROSCOPIC POLYANGIITIS (MPA)

DEFINITION & PATHOPHYSIOLOGY

Definition: A systemic necrotizing vasculitis affecting small blood vessels (capillaries, arterioles, venules) with few or no immune deposits. It is distinct from Wegener's Granulomatosis (WG) because it is non-granulomatous and differs from polyarteritis nodosa (PAN) because it does not cause renal or mesenteric aneurysm formation.

Pathophysiology: The initiating factor(s) responsible for the development of vasculitis is/are unknown. Endothelial cells are quickly activated and upregulate adhesion molecules, cytokines, growth factors, and receptors recruiting and activating components of the innate and adaptive immune systems. PMNs express antigens (MPO, PR3) on their surface and are activated through ANCA binding to these antigens. Activated PMNs release MPO, PR3, & reactive oxygen species further upregulating the immune response which may result in significant damage to endothelial cells

PRESENTATION

Identifying Data: Men: Women = 1.8:1; Most common between the ages of 30 and 50 but can present at any age

Onset: There are two typical clinical presentations: *(a) Hyper-acute onset:* Rapidly progressive glomerulonephritis (RPGN) manifest as oliguric renal failure with associated edema. Hypertension, anorexia, vomiting, and mental status changes may accompany the presentation. Pulmonary hemorrhage is present in 12% of hyper-acute presentations giving the pulmonary renal syndrome. *(b) Insidious onset:* A less common presentation which involves several years of constitutional symptoms including arthralgias, purpuric skin lesions, episodic bouts of hemoptysis, mild renal disease, and mononeuritis multiplex

Progression: Renal disease is rapidly progressive with 50% of patients requiring dialysis

Constitutional Features: Fatigue, fevers, anorexia, weight loss, night sweats & chills are common

Functional Status: Patients with hyper-acute onset may be severely disabled

RHEUMATOLOGIC REVIEW OF SYSTEMS

Musculoskeletal Involvement: Arthralgia, myalgia, arthritis

Mucocutaneous Involvement: Palpable purpura - leukocytoclastic vasculitis; Splinter hemorrhages; Sore throat, mouth ulcers, epistaxis, sinusitis - Involvement tends to be less severe than WG

Ocular Involvement: Episcleritis

Neurologic Involvement: Peripheral Neuropathy - Mononeuritis multiplex, mononeuropathy, distal sensory neuropathy; Central Nervous System - rare

Cardiac Involvement: Pericarditis

Respiratory Involvement: Present in over 50% of reported cases; (a) Pulmonary Hemorrhage: Diffuse alveolar hemorrhage is the most serious presentation with symptoms ranging from mild dyspnea to massive hemorrhage; Hemoptysis is absent in up to 1/3 of cases; Chest radiographs show fluffy alveolar infiltrates which can be confused with CHF or infection; Pathologic findings include a capillaritis, neutrophilic infiltrate, and leukocytoclasia; (b) Interstitial Fibrosis: Secondary to small repeated episodes of pulmonary hemorrhage

Gastrointestinal Involvement: Abdominal pain, diarrhea, and hepatomegaly

Renal Involvement: Usually presents as an RPGN

RISK FACTORS

No known risk factors

FAMILY HISTORY
No known association

RED FLAGS
Must always rule out sepsis as it can present as multi-organ failure and can mimic vasculitis. Refractory vasculitis is an infection until proven otherwise

DIFFERENTIAL DIAGNOSIS
Differential Diagnosis of Pulmonary-Renal Syndrome: (a) Goodpastures disease; (b) Wegener's granulomatosis; (c) Microscopic polyangiitis; (d) Systemic lupus erythematosus; (e) Henoch Schonlein purpura (rare)

Differential Diagnosis of Small Vessel Vasculitis: (a) ANCA Related (Wegener's granulomatosis; Churg-Strauss syndrome; Microscopic polyangiitis); (b) Immune Complex Related: Hypersensitivity vasculitis - Cutaneous leukocytoclastic vasculitis; Cryoglobulinemic vasculitis; Connective tissue disease associated vasculitis; Henoch-Schonlein purpura; Urticarial vasculitis; (c) Miscellaneous: Malignancy related vasculitis; Behcet's disease; Inflammatory bowel disease

PHYSICAL EXAMINATION
Vitals: Pulse: Normal to elevated; BP: Low if very ill to elevated if hypertensive with renal disease; RR: Normal to elevated; Temperature: May have accompanying fever

Cutaneous: Splinter hemorrhages & nail-fold infarcts; Palpable purpura

Head & Neck: Episcleritis; Sinusitis & epistaxis; Oral ulceration; Cranial nerve palsies

Respiratory: Reduced breath sounds, adventitious sounds, pleural friction rubs

Cardiovascular: CHF with renal failure, flow murmurs with anemia, pericardial friction rub with pericarditis

Gastrointestinal: Enlarged liver

Musculoskeletal: Muscle & joint tenderness; Inflammatory arthritis

Neurologic: Peripheral neuropathy (mononeuritis multiplex); Cranial nerve neuropathies

INVESTIGATIONS
CBC: Normochromic, normocytic anemia, leukocytosis - Can see eosinophilia in 14% of patients, thrombocytosis

Albumin: Low

Complement: Normal or elevated C3, C4

ESR/CRP: Elevated

Creatinine: Almost always elevated (85%)

Urinalysis: Microscopic hematuria, proteinuria in more than 90% of cases

ANCA: p-ANCA in 60% (myeloperoxidase); c-ANCA in 15-30% (proteinase-3)

Chest Radiographs: Alveolar infiltrates in the absence of pulmonary edema or infection

Renal Histology: Crescentic focal segmental glomerulonephritis without immune deposits. *Renal Immunofluorescence:* Pauci immune

MANAGEMENT
General: Education about the disease; Vocational counseling; Arthritis self management programs

Physical Therapy: Joint protection; Active and passive ROM; Strengthening; Weight loss

Occupational Therapy: Splints & braces; Assistive devices; Ambulatory devices - Canes; Orthotics

Supportive: Treatment of hyper-acute onset pulmonary-renal syndrome usually requires fluid resuscitation with hemodynamic and ventilatory support; Renal failure requires nephrology consultation as 40% require dialysis

High-Dose Corticosteroids: Pulsed methylprednisolone 1 gram IV over 60 minutes daily for 3-5 days. After 3 days give prednisone 1 mg/kg PO OD - This can be given in 3 - 4 divided daily doses for 7 - 10 days consolidating to a single morning dose by 2-3 weeks. As the patient improves clinically and the ESR normalizes the prednisone can be slowly tapered. *Example Tapering Regimens:* Taper to 50% original dose by decreasing by 2.5 mg q10days; Maintain at this dose for 3 weeks; Taper to 20 mg by decreasing by 2.5 mg qweekly; Taper to 10 mg by decreasing by 1 mg q2weeks; Maintain at 10 mg for 3 weeks; Taper to 0 by decreasing by 1 mg qmonthly OR Taper by 5 mg on alternate days qweekly gradually converting the treatment regimen to alternate daily prednisone; Thereby the prednisone is tapered by 2.5-5 mg each week until it is discontinued

Cyclophosphamide: Indications for Cyclophosphamide are as follows: (a) Five factor score > 0; (b) Severe pulmonary-renal disease; (c) Mononeuritis multiplex; (d) CNS disease; (e) RPGN; (f) Mesenteric vasculitis; (g) Cardiac involvement; (h) Alveolar hemorrhage

Pulsed IV Cyclophosphamide: Initial pulses may vary from 0.25 to 2.5 grams at intervals of 1 week to 1 month. In Europe, mini-pulses given more frequently are routinely used. Example orders see page 166.

Oral Cyclophosphamide: More effective (less relapses) and used second line when IV fails; Given as 1-2 mg/kg/day orally for a maximum of one year. Use cyclophosphamide as the induction agent aiming to stop it at 3-6 months and continue with one of the maintenance agents. The initial NIH regimen states to continue cyclophosphamide for one year after remission then taper by 25 mg every 2-3 months, however, they do state that the "necessary duration of treatment is open to question and our views have changed over the years".

Remission with Azathioprine: European Union Vasculitis Study Group used the CYCAZAREM regimen (2 studies one in abstract form in *A&R, 1999* and the other in *NEJM 349:1, 2003*); *Induction:* Oral cyclophosphamide 2 mg/kg/day for 3 months; *Remission:* Oral cyclophosphamide 1.5 mg/kg/day or azathioprine 2 mg/kg/day; *Results:* 93% remission rate with cyclophosphamide & prednisone; Mortality at 18 months ~ 5%; Relapse rate 14-15% (same in both CYC and AZA groups); Adverse events 21-26%

Methotrexate: Has been used for maintenance of remission in patients with Wegener's Granulomatosis (not MPA). Oral cyclophosphamide was used to initiate disease remission and weekly methotrexate was substituted given 1-2 days after the last dose of CYC.

Mycophenolate Mofetil: Also under investigation as a maintenance agent

IVIG: Conflicting results

Plasmapheresis/Plasma Exchange: Uncertain benefit & undeniable risks

PROGNOSIS

Risk Stratification for Poor Progression: Five Factor Score (total of 5 points): (a) Proteinuria > 1 gram/day (1 point); (b) Renal insufficiency with creatinine > 140 umol/L (1 point); (c) Cardiomyopathy (1 point); (d) Gastrointestinal tract involvement (1 point); (e) CNS involvement (1 point); 5 year mortality with the FFS is as follows: FFS = 0 (12%), FFS = 1 (26%), FFS > 1 (46%)

Prognosis: Relapses are common (up to 1/3 of patients); The overall 5 year survival rate is 65-80%

MIXED CONNECTIVE TISSUE DISEASE (MCTD)

DEFINITION & PATHOPHYSIOLOGY

Definition: A distinct connective tissue disease characterized by an overlap of clinical features found in systemic lupus erythematosus, inflammatory myositis, systemic sclerosis, and rheumatoid arthritis in the presence of high titers of antibodies to U1RNP

Pathophysiology: Patients with MCTD form high titers of antibodies to U1-RNP. U1-RNP is more commonly seen in SLE (in low titer) but can also be seen in systemic sclerosis (low titer). There is an association between HLADR2 and HLADR4 and antibodies to U1-RNP. The molecular mimicry hypothesis, based on an infectious or environmental trigger, is as follows: A genetically predisposed individual becomes infected or exposed to an environmental antigen; The foreign antigen contains amino acid sequences which are homologous to those found in the U1-RNP structure; An antibody response is mounted against the foreign antigen; Antibodies produced also cross react with U1-RNP because of the homologous sequences. Epitope spreading is another hypothesis to explain how a foreign antigen may induce multiple antibodies to a single pathogen

PRESENTATION

Identifying Data: Men: Women = 1:16; Typically onset is in younger people (30-40) but can affect any age

Onset: The initial presentation usually consists of non-specific symptoms including general malaise, myalgias, arthralgias, and occasionally a low-grade fever; Most patients initially receive other diagnoses such as systemic lupus erythematosus, systemic sclerosis, rheumatoid arthritis, or undifferentiated connective tissue disease as the features of MCTD may take years to evolve; However, common presentations of MCTD include the following: (a) Raynaud's Phenomenon: A common presenting feature in 90% of patients. It can be severe and debilitating with digital ulceration and ischemia. (b) Mild Edema and Sclerodactyly: Can be found in up to 70% at initial presentation. (c) Fever: Can present with fever of unknown origin. (d) Skin Rash: Malar rash and discoid lesions are indistinct from SLE. (e) Polyarthritis: A very common presenting feature (>90%) which is generally non-erosive with deformities that resemble rheumatoid arthritis. A minority of patients can have a destructive arthritis and even arthritis mutilans.

Progression: With time signs and symptoms of polymyositis, esophageal dysmotility, and pulmonary disease become more evident, It is unusual to develop severe CNS or renal disease

Constitutional Features: Fatigue, anorexia, weight loss, general malaise, and low-grade fevers

Functional Status: Patients may endure significant functional impairment largely secondary to arthritis, Raynaud's phenomenon, and fatigue

RHEUMATOLOGIC REVIEW OF SYSTEMS

Musculoskeletal Involvement: (a) Polyarthritis: Arthritis is common in MCTD with patients developing deformities similar to those found in rheumatoid arthritis, however, it is non-erosive and the radiographic findings usually do not show typical cartilage loss, cysts, or erosions; Occasionally, an erosive arthritis, even arthritis mutilans, can develop; ***(b) Inflammatory Myopathy:*** Clinically identical to polymyositis; Tends to come on as a flare of the disease

Mucocutaneous Involvement: Skin rashes (malar rash, photosensitivity, discoid) indistinguishable from SLE; Raynaud's phenomenon; Early hand edema and sclerodactyly; Oral/nasal ulceration; Sicca symptoms

Neurologic Involvement: Another hallmark of MCTD is the lack of severe CNS involvement. However, CNS involvement can occur with: Trigeminal neuropathy (like in systemic sclerosis); Headaches (migraine)

Cardiac Involvement: Pericarditis is the most common cardiac abnormality; Abnormal ECG; Inflammatory myositis of cardiac muscle

Respiratory Involvement: Episodic pleuritic chest pain; Interstitial lung disease; Pulmonary hypertension - primary cause of mortality; Aspiration

Gastrointestinal Involvement: GI involvement is similar to systemic sclerosis with: Reduced esophageal sphincter (upper and lower) tone; Esophageal dysmotility; Gastroesophageal Reflux Disease (GERD)

Renal Involvement: One of the hallmarks of MCTD is the lack of severe renal involvement. However, renal involvement does occur with: Membranous nephropathy; Rarely scleroderma renal crisis

RISK FACTORS
Silica exposure; Vinyl chloride exposure

FAMILY HISTORY
No known family history

RED FLAGS
Look for the presence of pulmonary hypertension

DIFFERENTIAL DIAGNOSIS
(a) Mixed Connective Tissue Disease; (b) Overlap syndromes; (c) Undifferentiated connective tissue disease; (d) Systemic Lupus Erythematosus; (e) Systemic Sclerosis; (f) Inflammatory myositis; (g) Rheumatoid arthritis; (h) Vasculitis

PHYSICAL EXAMINATION
Vitals: Pulse: May be elevated with pulmonary or cardiac involvement; BP: May be normal to elevated; RR: May be elevated with lung involvement; Temperature: Low-grade fever

Cutaneous: Raynaud's phenomenon with digital ulceration and pitting; Edema and sclerodactyly; Abnormal nailfold capillaroscopy, nailfold infarcts, splinter hemorrhages; Rashes similar to those found in SLE *(215)*

Head & Neck: Alopecia; Malar rash; Dry eyes and mouth; Oral/nasal ulceration

Respiratory: Reduced breath sounds, adventitious sounds (crackles), & dullness to percussion

Cardiovascular: Pulmonary hypertension with a loud P2, RV heave, pulmonary flow murmur, tricuspid regurgitation, and peripheral edema; Myositis with signs of CHF

Gastrointestinal: Abdominal tenderness

Musculoskeletal: Inflammatory polyarthritis with deformities; Proximal muscle weakness secondary to associated myositis

Neurologic: Trigeminal neuralgia

INVESTIGATIONS
CBC: Anemia (usually due to chronic disease but may see mild hemolysis) and leukopenia (primarily due to lymphopenia)

ESR/CRP: Elevated

SPEP: Hypergammaglobulinemia

RF: Positive in 50-60%

ANA: Positive in 100% and usually very high titer

ds-DNA: Negative

Antiphospholipid antibodies: Not as frequently found as in SLE

ENA Panel: *Anti-U1-RNP* - Positive in 100%; U1RNP is a spliceosome and functions to assist in splicing RNA to mature RNA, Present in high titers, *Ro/SSA* - Negative, *La/SSB* - Negative, *SCl-70* - Negative

Plain Radiographs: Evidence of an inflammatory arthritis which is usually non-erosive but may occasionally see erosions and rarely a mutilans variant; Radiographic findings do show deformities however, cysts, erosions, and cartilage loss are rare

MANAGEMENT

General Treatment Principles: Management of mixed connective tissue disease involves: (a) Determining the clinical activity of the disease and organ systems affected; (b) Determining the hematologic and serologic activity of disease; (c) Directing appropriate therapeutic interventions

Arthritis: Education; Physiotherapy; Occupational therapy; Simple analgesics such as acetaminophen; NSAIDs and COXIBs; Corticosteroids - Low dose prednisone; DMARDs (Anti-malarials - Hydroxychloroquine, Methotrexate, Gold)

Raynaud's Phenomenon: Avoid cold and keep warm (socks, hat, scarf, gloves); Stop smoking; Avoid estrogen containing compounds; Calcium channel blockers – Nifedipine XL 30 – 60; Topical nitroglycerin paste; IV iloprost

Gastrointestinal: Reduce caffeine and alcohol, stop smoking, elevate head of the bed, avoid foods which precipitate GERD, eat frequent small meals; Oral antacids, H2 blockers, and proton pump inhibitors; Metoclopramide, erythromycin, or domperidone for dysmotility; Broad spectrum antibiotics; Supplemental vitamins

Cardiopulmonary: Pleurisy: NSAIDs; Low-dose prednisone; Myocarditis: Corticosteroids and IV Cyclophosphamide; Interstitial Fibrosis: Consider treatment if Forced Vital Capacity (FVC) is reduced in early disease, a decreasing FVC, ground glass on High Resolution CT scan, polymorphonuclear cells or eosinophils on bronchoalveolar lavage (BAL), and no significant pulmonary hypertension; Treat with IV Cyclophosphamide and corticosteroids

Pulmonary Hypertension: Oxygen and warfarin for everyone; Calcium channel blockers; Bosentan – Endothelin receptor antagonist; Epoprostenol – Flolan; Treprostinil; Sildenafil; ACE-Inhibitors

Inflammatory Myopathy: Same treatment principles as treating the inflammatory myopathies

PROGNOSIS

Risk Stratification for Poor Progression: Development of pulmonary hypertension; Nailfold capillary abnormalities; Anti-cardiolipin antibodies

Prognosis: The ten year mortality ranges from 15-30% with a higher mortality seen in patients with predominant features of systemic sclerosis or myositis. However, the prognosis is regarded as better than SLE. The main causes of mortality include: Pulmonary hypertension; Myocarditis; Cerebral hemorrhage

NEUROPATHIC ARTHROPATHY

DEFINITION & PATHOPHYSIOLOGY

Definition: Neuropathic arthritis is a degenerative and destructive process affecting joints which have lost sensory innervation.

Pathophysiology: The exact etiology is not known, however, two theories exist: Neuropathic arthritis develops secondary to vasomotor changes; Neuropathic arthritis develops secondary to increased trauma which occurs due to the lack of sensation around the joint

PRESENTATION

Identifying Data: The typical patient is a long-standing diabetic with peripheral neuropathy; Most common in 60 & 70 year old patients

Onset: In diabetics, it typically begins as a monoarthritis affecting the ankle and foot (tarsal & tarso-metatarsal joints) with variable amounts of swelling, erythema, and pain. Swelling precedes pain. It may be bilateral (20%), although this is uncommon; The most striking features include: A relative lack of pain and loss of sensation in the affected limb. Patterns of Involvement include: (a) Tabes Dorsalis: Hips and knees; (b) Syringomyelia: Shoulders & elbows; (c) Diabetic neuropathy: Tarsal & tarso-metatarsal joints

Progression: Progression varies from a rapidly destructive course to a slow lingering evolvement; Progressive joint deformity and destruction is common; In diabetics, the arch of the foot will collapse ("rocker-bottom" foot) and bony prominences will form in unusual places

Constitutional Features: Usually none

Functional Status: Significant functional impairment may accompany a neuropathic arthropathy

RHEUMATOLOGIC REVIEW OF SYSTEMS

Associated Conditions: Associated peripheral neuropathy; Diabetes

RISK FACTORS

(a) Diabetes Mellitus: 0.1% - 0.5% of all diabetics; All have peripheral neuropathy; Tarsal & tarso-metatarsal joints most commonly affected; 20% of patients may be bilateral involvement; Usually a history of antecedent trauma; *(b) Tabes Dorsalis:* Tertiary syphilis affecting the posterior spinal column at the fasiculus gracilis; Declining due to rapid detection and improved antibiotics; Predominantly affects the knees, feet & ankles, and hips; *(c) Syringomyelia:* Up to 1/4 of patients with syringomyelia will develop a neuropathic arthritis; Predominantly affects the shoulders and elbows; *(d) Calcium Pyrophosphate Dihydrate Crystal Deposition Disease (CPPD):* Known as pseudo-neuropathic joint disease; Commonly affects the knees, shoulders, hips, and wrists; Other factors likely play a role; *(e) Intra-Articular Corticosteroid Injection:* Usually seen with frequent repeat injections into weight bearing joints with short-lived, relatively soluble preparations; *(f) Congenital Insensitivity to Pain;* *(g) Other Neurologic Disorders:* Multiple sclerosis; Spina bifida; Neurofibromatosis; Peripheral nerve trauma; *(h) Medication Related:* Alcoholism; Thalidomide; *(i) Other Systemic Diseases:* Pernicious anemia (B12); Charcot-Marie-Tooth disease; Amyloidosis; Leprosy; Yaws

FAMILY HISTORY

Family history of diabetes, patient may be undiagnosed

RED FLAGS

Think about a concomitant fracture; Think about associated osteomyelitis (especially in diabetics); Look for skin ulceration which may be infected; Corticosteroid injection into neuropathic joints is not recommended

DIFFERENTIAL DIAGNOSIS
(a) Neuropathic arthritis; (b) Septic arthritis; (c) Avascular necrosis; (d) Crystalline arthritis (gout & CPPD); (e) Osteoarthritis; (f) Malignancy; (g) Trauma

PHYSICAL EXAMINATION
Vitals: Pulse: Normal; BP: May be elevated with diabetes; RR: Normal; Temperature: Normal

Cutaneous: Vasculitic ulceration

Head & Neck: Diabetic retinopathy

Respiratory: No specific findings

Cardiovascular: No specific findings

Gastrointestinal: No specific findings

Musculoskeletal: Cervical spine with syringomyelia; May have shoulder and elbow involvement if syringomyelia; Foot and ankle involvement with evidence of deformity

Neurologic: Evidence of a distal peripheral neuropathy with loss of vibration, position, and sensation

INVESTIGATIONS
Bloodwork & Urinalysis: No specific findings on bloodwork or urinalysis

Plain Radiographs: (a) Early indistinct features: Joint effusion, soft-tissue swelling, and osteophyte formation; *(b) More advanced features:* Debris: Fragments of bone and cartilage collect in the synovial and peri-articular tissues; No Dominoralization: Ao cartilago woaro away the underlying bone becomes eburnated (ivory) which is accompanied by sclerosis; Disorganization; Destruction; Dislocation

Bone Scan (Tc99 labeled pyrophosphate): Non-specific findings of increased uptake in the flow phase and continued increased uptake seen on delayed images; Peripheral neuropathy alone and infection may give the same results

Indium-111 Labeled WBC Scanning: If osteomyelitis is associated, increased uptake on WBC scanning may be observed. However, there are other reasons for increased uptake on WBC scanning and it may be seen without infection. A negative scan indicates osteomyelitis is unlikely. A positive scan is less useful but may be compatible with infection

Magnetic Resonance Imaging (MRI): Can be very helpful in diagnosing osteomyelitis and looking for concomitant fractures

Synovial Fluid: A non-inflammatory synovial fluid (< 2000 WBC/mm3); May be hemorrhagic; CPPD & BCP crystals may be seen

MANAGEMENT
General: Rule out associated infection and fracture; Education; Non-weight bearing with elevation of the foot: It is imperative to reduce weight-bearing stress until edema and erythema subside and radiographic changes slow; A minimum of 8 weeks is advised, however, it may take up to 6 months for the arthropathy to heal; Proper footwear with orthotics; Bracing; Blood sugar control (if diabetic)

Pain control: Simple Analgesics - Acetaminophen; NSAIDs & COXIBs (Care in elderly diabetic patients); Amitriptyline, Cyclobenzaprine, & Gabapentin; Opioids

Surgical: Only used after inflammation has settled and have a high risk of failure due to non-union and infection; Surgery can be used to realign joints and increase stability with the goal to reduce pain and increase function

PROGNOSIS
Dependant on the severity of the arthropathy and the response to treatment; Unfortunately, amputation of limbs is sometimes required

OSTEOARTHRITIS (OA)

DEFINITION & PATHOPHYSIOLOGY

Definition: Osteoarthritis is a degenerative disease of the joint and the result of both mechanical and biologic events that de-stabilize the normal coupling of degradation and synthesis of articular cartilage and subchondral bone

Pathophysiology: Early in the process cartilage becomes edematous and loses its smooth surface with the appearance of micro-cracks. Chondrocytes initially try to proliferate to help fix the damage but they shift to produce type 1 and 3 collagen. The collagen fibrils become loosely packed and fragmented. Chondrocytes also release more degradative enzymes (matrix metallo-proteinases (MMPs)) such as collagenase, gelatinase, and stromelysin. With time, these enzymes break down proteoglycans faster than they can be secreted resulting in diminished proteoglycan content of the cartilage (up to 50%). Focal areas of chondrocyte loss are also observed. With time, the micro-cracks fissure and deepen. Vertical clefts form in the subchondral bone cartilage. Articular cartilage thins and softens. The fissures eventually lead to loss of fragments of cartilage creating osteocartilaginous loose bodies exposing the underlying subchondral bone. Synovial fluid can be forced, by the pressure of weight, into the subchondral bone resulting in cysts or geodes on x-ray. Remodeling or hypertrophy of the subchondral bone results in subchondral sclerosis

PRESENTATION

Identifying Data: Typical patient is overweight, middle-aged or elderly (usually > 40 years of age); More common in women over the age of 50 than in age-matched men (3:1); Symptomatic OA is present in 2-3% of the population

Onset: The initial symptoms of osteoarthritis include: ***(a) Monoarthritis–Oligoarthritis:*** Usually presents with symptoms in a single joint (knee or hip) but may present with hand involvement which could be an oligoarthritis-polyarthritis. The typical joints involved are: DIPs & PIPs; First CMC and trapezio-scaphoid articulation; AC joint of the shoulder; C-Spine – Discovertebral junction and zygoapophyseal joints; L-Spine – Discovertebral junction and zygoapophyseal joints; Hips; Knees; First MTP & TMT; ***(b) Pain:*** Insidious onset of pain, exacerbated by activity and relieved by rest. With progression of the disease, pain may persist at rest and occur during the night, a symptom more indicative of severe disease; ***(c) Stiffness:*** Morning stiffness is usually less than 30 minutes; Stiffness may occur after periods of inactivity ("gelling"); ***(d) Instability:*** True ligament laxity with ligaments stretched by a swollen joint capsule; Pseudolaxity occurs when one joint compartment wears faster than another resulting in narrowing of the joint space and a redundancy of the ligament; Joint swelling results in reflex inhibition of the quadriceps muscle reducing joint stability; ***(e) Joint Swelling:*** Synovial effusions may be present but erythema is usually absent or minimal; ***(f) Crepitus:*** Grinding noise made by joints which may be uncomfortable

Progression: With time the degenerative process continues leading to persistent pain which is not relieved by simple analgesics or NSAIDs

Constitutional Features: There are usually no constitutional features

Functional Status: Reduced functional status with difficulties with ADLs due to pain, limited ROM, and muscle weakness

RHEUMATOLOGIC REVIEW OF SYSTEMS

Usually none unless associated with systemic disease (secondary osteoarthritis)

RISK FACTORS

Primary Osteoarthritis: (a) Genetic: Hereditary factors; (b) Advanced age: The strongest risk factor; (c) Female gender: Increased risk of OA; (d) Obesity: Increased risk of knee OA and hand OA. Hip OA is less convincingly associated; (e) Lack of osteoporosis; (f) Weak quadriceps in knee OA; (g) Smoking;

Secondary Osteoarthritis: (a) Congenital abnormalities: Congenital hip dysplasia; (b) Previous trauma to a joint; (c) Inflammatory arthritis: End result of inflammatory disease; (d) Metabolic diseases: Hemochromatosis, ochronosis; (e) Endocrine diseases: Hyperparathyroidism, acromegaly, hypothyroidism; (f) Neuropathic joints; (g) Septic joints; (h) Paget's disease; (i) Avascular necrosis

FAMILY HISTORY

Heritability of primary OA of the hands has been reported to be has high as 65%

RED FLAGS

Think about secondary causes of osteoarthritis

DIFFERENTIAL DIAGNOSIS

(a) Chronic infection (monoarthritis with Tb); (b) Calcium pyrophosphate deposition (CPPD); (c) Seronegative arthritis (mono or oligoarthritis); (d) Secondary osteoarthritis *(see above)*; (e) Neoplasms; (f) Avascular necrosis

PHYSICAL EXAMINATION

Vitals: Pulse: Normal; BP: Normal; RR, Normal

Cutaneous: No specific findings

Head & Neck: No specific findings

Respiratory: No specific findings

Cardiovascular: No specific findings

Gastrointestinal: No specific findings

Musculoskeletal: **(a) Hands:** Bony enlargement of the DIPs – Heberden's nodes with flexion or angulation deformities and loss of range of motion. They may be tender to palpate. Bony enlargement of the PIPs – Bouchard's nodes with flexion or angulation deformities and loss of range of motion. They may be tender to palpate and mildly swollen. Loss of the ability to abduct the thumb with squaring of the first CMC joint as the thumb falls toward the palm; **(b) Hips:** Pain is predominantly felt in the groin; Pain with walking and a Trendelenburg gait due to weak hip abductors on the affected side; Positive Trendelenburg test; The affected limb may be held in mild external rotation; Hip flexion deformities with resulting hyperlordosis of the lumbar spine; Reduced ROM – Internal rotation > abduction > flexion; **(c) Knees:** Swelling and bony enlargement; Wasting of the quadriceps muscle; Genu varus (more common) or valgus alignment; Abnormal gait with a short "stance phase" on the affected limb; Mild flexion contracture with loss of passive extension; Pain on palpation of the joint line (osteophytes); Evidence of effusion (Patellar tap, ballottement, fluid wave); Reduced range of motion with crepitus and pain; Increased laxity of ligamentous structures (pseudolaxity of MCL/LCL); **(d) Feet:** First MTP bony enlargement; Hallux valgus with bunion formation; Hallux rigidus with loss of ROM; Mobile first ray and degeneration at the first TMT joint; **(e) Axial:** Cervical and lumbar spine involvement with reduced ROM

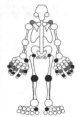

INVESTIGATIONS

Bloodwork & Urinalysis: Blood work and urinalysis should be normal in primary OA

Synovial fluid Analysis: WBC count is less than 2000 cells/mm3

Radiology: The major radiographic findings of osteoarthritis are: (a) Non-uniform joint space narrowing; (b) Subchondral sclerosis; (c) Osteophyte formation; (d) Subchondral cyst formation

MANAGEMENT

General: Education; Arthritis self-management programs; Social support & group programs

Physiotherapy: Pain relieving strategies and interventions; Mobility aids (canes & walkers) and braces; Exercise to improve ROM, muscle strength, aerobic conditioning, and core stability training; Weight loss; Manual therapy (manipulation) when appropriate

Occupational Therapy: Splints and orthotics; Joint protection measures and energy conservation; Assistive devices; Lifestyle management

Topical Treatment: Topical Capsaicin; Topical NSAIDs and salicylates

Systemic Treatment: Acetaminophen up to 4 grams per day (1000 mg QID); Non-Steroidal Anti-Inflammatory Drugs and COXIBs; Narcotic Analgesics

Intra-Articular Treatment: Intra-Articular Corticosteroids; Intra-Articular Viscosupplementation

Complementary/Alternative Treatments: Glucosamine Sulfate

Surgical: Most commonly used in OA of the hips and knees, however, CMC & MTPs can also be surgically corrected; The goal of surgery is to reduce pain and improve function

PROGNOSIS

In most people, osteoarthritis is slowly progressive. However, the rate of progression is highly variable, and the disease may remain stable in some individuals. Osteoarthritic progression is seen with discrete "flares" of the disease between periods of stability. With each "flare" the disease progresses. **Risk factors for progression of hip OA include:** (a) Pain at night; (b) Lower functional capacity; (d) Female gender; **Risk factors for progression of knee OA include:** (a) Increased body mass index; (b) Generalized OA. There are no known measures to prevent the development or slow the progression of osteoarthritis, however, the best preventative measures with existing osteoarthritis include: (a) Education; (b) Weight loss; (c) Physiotherapy to improve muscle function around affected joints; (d) Appropriate exercise program which does not "flare" the disease

OSTEOPOROSIS (OP)

DEFINITION & PATHOPHYSIOLOGY

Definition: Osteoporosis is a disease of the skeleton characterized by two things that lead to an increased risk of fracture: Low bone mass; Disruption of the normal microarchitecture of bone; Osteoporosis is defined by the World Health Organization as a bone mineral density less than 2.5 standard deviations below the mean bone density of a healthy 30 year old Caucasian woman. Remember that bone mineral density only takes into account the bone mass and not the structural integrity of the bone. See the WHO Criteria for Osteoporosis *(244)*

Pathophysiology: A decrease in bone mass can be due to: (a) Failure to attain an adequate peak bone mass, (b) excessive resorption of bone, or (c) reduction in bone formation during the remodeling process; Failure to attain an adequate peak bone mass with genetics likely play the largest role in determining peak bone mass, however, no single gene has been found to be responsible; Calcium intake, adequate vitamin D, and exercise all play a role in determining peak bone mass. Excessive resorption of bone. Bone resorption does not actually need to be excessive, it simply needs to affect the underlying architecture of the bone and be greater than bone formation. Reduction in bone formation. In some circumstances, osteoporosis may result from decreased osteoblastic activity.

PRESENTATION

Identifying Data: In all patients, the presence of a vertebral fracture on radiographs or fragility fractures should be considered as identifiers of those with an increased risk for fracturing. This is probably a better predictor of fracture risk than osteoporotic BMD measurements. *Women* (all Caucasian women, age > 50): Measure total hip BMD: 17% have osteoporosis (WHO definition); 42% have osteopenia; Lowest value of hip, spine, or radius BMD: 30% have osteoporosis (WHO definition); 54% have osteopenia. *Men* (All Caucasian men, age> 50): Measure total hip BMD: 4% have osteoporosis; 33% have osteopenia

Onset: Most patients with osteoporosis are asymptomatic or they may present with: (a) Fragility fracture: Any fracture which occurs due to a fall from a distance no greater than the individual's standing height or with normal use. Common sites include vertebrae, hip, and radius; (b) Bone pain incl. back pain; (c) Loss of height (>3-4 cm) with increasing thoracic kyphosis; (d) Asymptomatic (most common)

Progression: A progressive disorder with continued loss of bone mass with time

Constitutional Features: Anorexia and weight loss may accompany osteoporosis

Functional Status: Chronic back pain with increased thoracic kyphosis may reduce functional status and self-confidence due to concerns about appearance; Abdominal protuberance and kyphosis are patient concerns; Compromised respiratory function may occur in those with multiple vertebral fractures; Vertebral and hip fractures may lead to chronic pain, a decrease in mobility, and fear of falling

RHEUMATOLOGIC REVIEW OF SYSTEMS

Associated Conditions: (a) Vertebral Fracture: Women: Found in 5-10% at age 55 and 30-40% at age 80; Men: Lifetime risk of 5%; 66% are asymptomatic and diagnosed on plain radiographs; Typically occur with minimal trauma; If symptomatic, acute pain typically lasts 4-6 weeks. It may be replaced by a chronic dull pain which can be quite prolonged; Symptoms of successive fractures include: Loss of height; Increased thoracic kyphosis; Abdominal protrusion; Pain over the iliac crests - ribs rubbing on the iliac crests; Difficulty looking forward (severe thoracic kyphosis) & neck pain; Dyspnea - extrathoracic restriction; If a patient has sustained an osteoporotic vertebral fracture, the risk of re-occurrence is up to 19%

in the following year. *(b) Hip Fracture:* Women: Overall a 15% lifetime risk; Men: Overall a 5% lifetime risk; Over 90% are associated with falls

RISK FACTORS

Major Risk Factors: (a) Low bone mineral density; (b) Age > 65; (c) Vertebral compression fracture; (d) Fragility fracture after age 40; (e) Family history of osteoporotic fracture (especially maternal hip fracture); (f) Systemic glucocorticoid therapy of > 3 months duration; (g) Malabsorption syndrome; (h) Primary hyperparathyroidism; (i) Propensity to fall; (j) Osteopenia apparent on radiograph; (k) Hypogonadism; (l) Early menopause (before age 45)

Minor Risk Factors: (a) Rheumatoid arthritis; (b) Past clinical history of hyperthyroidism; (c) Chronic anticonvulsant therapy; (d) Low dietary calcium intake; (e) Smoking; (f) Excessive alcohol intake; (g) Excessive caffeine intake; (h) Weight < 57 kg or Weight loss > 10% of weight at age 25; (i) Chronic heparin therapy

FAMILY HISTORY

Family history of osteoporotic fracture is a major risk factor for future fracture risk

RED FLAGS

Rule out secondary causes of osteoporosis

DIFFERENTIAL DIAGNOSIS

Secondary Causes of Osteoporosis: (a) Chronic inflammatory conditions: Rheumatoid arthritis, SLE, psoriatic arthritis; Inflammatory bowel disease; Mastocytosis; *(b) Endocrinopathies:* Cushing's syndrome; Hyperthyroidism; Hyperparathyroidism; Hypogonadism; *(c) Organ Dysfunction:* Liver Disease; Renal Disease; *(d) Medications & Toxins:* Corticosteroids; Anti-convulsants; Heparin; Thyroxine; Alcohol; *(e) Malabsorption/Malnutrition diseases:* Celiac disease; IBD; Anorexia nervosa; Vit. D deficiency; *(f) Malignancy:* Metastases; Multiple myeloma

PHYSICAL EXAMINATION

Vitals: Pulse: Normal to elevated with pain; BP: Normal to elevated with pain; RR: May be elevated with vertebral fractures and pain; Temperature: Normal

Cutaneous: Ehlers-Danlos syndrome seems to increase risk for osteoporosis

Head & Neck: Increased thoracic kyphosis with a forward set head posture and difficulty looking forwards resulting in extension of the cervical spine; Examine for thyroid abnormalities; Bue sclera (osteogenesis imperfecta); Loss of height

Respiratory: Reduced chest expansion

Cardiovascular: No specific findings

Gastrointestinal: Protuberant abdomen due to vertebral compression fractures; Pain over the iliac crests

Musculoskeletal: Reduced range of motion with pain on axial exam; Loss of height; Point tenderness over recent fracture sites

Neurologic: No specific findings

INVESTIGATIONS

Screening bloodwork for secondary causes: (a) CBC with differential - Evidence of inflammatory diseases; (b) Creatinine & urinalysis - Look for renal dysfunction; (c) Liver enzymes - AST, ALT, ALP, albumin - Look for hepatic dysfunction; (d) Calcium, phosphorous, alkaline phosphatase, PTH - Rule out hyperparathyroidism; (e) 25-Hydroxyvitamin D - Rule out vitamin D deficiency or osteomalacia; (f) TSH - Rule out thyroid abnormalities; (g) Serum & urine protein electrophoresis - Multiple myeloma; (h) Serum testosterone - In men (optional)

Biochemical markers of bone turnover: (a) Bone formation markers (osteoblasts): Osteocalcin (OC); Bone specific alkaline phosphatase (BSALP); Procollagen 1 carboxyterminal propeptide (P1CP); *(b) Bone degradation markers*

(osteoclasts): Urinary Pyridinoline (PYR); Urinary Deoxypyridinoline (D-PYR); Collagen type 1 cross-linked N-telopeptide (NTX); Collagen type 1 cross-linked C-telopeptide (CTX). Not yet used routinely in clinical management but will likely become an important marker of fracture risk and management in the future

Bone Mineral Densitometry: *(a) Technique:* Most widely used technique to measure BMD is by dual energy x-ray absorptiometry (DXA) of the hip and lumbar spine; The most effective technique to estimate fracture risk in post-menopausal Caucasian women; DXA is reported as a "T-score" which represents the number of standard deviations below or above the mean value for a healthy young adult. *(b) Precision:* Measurement precision is affected by the clinical setting, patient population, device used, and the site of measurement. The BMD lab should be able provide internal precision estimates The variability in precision is about 1-2%. A 3% increase in the spine and a 6% increase in the hip is considered significant to overcome the variability inherent in the test. *(c) Use:* Since osteoporosis is often asymptomatic there is considerable debate over screening protocols; The National Osteoporosis Foundation (USA) suggests the following reasons for ordering a BMD: All women age 65 and older regardless of risk factors; Younger post-menopausal women with one or more risk factors; Post-menopausal women who present with fractures; The Canadian Guidelines suggest the following reasons for ordering a BMD: All women age 65 and older regardless of risk factors; Individuals with 1 major risk factor (see risk factors below); Individuals with 2 minor risk factors (see risk factors above). *(d) Estimation of Fracture Risk (data adapted from Kanis et al Osteoporosis Int 2001;12:989-995):* **Men:** The 10 year probability of sustaining any osteoporotic fracture varies from 2.3% at age 45 to 7.5% at age 85 provided there is a T-score of 0 at the femoral neck: T-Score -1 increases the risk 1.5 times; T-Score -2 increases the risk 2 times; T-Score -2.5 increases the risk 2.25-2.75 times; T-Score -3 increases the risk 2.6-3.3 times; T-Score -4 increases the risk 3.5-4.9 times. **Women -** The 10 year probability of sustaining any osteoporotic fracture varies from 2.8% at age 45 to 7.4% at age 85 provided there is a T-score of 0 at the femoral neck: T-Score -1 increases the risk 1.5 times; T-Score -2 increases the risk 2.4 - 2.6 times; T-Score -2.5 increases the risk 2.9 - 3.2 times; T-Score -3 increases the risk 3.6 - 4 times; T-Score -4 increases the risk 5.4-5.8 times

Calcaneal Ultrasound: Good evidence to show it is effective in predicting fracture risk in elderly populations; However, it is not been shown to be useful for monitoring response to treatment

MANAGEMENT

General: (a) Weight bearing exercise: Individual programs designed by physical therapists aimed at improving muscle strength and balance has been shown to reduce the risk of falls and fracture; Moderate exercise for 30 minutes 3 times per week is recommended; (b) Smoking cessation; (c) Limit alcohol; (d) Limit caffeine: > 4 cups of coffee/day is associated with hip fracture; (e) Adequate nutrition

Calcium: Recommended daily elemental calcium intake from all sources based on age and gender: (a) Pre pubertal children (age 4 - 8): 800 mg per day; (b) Adolescents (age 9 - 18): 1300 mg per day; (c) Women (age 19 - 50): 1000 mg per day (500 mg PO BID); (d) Women (age >50): 1500 mg per day (500 mg PO TID); (e) Men (age 19 - 50): 1000 mg per day; (f) Men (age >50): 1500 mg per day

Vitamin D: In the elderly and those who have sustained a hip fracture, vitamin D deficiency is probably the most important cause of bone loss. 25-Hydroxyvitamin D levels should be greater than 40. Recommended daily vitamin D intake based on age and gender: (a) Women (age 19 - 50): 400 IU/day; (b) Women (age >50): 800 IU/day; (c) Men (age 19 - 50): 400 IU/day; (d) Men (age >50): 800 IU/day

Who To Treat: The **National Osteoporosis Foundation (USA)** suggests the following patients be considered for treatment: (a) T-Scores < -2.0 by DEXA with no other risk factors; (b) T-Scores <-1.5 by DEXA with 1 additional risk factor; (c) Prior vertebral or hip fracture. The **Canadian Guidelines** suggest the following patients be considered for treatment: (a) History of fragility fracture after age 40 and T-score < -1.5; (b) Non-traumatic vertebral compression deformities and T-score < -1.5; (c) 1 Major or 2 minor clinical risk factors and a T-score <-1.5; (d) BMD by DEXA T-score < -2.5; (e) Long-term glucocorticoid therapy (>7.5 mg/day for 3 m or more)

Treatment Rationale: While there is a relationship between pre-treatment BMD and fracture risk, evidence suggests that BMD measurements reflect only 1 component of bone strength. For example, small changes in BMD produced by osteoporosis treatments do not fully explain the reductions in fracture risk observed after initiation of therapy, and substantial fracture risk reduction is observed before peak increases in BMD are achieved. Osteoporosis therapies have recently been shown to have positive effects on bone strength independent of BMD, due to changes in other important factors (e.g. microarchitecture, mineralisation, bone turnover).

Possible Treatment Algorithm: (1) All Patients: Calcium, Vitamin D, exercise, and education;(2) Patients WITHOUT Fragility Fracture: (a) With vasomotor symptoms: First Line: Hormone replacement therapy; Second Line: Alendronate, risedronate, raloxifene, calcitonin. (b) Without vasomotor symptoms: First Line: Alendronate, risedronate, raloxifene; Second Line: Calcitonin, etidronate, HRT, teriparatide. (3) Patients WITH Fragility Fracture: (a) First Line: Alendronate, risedronate, raloxifene; (b) Second Line: Calcitonin, etidronate, HRT, teriparatide

Alendronate: (a) Bone mineral density: Lumbar spine: Increase of 7-8% over 3-4 years; Hip: Increase of 3-4% over 3-4 years; **(b) Fracture risk with WITH previous vertebral fracture:** Black et al - FIT Trial (Lancet 1996) - Post-menopausal women - group with prior vertebral fractures treated with alendronate for 3 years. Vertebral fractures: 8% vs 15% (NNT of 9) & Hip fractures: 1.1% vs 2.2% (NNT of 91); **(c) Fracture risk WITHOUT previous vertebral fracture:** Cummings et al - FIT Trial (JAMA 1998) - Post-menopausal women - group without prior vertebral fractures treated with alendronate for 3 years. Vertebral fractures: 2% vs 4% (NNT of 60) & Hip fractures: 0.9% vs 1.1% (p = NS). Liberman et al - (NEJM 1995) - Subgroup analysis since 20% of patients had vertebral fracture. Vertebral fractures: 3% vs 6% (NNT of 33) & Hip fractures: 0.2% vs 0.8% (p = NS)

Etidronate: (a) Bone mineral density: Lumbar spine: Increase of 4.5-5.3% over 2-3 years; Femoral Neck: Increase of 3% over 2 years; (b) **Fracture risk WITH previous vertebral fracture:** Watts et al (NEJM 1990) - Post-menopausal women with prior vertebral fractures treated with etidronate for 2 years - Primary analysis was BMD so fracture data is subgroup (n = 429). Vertebral fractures: 63% vs 30% per 1000 patient years (NNT = 20) & Hip fractures: NA; Storm et al (NEJM 1990) - Post-menopausal women with prior vertebral fractures treated with etidronate for 3 years - Primary analysis was BMD so fracture data is subgroup (n = 66). Vertebral fractures: 43% vs 18% per 1000 patient years & Hip fractures: NA

Ibandronate: (a) Bone mineral density: Lumbar spine: Increase of 6.4% over 3 years; Femoral Neck: Increase of 2.6% over 3 years; **(b) Fracture risk WITH previous vertebral fracture:** BONE (JBMR 2004) - Post-menopausal women with prior vertebral fractures treated with ibandronate for 3 years . Vertebral fractures: 4.7% vs 9.6% (NNT of 20); Non-Vertebral (including hip): 9.1% vs 8.2% (p=NS).

Risedronate: ***(a) Bone mineral density:*** Lumbar spine: Increase of 5.4 - 7.5% over 3 years; Hip: Increase of 1.6 - 2.2% over 3 years; ***(b) Fracture risk WITH previous vertebral fracture:*** Harris et al - VERT-NA Trial *(JAMA 1999)* - Post-menopausal women - group with prior vertebral fractures treated with risedronate for 3 years. Vertebral fractures at 1 year: 2.4% vs 6.4% (NNT of 25); Vertebral fractures at 3 years: 11% vs 16% (NNT of 20); Non-Vertebral (including hip) fractures at 3 years: 5.2% vs 8.4% (NNT=31). Reginster et al - VERT-MN *(Osteoporosis Int 2000)* - Post-menopausal women with at least 2 prior vertebral fractures treated with risedronate for 3 years. Vertebral fractures at 1 year: 5.6% vs 13% (NNT of 13.5); Vertebral fractures at 3 years: 18% vs 29% (NNT of 10); Non-Vertebral (including hip) fractures at 3 years: 10.9% vs 16% (p=NS). McClung et al *(NEJM 2001)* - Post-menopausal women with low BMD and vertebral fracture at baseline (sub-group analysis) treated with risedronate for 3 years. Hip fractures: 2.3% vs 5.7% (NNT of 29); ***(c) Fracture risk WITHOUT previous vertebral fracture:*** McClung et al *(NEJM 2001)* - Post-menopausal women with low BMD without vertebral fracture at baseline (sub-group) treated with risedronate for 3 years. Hip fractures: 1.0% vs 1.6% (p=NS). Heaney et al *(Osteoporosis Int 2002)* - Post-menopausal women with low BMD without vertebral fractures at baseline treated with risedronate for 3 years. Vertebral fractures: 2.6 % vs 9.4% (NNT of 15).

Estrogen: ***(a) Bone mineral density:*** Lumbar spine: Increase of 3.5 - 5% over 3 years; Hip: Increase of 1.7% over 3 years; ***(b) Fracture risk WITHOUT previous vertebral fracture:*** Women's Health Initiative *(JAMA 2002)* - Post-menopausal women without vertebral fracture at baseline treated with premarin 0.625 mg and progesterone 2.5 mg for an average of 5.2 years. Vertebral fractures: 0.09% vs 0.15% (NNT of 1667) & Hip fractures: 0.10% vs 0.15% (NNT of 2000).

Raloxifene: ***(a) Bone mineral density:*** Lumbar spine: Increase of 3 - 3.5% over 3 years; Hip: Increase of 2 - 2.5% over 3 years; ***(b) Fracture risk WITH previous vertebral fracture:*** Ettinger et al - MORE Trial (JAMA 1999) - Post-menopausal women - group with prior vertebral fractures treated with raloxifene for 3 years. Vertebral fractures: 21% vs 15% (NNT of 16) & Hip fractures: 0.7% vs 0.8% (p = NS) - subgroup analysis; ***(c) Fracture risk WITHOUT previous vertebral fracture:*** Ettinger et al - MORE Trial *(JAMA 1999)* - Post-menopausal women - group without prior vertebral fractures treated with raloxifene for 3 years. Vertebral fractures: 4.5% vs 2.3% (NNT of 16) & Hip fractures: 0.7% vs 0.8% (p = NS) - subgroup analysis.

Calcitonin: ***(a) Bone mineral density:*** Lumbar spine: Increase of 1 - 1.5% over 5 years; Hip: No significant increase at femoral neck or trochanter; ***(b) Fracture risk WITH previous vertebral fracture:*** Chesnut et al - PROOF Trial (American J Med 2000) - Post-menopausal women with prior vertebral fractures treated with calcitonin for 3-5 years. Vertebral fractures; 26% vs 20% (NNT of 17)

Teriparatide: ***(a) Bone mineral density:*** Lumbar spine. Increase of 9.7% over 2 years with 20 mcg dose & 13.7% with 40 mcg dose; Hip: Increase of 2.6% over 2 years with 20 mcg dose & 3.6% with 40 mcg dose; ***(b) Fracture risk WITH previous vertebral fracture:*** Neer et al - (NEJM 2001) - Post-menopausal women - prior vertebral fractures treated with teriparatide for 2 years. Vertebral fractures: 14% vs 4-5% (NNT of 11) & Hip fractures: 0.7% vs 0.8% (p=NS) - subgroup analysis.

PROGNOSIS

Risk Stratification for Poor Progression: Multiple fractures at presentation; Older, frail individuals; High risk for falling

Prognosis: Variable depending upon patient age, degree of bone loss, and response to treatment

POLYMYALGIA RHEUMATICA (PMR) & GIANT CELL ARTERITIS (GCA)

DEFINITION & PATHOPHYSIOLOGY

Definition: Giant cell arteritis is a chronic granulomatous vasculitis affecting large arteries in patients over 50 years of age; See the Classification Criteria for Giant Cell Arteritis (241); See the Criteria for the Diagnosis of Polymyalgia Rheumatica (245)

Pathophysiology: Early pathogenic mechanisms of giant cell arteritis are unknown. What is known is the following: The disease is limited to blood vessels with an internal elastic lamina; A clonal population of CD-4 T-cells can be found within the arterial wall suggesting in-situ activation; Interleukin-2 and interferon-gamma are produced within the vascular wall; Activated macrophages within the vessel wall produce IL-1 beta, IL-6 and TGF-beta; Giant cells are large multi-nucleated cells usually formed by a coalescence of epithelioid cells (modified macrophages)

PRESENTATION

Identifying Data: Patient age > 50 (most are > 60 with average age ~ 70); Women: Men = 2:1; Mainly people of northern European descent

Onset: (a) Polymyalgia Rheumatica: Pain & stiffness usually insidious in onset and profound involving at least 2 of three areas including the muscles of the neck, shoulder girdle, and pelvic girdle; Occasionally the onset can be very abrupt or the initial symptoms can be unilateral; Symptoms present for at least one month; Morning stiffness is usually dramatic; Fever, sweats, malaise, and weight loss all may occur with PMR alone; May have an associated peripheral arthritis (usually oligoarticular); ***(b) Giant Cell Arteritis:*** May present in one of 4 different ways: (1) Polymyalgia Rheumatica (15%) - See above; (2) Large Vessel GCA (10-15%) - Symptom presentation is dependant on vessel involvement: Subclavian - Arm claudication; Iliac/femoral - Leg claudication; Aortic arch involvement - Claudication of the arms, paresthesias, Raynaud's phenomenon, and occasionally digital gangrene; Aortic insufficiency - Aortitis; Renal artery - Hypertension; Pulmonary artery – Cough, SOB, hoarseness, chest pain; (3) Cranial Arteritis (70%): Headache – Temporal region most common, frontal or occipital with neck pain; Scalp tenderness – Temporal or occipital; Jaw & tongue claudication; CNS ischemia (stroke like or vertigo (vertebral)) in 20-30%; Diplopia; Loss of vision (ophthalmic – ischemic optic neuritis) – 15-20% in most series; (4) Fever of Unknown Origin

Progression: (a) Giant cell arteritis: Generally progresses until treatment is initiated. Thought to run a self-limited course over several months to several years, however, smoldering disease activity is more common than thought. ***(b) Polymyalgia rheumatica:*** Generally persists with treatment for a median of 2 years

Constitutional Features: Fever, fatigue, anorexia, weight loss, night sweats, general malaise, and weakness

Functional Status: Given the age of patients affected, decline in functioning may be rapid and severe. Prompt intervention is important to prevent functional decline.

RHEUMATOLOGIC REVIEW OF SYSTEMS

Musculoskeletal Involvement: ~ 40% with GCA will have concomitant PMR

Vascular Involvement: Subclavian or Iliac artery - Claudication of lower extremities

Ocular Involvement: Retinal vasculitis with ischemic optic neuropathy

Neurologic Involvement: CVA

Cardiac Involvement: Myocardial ischemia; myocardial infarction; Aortic regurgitation with aortitis

Gastrointestinal Involvement: Mesenteric vasculitis with abdominal pain

Renal Involvement: Hypertension due to renal artery vasculitis

RISK FACTORS
(a) Age; (b) Female sex; (c) Northern European descent; (d) Siblings of a patient are at a 10-fold increase of getting GCA

FAMILY HISTORY
Siblings are at increased risk of developing GCA

RED FLAGS
(a) Look for symptoms suggestive of visual loss and stroke; (b) Examine all pulses: Giant cell arteritis can involve a multitude of large vessels; 10-15% of patients presenting with polymyalgia rheumatica, with nothing to suggest associated vasculitis, have positive temporal artery biopsies; (c) Polymyalgia rheumatica may be part of the presentation of a paraneoplastic syndrome; (d) About 10-15% of patients may present with a normal ESR (some reports suggest as high as 25%)

DIFFERENTIAL DIAGNOSIS
(a) GCA; (b) PMR; (c) Seronegative RA; (d) Hypothyroidism; (e) Bacterial endocarditis; (f) Polymyositis; (g) Amyloidosis; (h) Malignancy; (i) Fibromyalgia

PHYSICAL EXAMINATION
Vitals: Pulse: May be elevated in severe disease; Feel both radials, carotids, femorals, posterior tibials and dorsalis pedis; Listen over the carotids, subclavians, temporals, abdominal aorta, renal, and femorals for bruits; BP: Measure the blood pressure in both arms; RR: May be elevated; Temperature: May be elevated

Cutaneous: Scalp necrosis

Head & Neck: Inspect for scalp necrosis, visible swelling or erythema over the temporal arteries; Palpate the temporal artery for tenderness, thickening, and the presence of a pulse; Palpate the occipital arteries for tenderness and thickening; Palpate the carotid arteries for a pulse and tenderness; Auscultate the carotids, occipital, and over the orbits for bruits; Ocular exam: Extra-ocular movements, visual fields, visual acuity, fundoscopy; Oropharyngeal: Look for erythema, occasionally presents with intensely sore throat; Feel for adenopathy and thyroid enlargement/nodules as occasionally PMR/GCA is associated with malignancy

Respiratory: Examine for reduced breath sounds and adventitious sounds as occasionally patients can present with pulmonary infiltrates

Cardiovascular: Murmur of aortic regurgitation

Gastrointestinal: Aortic pulse & listen for bruit; Listen for renal bruits

Musculoskeletal: Look for evidence of synovitis (especially at the wrists) but also other small joints; Examine the elbows and shoulders; Palpate the muscles of the shoulder and hip girdle for tenderness

Neurologic: Signs suggestive of CVA

INVESTIGATIONS
CBC: Normocytic anemia representing chronic inflammation, reactive thrombocytosis, usually a normal WBC count

Liver enzymes: May be elevated (particularly AST, ALP) in PMR

ESR: It is usually >50 (80-100), however it may be normal in up to 25% of cases

CRP: Elevated and may be more sensitive than ESR

Urinalysis: Microscopic hematuria

Complement (C3, C4): May be elevated

ANA: May be positive

Anticardiolipin antibodies: May be present increasing risk of thrombosis

Ultrasound of the Temporal Arteries: Abnormal U/S findings in 93% of those with biopsy positive GCA; The presence of a "halo" was very specific (100%)

Temporal Artery Biopsy: Need at least a 3-5 cm segment of temporal artery due to "skip lesions"; Biopsy is positive in 60-80% of cases; Biopsy performed on the contralateral side increases the yield; Biopsy should be performed within 2 weeks of initiation of corticosteroids; Biopsy pathology includes: A granulomatous infiltration and inflammatory response in the media of the vessel; Disruption of the internal elastic lamina; Mononuclear cellular infiltrate with multinucleate giant-cells; Occasionally, a non-specific panarteritis is seen

MANAGEMENT

General: Education; Vocational counseling; Arthritis self management programs

Physiotherapy: Pain relieving strategies and interventions; Mobility aids (canes & walkers) and braces; Exercise to improve ROM, muscle strength, aerobic conditioning, and core stability training; Weight loss

Occupational Therapy: Splints and orthotics; Joint protection measures and energy conservation; Assistive devices; Lifestyle management

Corticosteroids: **(a) Giant Cell Arteritis:** If patient has recent visual loss should consider IV Methylprednisolone; Otherwise, initiate Prednisone 1 mg/kg/day (40-60 mg) which can be given in divided doses (i.e. 20 mg PO TID); Increase the dose if the patient does not respond promptly; Continue the initial dose until all symptoms have disappeared and laboratory parameters have normalized (ESR/CRP); Slowly begin a tapering regimen such as: Reduce slowly by 5 mg every other week to 20 mg/day if the ESR remains normal; Below 20 mg reduce by 2.5 mg every 2-4 weeks as tolerated by symptoms and ESR; Below 10 mg reduce by 1 mg every 4 weeks as tolerated by symptoms and ESR; At doses of 10-20 mg per day reductions may be hampered by elevations in the ESR or CRP; **(b) Polymyalgia Rheumatica:** Prednisone 10-20 mg/day as a starting dose continued for one month until symptoms controlled and ESR/CRP normalized. Some evidence to suggest an initial dose of 20 mg may reduce the risk of relapse. Tapering Regimen: Below 20 mg reduce by 2.5 mg every 2-4 weeks as tolerated by symptoms and ESR; Below 10 mg reduce by 1 mg every 4 weeks as tolerated by symptoms and ESR

Osteoprotection: Given the dose and expected duration all patients should be placed on osteoprotective measures: (a) Education about glucocorticoid induced bone loss; (b) Encourage to exercise, stop smoking, and avoid excessive alcohol and caffeine; (c) Calcium & Vitamin D supplementation; (d) Bisphosphonates

Methotrexate: Controversial evidence on whether methotrexate can act as a steroid sparing agent as controlled trials have reached opposite conclusions; Regardless, it is often tried as a steroid sparing agent in patients with refractory disease

Other Immunosuppressants: Cyclophosphamide, azathioprine, & mycophenolate mofetil have been helpful in some reported cases

Biologics: Infliximab and etanercept used to treat refractory GCA with good results

PROGNOSIS

Risk Stratification for Poor Progression: (a) Vision loss as a presenting feature; (b) Require > 10 mg prednisone at 6 months

Prognosis: The average duration of corticosteroids for patients with PMR or GCA is 2.4 years. Up to 50% of patients will have discontinued treatment at 2 years. There is a subgroup of patients with GCA who continue to have smoldering disease activity for much longer (7 - 10 years). Thoracic aneurysms can occur up to 15 years after the initial diagnosis of GCA. The most significant complications of GCA include: Optic neuritis with visual loss and Malperfusion of the CNS resulting in CVA. Mortality is usually due to vascular complications related to inflammation.

PAGET'S DISEASE

DEFINITION & PATHOPHYSIOLOGY
Definition: A localized disorder of hyperactive bone remodeling where abnormal osteoclasts accelerate the process of normal bone turnover. Results in the production of bone that is disorganized, thickened, weak, and often hypervascular.

Pathophysiology: (a) Stage 1 - Increased osteoclastic activity: Initial phase involves an increase in osteoclastic activity with increased numbers of osteoclasts, increased resorption surface, and increased depth of the resorption areas; Pagetic osteoclasts become quite large and contain more than the usual 3-4 nuclei; (b) Stage 2 - Vascular hypertrophy and medullary fibrosis; (c) Stage 3 - Repair: The normal coupling of resorption and formation of bone is still in place. Osteoblasts are stimulated to fill in the resorption pits. The quantities of osteoid are often inadequate and osteoblasts may synthesize and secrete collagen into cavities with markedly irregular surfaces. The resulting bone is disorganized with thickened trabeculae and a haphazard appearance of woven bone with shortened lamellar collagen fibrils. The remaining bone becomes heavily calcified and sclerotic.

PRESENTATION
Identifying Data: More common in older individuals (>50); Prevalence of 2% in general population; Female: Male = 1:2 (more common in men)

Onset: The common presentations include: *(a) Pain:* Most common presentation; Back pain is common; Periarticular involvement may result in hip or knee pain; Pain is worse with weight bearing and may worsen at night; Pain is secondary to: Pagetic bone; Fracture; Degenerative arthritis; Nerve impingement; *(b) Asymptomatic:* Incidental finding on routine radiographs; Elevated alkaline phosphatase; *(c) Bony Deformity:* Tibial bowing; Skull thickening; Spontaneous fractures of the femur, tibia, humerus, and forearm; *(d) Neurologic Manifestations*

Progression: Most commonly involved sites are: Pelvis, lumbar spine, femur, thoracic spine, sacrum, skull, tibia, & humerus; Monostotic (20%); Polyostotic (80%)

Constitutional Features: Usually little

RHEUMATOLOGIC REVIEW OF SYSTEMS
Associated Conditions: Malignancies Including Osteogenic sarcoma (0.2-1%) and Fibrosarcoma; Benign giant-cell tumors

Musculoskeletal Involvement: Fracture; Excessive bleeding after a fracture due to hypervascularity; Deformity

Vascular Involvement: Vascular steal syndrome

Neurologic Involvement: Deafness: Ossification of stapedius tendon or auditory nerve entrapment; Nerve entrapment: Cranial or spinal nerve roots; Spinal stenosis; Platybasia resulting in basilar invagination, hydrocephalus, and headaches; Stroke from blood vessel compromise

Cardiac Involvement: Congestive heart failure; Hypertension

Renal Involvement: Nephrocalcinosis

Endocrine Involvement: Hypercalcemia & Hypercalciuria

RED FLAGS
Don't assume pain is secondary to Pagetic bone – Look for other causes!

FAMILY HISTORY
15-25% of family members eventually contract the disease; First-degree relatives have a 7-fold increased risk; Risk is further increased if affected relative had severe disease or disease at a young age

RISK FACTORS
Family history

DIFFERENTIAL DIAGNOSIS
(a) Paget's disease; (b) Primary malignancy; (c) Metastatic malignancy; (d) Infection

PHYSICAL EXAMINATION
Vitals: Pulse: Usually normal may be tachycardic; BP: Usually normal may be hypertensive; RR: Elevations in RR may be an indicator of high output CHF

Cutaneous: No specific findings

Head & Neck: Bony deformity of the skull

Respiratory: Pulmonary edema & pleural effusions suggesting associated CHF

Cardiovascular: Elevated JVP and peripheral edema suggesting CHF

Gastrointestinal: No specific findings

Musculoskeletal: Deformity – femoral or tibial bowing; Degenerative arthritis

Neurologic: Cranial neuropathies; Findings secondary to spinal stenosis; Neuropathy secondary to nerve impingement; Hearing loss

INVESTIGATIONS
Alkaline Phosphatase: 85% of people have increased ALP – up to 10 times normal

Calcium, Phosphorous: Typically normal (hypercalcemia with # or immobilization)

Vitamin D: Typically normal

PTH: Normal

Radiology: Commonest sites of involvement: Skull, vertebrae, pelvis, sacrum, and bones of the lower extremities

Bone Scan (99Tc labeled bisphosphonate): Most sensitive test for Paget's disease; Produces areas of focal increased uptake due to elevated metabolic rates; Useful for determining the extent of disease

Plain Radiographs: Usually shows mixed areas of osteolysis and sclerosis; Characteristic Pagetic lesions include: "Cortical thickening"; "Blade of grass" appearance on long bones; Due to the expanding lytic front; "Osteoporosis circumscripta": Extensive lytic involvement in the skull

MANAGEMENT
Consider treatment for: (a) Bone or joint pain; (b) Bone deformity; (c) Neurologic complications; (d) Asymptomatic disease if: Disease is moderately active and present at sites where complications could occur (weight bearing joints, spinal involvement etc); (e) Preparation for surgery to reduce hypervascularity and blood loss; (f) Patients with extensive skull involvement

Treatment outcome measures: Symptomatic improvement; Normalization of ALP

General: Education & Physiotherapy

Analgesics: Symptomatic relief

NSAIDs and COXIBs: Have analgesic and anti-inflammatory properties especially when the patient has concomitant osteoarthritis

Bisphosphonates: Treatment of choice due to their efficacy and prolonged duration of response; Most courses are higher dose and of shorter duration; Therapy will normalize ALP levels in 50-66% of patients; Consider re-treatment if ALP levels do not fall or rise because these patients are at increased risk of complications

Calcitonin: An alternative to bisphosphonate therapy; Used with extensive lytic disease, severe pain, rapid response, or intolerable to bisphosphonates

Surgical: To repair deformities, relieve nerve compression, & increase joint mobility

PROGNOSIS
Paget's disease does not spread to adjacent bone or metastasize to distant bone. The lesions are typically in fixed locations. Development of a new lesion over time should raise suspicion. The progression of each lesion is individual and highly variable

POLYARTERITIS NODOSA (PAN)

DEFINITION & PATHOPHYSIOLOGY

Definition: Polyarteritis Nodosa (PAN) is a necrotizing vasculitis affecting small and medium sized arteries without glomerulonephritis or vasculitis in arterioles, venules, or capillaries. See the Classification criteria for PAN 244

Pathophysiology: The mechanism of vascular inflammation is theorized to be immune complex induced. Immune complexes activate the complement cascade and, in turn, attract and activate neutrophils.

PRESENTATION

Identifying Data: Affects males and females equally; Can affect people of any age but typically presents between the ages of 40-60; Rare 5-10 cases per million

Onset: Majority of patients present with non-specific constitutional features of malaise, anorexia, weight loss, fever, and appear ill. Organ systems more commonly involved at presentation include: (a) Musculoskeletal involvement: Myalgias and arthralgias; (b) Peripheral nerve involvement: Mononeuritis multiplex is the most frequent finding. It tends to affect the lower extremities more commonly with sciatic, peroneal, and tibial nerve involvement. (c) Skin involvement: Palpable purpura is the most common finding; (d) Gastrointestinal tract Involvement: Abdominal pain; (e) Limited PAN: Occasionally PAN is limited to a single organ (appendix, gallbladder, uterus, testis, and skin). 10% progress to systemic PAN.

Progression: The disease may progress to fulminant multi-organ involvement. The majority of patients have severe manifestations and appear unwell.

Constitutional Features: Fever, fatigue, anorexia, weight loss, and malaise

Functional Status: Severely impaired function with severe disease

RHEUMATOLOGIC REVIEW OF SYSTEMS

Musculoskeletal Involvement: Myalgias & arthralgias; Asymmetric arthritis predominantly affecting the joints of the lower extremity

Mucocutaneous Involvement: Ear, nose, & throat involvement

Ocular Involvement: Retinal vasculitis; Retinal detachment; Cotton-wool spots

Neurologic Involvement: Peripheral Nervous System: Mononeuritis multiplex with motor and sensory deficits; May progress to look like a distal polyneuropathy; Affects the lower limbs predominantly (sciatic, peroneal, & tibial nerves); Cranial nerve palsies (rare); Central Nervous System - Strokes & brain hemorrhages

Cardiac Involvement: Coronary artery vasculitis: Myocardial infarction rare complication

Respiratory Involvement: Rare

Gastrointestinal Involvement: Mesenteric vasculitis: Abdominal pain may be the first symptom; Ischemia is more common in the small bowel and rare in the stomach and colon; GI bleeding and perforation can occur; Can see vasculitis of the appendix or gallbladder - may be an isolated finding; Hepatic involvement with necrosis (even in the absence of hepatitis B)

Renal Involvement: If glomerulonephritis it is classified as microscopic polyangiitis, otherwise: Vascular nephropathy (Hypertension, Renal infarcts with varying degrees of renal dysfunction)

Genitourinary Involvement: Orchitis - Good location for biopsy; Breast and uterine involvement

RISK FACTORS

Hepatitis B infection (7-10% of cases); Hairy cell leukemia

FAMILY HISTORY

No known association

RED FLAGS
Must always rule out sepsis as it can present as multi-organ failure and can mimic vasculitis

Refractory vasculitis is an infection until proven otherwise

DIFFERENTIAL DIAGNOSIS
Differential Diagnosis of Medium Vessel Vasculitis: PAN; Kawasaki disease

Differential Diagnosis of Small Vessel Vasculitis: *(See page 3)*

Differential Diagnosis of Aneurysms on Mesenteric Angiography: (a) PAN; (b) Segmental mediolytic arteriolopathy; (c) Ehlers Danlos, type IV; (d) Fibromuscular dysplasia; (e) Pseudoxanthoma elasticum; (f) Neurofibromatosis; (g) Atrial myxoma

PHYSICAL EXAMINATION
Vitals: Pulse: Normal to elevated; BP: Low if very ill to elevated if hypertensive with renal disease; RR: Normal to elevated; Temp: May have accompanying fever

Cutaneous: Subcut. nodules; Distal gangrene; Livedo reticularis; Palpable purpura

Head & Neck: Retinal detachment, cotton wool spots

Respiratory: Reduced breath sounds, adventitous sounds, pleural friction rubs

Cardiovascular: CHF with renal failure, flow murmurs with anemia

Gastrointestinal: Peritoneal signs if perforation of bowel; Diffuse abdominal pain, Rebound tenderness; GI bleeding; Testicular tenderness with orchitis

Musculoskeletal: Myalgias and muscle weakness; Inflammatory arthritis in an oligoarticular pattern

Neurologic: Cranial nerve palsies; Neuropathic changes (mononeuritis multiplex)

INVESTIGATIONS
CBC: Normochromic normocytic anemia, leukocytosis with occasional hypereosinophilia, thrombocytosis

ESR & CRP: Elevated inflammatory markers

Albumin: Low

Creatinine: May be elevated

Hepatitis B Surface Antigen (HepBsAg): Positive in 10%

ANCA: p-ANCA in 20-25% without hepatitis B (HBV) and 10% of patients with HBV

Angiography: Microaneurysms and stenosis in medium sized vessels predominantly found in the mesentery, kidney, and liver

Aspiration & Pathology: Diagnosis is best made via biopsy of an affected organ. The most fruitful biopsy sites include muscle, peripheral nerve, testis, skin, or kidney. Pathologic findings include: (a) A focal segmental necrotizing vasculitis; (b) Fibrinoid necrosis and mixed cellular infiltrate (PMNs, lymphocytes, & eosinophils) of the vessel wall; (c) Disruption of the normal architecture of the vessel wall (elastic lamina); (d) Thrombosis and aneurysmal dilatation; (e) Evidence of healing is seen with areas of fibrosis within the vessel wall

MANAGEMENT
General: Education; Vocational counseling; Arthritis self management programs

Physiotherapy: Pain relieving strategies and interventions; Mobility aids; Exercise to improve ROM; muscle strength; aerobic conditioning; Core stability training; Wt loss

Occupational Therapy: Splints and orthotics; Joint protection; energy conservation

Supportive: Supportive treatment of serious manifestations including gastrointestinal, nerve, cardiac, and renal lesions; Treat hypertension with ACE-Inhibitors; Renal failure requires nephrology consultation

Treatment of PAN WITH Hepatitis B Infection: (a) Initial high dose Corticosteroids (see below) for the first few weeks of disease to control severe life-threatening manifestations. Conventional immunosuppression treatment enhances the viruses ability to replicate and may jeopardize the patients outcome. Instead a combination of plasma exchange and anti-viral agents seems to be effective. *(b) Plasma Exchange:* To remove circulating immune complexes (9-12 exchanges over 3 wks). *(c) Anti-Viral Agents:* Interferon-alpha-2b or lamivudine; A good prognostic sign is conversion from HBeAg to HBeAb

Treatment of PAN WITHOUT Hepatitis B Infection: High-Dose Corticosteroids: Found to be beneficial in some patients with the response usually coming within 3 months. Many patients remain steroid dependant. Pulsed methylprednisolone 1 gram IV over 60 minutes daily for 3-5 days; After 3 days give prednisone 1 mg/kg PO OD - This can be given in 3 - 4 divided daily doses for 7 - 10 days consolidating to a single morning dose by 2-3 weeks; As the patient improves clinically and the ESR normalizes the prednisone can be slowly tapered. *Example Tapering Regimens:* Taper to 50% original dose by decreasing by 2.5 mg q10days; Maintain at this dose for 3 weeks; Taper to 20 mg by decreasing by 2.5 mg qweekly; Taper to 10 mg by decreasing by 1 mg q2weeks; Maintain at 10 mg for 3 weeks; Taper to 0 by decreasing by 1 mg qmonthly *OR* Taper by 5 mg on alternate days qweekly gradually gradually converting the treatment regimen to alternate daily prednisone; Thereby the prednisone is tapered by 2.5-5 mg each week until it is discontinued

Cyclophosphamide: Indications for cyclophosphamide are as follows: Five factor score > 0; Mononeuritis multiplex; CNS disease; Renal vasculitis; Mesenteric vasculitis; Cardiac involvement;

Pulsed IV Cyclophosphamide: Initial pulses may vary from 0.25 to 2.5 grams at intervals of 1 week to 1 month. In Europe, mini-pulses given more frequently are routinely used. Example orders for cyclophosphamide see page 166.

Oral Cyclophosphamide: More effective (less relapses) and used second line when IV fails; Given as 1-2 mg/kg/day orally for a maximum of one year. Use cyclophosphamide as the induction agent aiming to stop it at 3-6 months and continue with one of the maintenance agents. The initial NIH regimen states to continue cyclophosphamide for one year after remission then taper by 25 mg every 2-3 months, however, they do state that the "necessary duration of treatment is open to question and our views have changed over the years".

Remission with Azathioprine: European Union Vasculitis Study Group used the CYCAZAREM regimen (2 studies one in abstract form in *A&R, 1999* and the other in *NEJM 349:1, 2003*); *Induction:* Oral cyclophosphamide (CYC) 2 mg/kg/day for 3 months; *Remission:* Oral CYC 1.5 mg/kg/day OR azathioprine 2 mg/kg/day; Results: 93% remission rate with CYC & prednisone, Mortality at 18 months ~ 5%, Relapse rate 14-15% (same in both CYC and AZA groups), Adverse events 21-26%

Methotrexate: Used for maintenance of remission in patients with Wegener's Granulomatosis (not PAN). Oral CYC was used to initiate disease remission and weekly methotrexate was substituted given 1-2 days after last dose of CYC.

IVIG: Conflicting results

Plasmapheresis/Plasma Exchange: Uncertain benefit & undeniable risks

PROGNOSIS

Risk Stratification for Poor Progression: Five Factor Score (total of 5 points): Proteinuria > 1 gram/day (1 point); Renal insufficiency with creatinine > 140 umol/L (1 point); Cardiomyopathy (1 point); Gastrointestinal tract involvement (1 point); CNS involvement (1 point); 5 year mortality with the FFS is as follows: FFS = 0 (12%), FFS = 1 (26%), FFS > 1 (46%)

Prognosis: The overall 5 year survival is 80%; Most deaths occur with severe disease in the initial 18 months

PSORIATIC ARTHRITIS (PsA)

DEFINITION & PATHOPHYSIOLOGY

Definition: Psoriatic arthritis is an inflammatory arthritis associated with psoriasis affecting both the peripheral and axial joints

Pathophysiology: **(a) Genetic Factors:** Monozygotic twin concordance with psoriasis is 70%; Family studies suggest a 50-fold increase risk of PsA in 1st degree relatives; Fathers twice as likely to transmit the disease; HLA-B27 +ve 50%; **(b) Environmental Factors:** Infectious agents; Trauma (Koebner phenomenon); **(c) Immunologic Factors:** T-cell activation with skewing of TCR repertoire consistent with an ongoing Th1 phenotype; CD8 T-cells also play an important role

PRESENTATION

Identifying Data: Psoriasis occurs in 1-3% of the population (Caucasians much more common); 6-42% of patients with psoriasis will get psoriatic arthritis; Overall prevalence is about 0.1% (1 in 1000); Onset ages 30-50

Onset: Some patients will present after a traumatic event; Peripheral Joints: Patients most commonly present with an inflammatory mono or oligoarthritis; Can affect the DIPs (associated with nail changes); Associated tenosynovitis resulting in dactylitis; Axial Joints: Spine symptoms rarely are a presenting feature; Sacroiliitis in 1/3 of patients is unilateral and asymptomatic; Spondylitis may affect any portion of the spine in a random fashion; Relationship to Skin Disease: Psoriasis present before the onset of arthritis (70%); Psoriasis and arthritis come together (15%); Psoriatic arthritis sine psoriasis (15%) - Psoriasis develops later

Progression: 1/3 to 1/2 evolve into an inflammatory polyarthritis like RA, however, 50% will have DIP involvement which would be unusual for RA; Axial disease usually manifests itself after several years of peripheral arthritis; Risk factors for progression: Active and severe disease at presentation; >5 joints involved; use of immunomodulating medications. Psoriatic arthritis can progress to destroy joints; Patterns of Disease: Mono or oligoarthritis (40-50%); Symmetric polyarthritis (30-50%); Predom. axial disease (5%); DIP involvement (5-10%); Arthritis mutilans (5%)

Constitutional Features: Associated fatigue

Functional Status: Up to 20% will experience significant functional limitations

RHEUMATOLOGIC REVIEW OF SYSTEMS

Musculoskeletal Involvement: Enthesitis: Achilles & plantar fascia

Mucocutaneous Involvement: Psoriasis: Sharply demarcated erythematous plaques with a well-marked, silvery scale; Nail Involvement: Pitting, onycholysis, transverse depression (ridging), brown-yellow discoloration, and leukonychia

Ocular Involvement: Conjunctivitis in 20% and iritis in 7% (assoc. with axial disease)

RISK FACTORS

Family history of psoriasis; Presence of psoriasis and nail lesions

FAMILY HISTORY

Monozygotic twin concordance with psoriasis is 70%; A 50-fold increase risk of PsA in 1st degree relatives; Fathers twice as likely to transmit disease

RED FLAGS

Examine for the presence of cervical spine disease; Think about HIV in a patient who presents with acute severe arthritis (especially in young males)

DIFFERENTIAL DIAGNOSIS

(a) Septic arthritis; (b) HIV related arthritis (HIV +ve test); (c) Polyarticular gout; (d) Rheumatoid arthritis (differs from PsA in that it lacks dactylitis, lacks enthesitis, no lumbar/sacral axial disease, rare DIP involvement, no psoriasis (a patient with RA may have psoriasis though), no nail changes, and the RF is positive in 70-85% of established cases); (e) Ankylosing spondylitis - Differs from PsA in that it usually begins earlier in life, has more severe spinal disease, a lack of psoriasis, a lack of nail changes, and prominent asymmetry; (f) Reactive arthritis - Differs from PsA in that it has a prodromal illness, no psoriasis; different rashes (keratoderma blenorrhagicum, oral ulceration, circinate balanitis), and is less likely to affect the upper extremity; (g) IBD - Differs from PsA in that it has symptoms suggestive of IBD and has a predilection for joints of the lower extremity; (h) Other connective tissue diseases

PHYSICAL EXAMINATION

Vitals: Pulse: Usually normal; BP: Usually normal; RR: Usually normal

Cutaneous: Nail changes such as pits, onycholysis, or psoriatic nails; Palmar erythema; Psoriatic lesions behind the ears (often missed), on extensor surfaces of forearms, umbilicus (often missed), gluteal fold, and knees

Head & Neck: Conjunctivitis; C-spine involvement with instability

Respiratory: Costochondritis (sternomanubrial joint disease)

Cardiovascular: No specific findings

Gastrointestinal: No specific findings

Musculoskeletal: Involvement of the DIPs; Arthritis mutilans with telescoping digits; Typically an oligoarticular pattern (early in the course) more often affecting the PIPs and wrists; PIPS: Fusiform swelling, pain, tenderness to palpate, flexion deformities, swan-neck deformities, boutonniere deformities, ligamentous instability; MCPs: Swelling, pain, tenderness to palpate, flexion deformities, ulnar drift, subluxation, fusion (ankylosis); Wrists: Dorsal swelling, pain, tenderness, radial deviation, volar subluxation, carpal tunnel syndrome, and interosseous wasting; Flexor tendon thickening with nodules and trigger finger; Elbow and shoulder involvement; Achilles tendonitis; Plantar fasciitis; Inflammatory arthritis affecting knees, ankles, and MTPs

Axial Examination: Features to suggest an inflammatory arthritis such as: Flattening of the lumbar lordosis; Loss of lumbar extension and lateral flexion; Reduced lumbar forward flexion with increased finger tip to floor distance and abnormalities of the modified Schober test and modified modified Schober test; Positive sacroiliac compression testing; Hip involvement with hip flexion contractures found on the Thomas test; Reduced chest expansion; Increased thoracic kyphosis with increased occiput to wall distance; Reduced ROM of cervical spine

Neurologic: Spinal cord and nerve root signs secondary to thick syndesmophytes and vertebral instability

INVESTIGATIONS

CBC: Anemia of chronic inflammation, blood loss (NSAIDs), & bm suppress. DMARD

ESR/CRP: Elevated in about 50% of patients

Synovial Fluid: Inflammatory cellular picture 2000 – 10,000 cells/mm

Radiology of Peripheral Joints: Dactylitis; DIP swelling; Fusiform swelling around other joints; Alignment: Malalignment secondary to deformities; Bones: (a) Evidence of new bone formation: Normal mineralization (lack of periarticular osteopenia); Periostitis (fluffy); Ankylosis of joints; (b) Evidence of bone resorption: Acro-osteolysis (resorption of the distal tufts); Erosions – paramarginal ("Mickey Mouse Ears"); Osteolysis of bone (mutilans deformities); *Cartilage:* Joint space may widen due to interposition of fibrous tissue as adjacent periarticular bone is resorbed; Narrowing of the joint space; *Distribution:* Bilateral but asymmetric; Distributed in a "ray-Like" fashion (all joints of one finger); Oligoarticular

Radiology of Axial Joints: Alignment: Loss of normal lumbar lordosis; Cervical spine abnormalities, syndesmophytes, and subluxation; *Bones:* Generalized osteoporosis of the spine; Fractures; Paravertebral ossification (thicker than syndesmophytes, runs from midbody to mid-body and may contain an unmineralized cleft between itself and the adjacent vertebral body); Whiskering of periostium (iliac crests, ischial tuberosities, greater trochanters); Squaring of vertebrae; Osteitis and erosion adjacent to the vertical endplate; Anterior longitudinal ligament mineralization may fill in the normal anterior concavity of the vertebral body; Syndesmophytes; Gracile ossification of the outer fibers of the annulus fibrosus; With maturation they create a bamboo spine; *Cartilage:* Asymmetric sacroiliitis: Stage 1: Pseudowidening due to erosions of subchondral bone with loss of joint margins, superficial erosions, and surrounding osteopenia; Stage 2: Stage 1 & sclerosis; Stage 3: Erosions; Stage 4: Ankylosis of SI joints; Apophyseal joint Involvement: Destruction then ankylosis; *Distribution:* Segmental asymmetrical process; Patchy involvement of SI, L, T, and C spines

MANAGEMENT

General: Education; Vocational counseling; Arthritis self management programs

Physiotherapy: Pain relieving strategies and interventions; Mobility aids ; Exercise to improve ROM, muscle strength, aerobic conditioning, and core stability training; Weight loss; Manual therapy (manipulation) when appropriate; Assistive devices

Occupational Therapy: Splints and orthotics; Joint protection & energy conservation

NSAIDs and COXIBs: Analgesic & anti-inflammatory properties; Not alter the course of disease or prevent joint destruction; Not to be used alone for the treatment of PsA

DMARDs: All patients are candidates for DMARD therapy; Have the potential to reduce or prevent joint damage, preserve joint integrity and function, reduce health costs, and maintain economic productivity; Initiate within 3 months of diagnosis.

Mild to Moderate Disease: Hydroxychloroquine; Sulfasalazine

Moderate to Severe Disease: (> 5 joints, reduced functional capacity, anemia, hypoalbuminemia, and erosions on radiographs): Methotrexate: Standard of care due to its efficacy, low toxicity, low cost, & established track record. Patients are more likely to stay on MTX (50% at 3 years) and if they do discontinue it is usually due to adverse effects. Little effect on spinal involvement. Sulfasalazine; Leflunomide: May be beneficial in 40% of patients; Gold

Severe Disease not controlled by initial DMARD (3-6 months): The options are as follows: Maximize the dose of monotherapy; Combination therapy: Methotrexate & Sulfasalazine; Methotrexate, Sulfasalazine, & Hydroxychloroquine; Methotrexate & Leflunomide; Methotrexate & Gold

Corticosteroids: Low dose glucocorticoids (<10 mg/day) are highly effective in controlling symptoms in patients with active PsA; The benefits of low-dose steroids should always be balanced against the risks; Options for Glucocorticoid use include: Intra-articular Steroid injections into the most symptomatic joints; Intra-muscular injection of 80 mg depo-medrol: Has the benefit of lasting 2-3 weeks and can be used nicely as bridge therapy while waiting for DMARD to work.

Biologics: Etanercept & Infliximab: Effective in patients with active PsA who had failed previous DMARD therapy; Used early in the course of disease if possible

PROGNOSIS

Risk Stratification for Poor Progression: (a) Younger age of onset; (b) Female gender; (c) Acute onset of arthritis; (d) Polyarticular disease (> 5 joints); (e) High ESR at presentation and a persistently elevated ESR; (f) Need for high levels of medications (suggesting more severe disease); (g) Certain HLA antigens (B27 in the presence of DR7, B39, and DQw3 in the absence of DR7)

Prognosis: Prognosis of the arthritis depends upon the risk stratification for poor progression. Increased mortality in patients with psoriatic arthritis

RAYNAUD'S PHENOMENON (RP)

DEFINITION & PATHOPHYSIOLOGY

Definition: Raynaud's phenomenon is defined as vasospasm of the arteries or arterioles causing pallor and at least one other color change upon reperfusion such as cyanosis or redness; Two categories of Raynaud's phenomenon include: Primary RP: No associated underlying illness (Raynaud's disease); Secondary RP: Associated underlying illness (usually a connective tissue disease)

Pathophysiology: The three pathophysiological mechanisms thought to play a role in the development of Raynaud's phenomenon include: (a) Endothelial Cell Dysfunction: Endothelial-dependant and independent vasodilatory responses are disrupted jeopardizing vascular control; Nitric oxide (major endothelial vasodilator) synthesis is reduced further impairing vascular control; (b) Neurogenic Mechanisms: Abnormalities of neurogenic mechanisms have not been clearly elucidated; Speculated that hypersensitive parasympathetic responses and sympathetic dysfunction result in increased cold-induced vasoconstrictor response (i.e. inappropriate vasospasm); (c) Abnormal Immune Responses: Speculated based on the association of Raynaud's phenomenon with other autoimmune diseases (only in a subset of patients with secondary RP); In systemic sclerosis, Raynaud's phenomenon is secondary to both vasospastic attacks and intimal proliferation

PRESENTATION

Identifying Data: More common in women than men 2:1; Primary RP tends to occur in younger women (15-45) whereas secondary RP occurs in slightly older individuals; Prevalence in the population varies from 3-4%

Onset: Usually begins quite abruptly with changes involving the hands, however, the feet, ears, and nose may also be affected. Attacks are predominantly triggered by cold exposure. Other triggers include emotional changes, trauma, hormonal changes, and smoking. The attacks classically result in a "triphasic" color pattern: Pallor due to vasoconstriction; Cyanosis due to ischemia which may be associated with numbness, pain, and a reduction in temperature; Rubor secondary to reactive hyperemia which may be associated with a burning sensation and increased sweating

Progression: Primary RP: Does not typically result in serious morbidity. Necrosis, as a result of ischemia, can occur but it is rare. Patients with RP for 2 years with no associated features of an underlying connective tissue disease (especially negative ANA and no superficial dilated nailbed capillaries) are at low risk for developing an autoimmune disease; Secondary RP: RP may precede the onset of connective tissue disease by years. Secondary RP tends to be more severe than primary more often resulting in debilitating symptoms including pain and digital ischemia

Constitutional Features: May occur in secondary RP associated with a connective tissue disease

Functional Status: Functional status is dependant upon the frequency and severity of ischemic attacks

RHEUMATOLOGIC REVIEW OF SYSTEMS

Associated Conditions: Findings associated with secondary RP which depend upon the underlying disease

RISK FACTORS

Causes of secondary RP include: (a) Trauma: Vibrational tools - Dentists, Jack hammer operators, lumberjacks; (b) Hyperviscosity (rare): Polycythemia; Cryoglobulinemia; Leukemia; Thrombocytosis; Arterial occlusive disease; Arterial thrombosis; (c) Drugs and Toxins: Chemotherapeutics: Vinblastine, vincristine;

Estrogens & ergots; Smoking; Environmental Toxins: Vinyl chloride; (d) Systemic Disease: Connective Tissue Diseases (Systemic sclerosis - 90-95%; Mixed connective tissue disease - 85%; SLE - Up to 45%; Anti-phospholipid antibody syndrome; Rheumatoid arthritis - 10%; Sjogren's syndrome - 30%; Inflammatory myopathies - 20%); Vasculitis; (e) Hepatitis; (f) Pulmonary hypertension; (g) Cryoglobulinemia

FAMILY HISTORY
Primary RP has a genetic predisposition

RED FLAGS
Think of secondary RP in the following situations: RP in a male; New onset RP in an individual > 30 yrs of age; Severe attacks; Digital pits or ulceration associated with RP

DIFFERENTIAL DIAGNOSIS
(a) Acrocyanosis; (b) Chronic regional pain disorder; (c) Thoracic outlet syndrome; (d) Thromboangiitis obliterans; (e) Cryoglobulinemia; (f) Atherosclerosis; (g) Vasculitis; (h) Thromboembolic disease; (i) Acrocyanosis; (j) Chilblains

PHYSICAL EXAMINATION
Vitals: Pulse: Usually normal; BP: Usually normal (may be elevated if associated with systemic sclerosis); RR: Usually normal; Temperature: Usually normal

Cutaneous: Sclerodactyly; Digital pits and ulceration; Dilated periungual capillary loops with or without dropout (increases the likelihood of secondary RP associated with connective tissue diseases); Digital calcinosis with systemic sclerosis; Loss of digital tufts; Livedo reticularis

Head & Neck: Raynaud's phenomenon in the ears; Findings of other connective tissue disease (i.e. systemic sclerosis)

Respiratory: No specific abnormalities in primary RP, may find if RP associated with other conditions

Cardiovascular: No specific abnormalities in primary RP, may find if RP associated with underlying conditions; Angina secondary to coronary vasospasm; Look for evidence of associated pulmonary hypertension (Loud P2, RV heave, pulmonary flow murmur, pulmonary regurgitation, tricuspid regurgitation, elevated JVP with prominent V waves due to TR)

Gastrointestinal: No specific abnormalities unless associated with an underlying condition

Musculoskeletal: Inflammatory arthritis in patients with secondary RP

Neurologic: No specific abnormalities in primary RP, may find if RP associated with other conditions

INVESTIGATIONS
CBC: Anemia (normochromic, normocytic in patients with secondary RP)

ESR, CRP: Should be normal in primary RP. If abnormal think of an underlying cause

Creatinine & urinalysis: To look for evidence of connective tissue disease

Glucose: Underlying diabetes

Rheumatoid factor: Look for underlying connective tissue disease

ANA: Look for underlying connective tissue disease

TSH: Look for evidence of thyroid dysfunction

May also consider (if history suggests CTD): Anti-centromere and anti-topoisomerase (Scl-70) antibodies in patients suspected of having systemic sclerosis; Anti-Ro & La antibodies can be found in patients with Sjogren's syndrome & SLE; Cryoglobulins; von-Willebrand factor may be increased in patients with secondary RP

Radiology: A chest x-ray may be useful to look for the presence of a cervical rib or associated lung fibrosis

MANAGEMENT

General: Education; Smoking cessation; Withdrawal of medication associated with vasospasm. Protection from the cold: Keep core body temperature warm - sweaters, hats, mittens; Keep extremities warm

ASA: Consider ASA in patients with a history of ischemic ulcers

Calcium channel blockers: Reduces the frequency and severity of ischemic attacks; Long acting agents such as nifedipine XL 30 mg OD are better tolerated than short acting ones; Other options include diltiazem and amlodipine although the evidence is not as readily available for these compounds

Other Vasodilators: The evidence for other vasodilators remains thin; Prazosin, losartan, fluoxetine have all been shown to produce some benefit in small trials

Topical Nitrates: Can be used on the most severely involved digits; Apply 0.5 - 1 cm of 2% nitropaste to the proximal portion of the affected digit twice daily; Remove the nitropaste for 12 hours in the evening

Intravenous Iloprost: A vasodilator and platelet inhibitor; Used in most severe cases to prevent and heal digital ulceration and reduce the frequency and severity of RP attacks; Given as an infusion starting at 0.5 ng/kg/min increasing by 0.5 ng/kg/hr every 30 minutes until the maximum tolerable dose is achieved; Infusions are given daily for 5 days

Surgical Sympathectomy & Ganglion Blocks: May be considered when all other options have been exhausted; It can be performed in the cervical, thoracic, or digital regions; A chemical sympathectomy (bupivicaine) may be useful prior to surgery to demonstrate efficacy; The duration and degree of improvement with sympathectomies has been unpredictable. They have not been shown to provide long lasting relief in most patients.

PROGNOSIS

Risk Stratification for Poor Progression: (a) Secondary RP; (b) Presence of digital pits and necrosis; (c) Frequent severe attacks; (d) New onset RP in an older individual or a very young child (usually secondary RP); (e) Asymmetric attacks; (f) Sclerodactyly; (g) Presence of autoantibodies

Prognosis: The prognosis is dependant upon the frequency and severity of ischemic attacks, the presence ischemic attacks resulting in necrosis, and the presence of an underlying systemic disease; Primary RP is usually episodic, does not result in significant impairment, and rarely requires pharmacologic treatment in most individuals. Approximately 5-10% of patients with primary RP may progress to a connective tissue disorder; Secondary RP is usually more severe than primary RP and can result in significant disability and impairment

REACTIVE ARTHRITIS (ReA)

DEFINITION & PATHOPHYSIOLOGY

Definition: An infection-induced systemic illness characterized by an inflammatory synovitis from which viable microorganisms cannot be cultured

Pathophysiology: Reactive arthritis is thought to occur in a genetically predisposed individual who comes in contact with an infectious trigger; Genetic predisposition comes in the form of HLA-B27 positivity (80%); The initial event is infection with an enterogenic or urogenital organism. Common infections include: Enterogenic: Salmonella; Shigella; Campylobacter; Yersinia; Urogenital: Chlamydia; Theories on pathogenesis include: (a) Molecular mimicry: A genetically predisposed individual becomes infected; The foreign antigen contains amino acid sequences which are homologous to those found on self proteins; An antibody response is mounted against the foreign antigen; Antibodies produced also cross react with self proteins; (b) Aberrant folding of the heavy chain of HLA-B27 blunting the immune response; (c) Arthritogenic peptides: In generating a response to the foreign antigen, HLA-B27 positive individuals present arthritogenic peptides while mounting a T-cell mediated response; HLA-B27 itself may be the source of the "arthritogenic" peptides

PRESENTATION

Identifying Data: Typical patient is a young male or young adult aged 20-40; Enterogenic ReA is equally distributed, however, urogenital ReA occurs predominantly in men

Onset: Begins 2-4 weeks after venereal infection or bout of gastroenteritis but no more than 6 weeks; Additive symmetric oligoarthritis (average 4 joints) predominantly affecting the lower limbs (ankles, knees, small joints of the feet); Joints involved are warm, swollen, tender and may be slightly erythematous and exquisitely tender suggestive of a septic joint; Low back pain occurs in 50% of patients and caused primarily by sacroiliac (unilateral) or other spinal joint involvement; Morning stiffness > 60 minutes – characterized by prolonged stiffness throughout the day; Sleep - Impaired sleep due to pain and stiffness is a definite contributor to fatigue

Progression: The arthritis is typically persistent until treated and worse with immobility such as overnight rest. Activity may improve stiffness but can aggravate pain. Enthesitis is a common feature in 60% presenting as heel pain (Achilles), metatarsalgia (plantar fascia), or sausage digits (dactylitis)

Constitutional Features: Low-grade fever and weight loss. Fatigue may be prominent due to sleep difficulties.

Functional Status: Reduced functional status and difficulties with ADLs; Difficulty at work; Loss of libido; Depression

RHEUMATOLOGIC REVIEW OF SYSTEMS

Associated Conditions: HIV Infection - ReA frequently reported in HIV patients, likely related to other STDs that are common to both ReA and HIV

Musculoskeletal Involvement: Enthesitis occurs at insertions of the: Plantar fascia; Achilles tendon; Pelvis; Costochondral junction; Patella; Rotator cuff

Mucocutaneous Involvement: Keratoderma blenorrhagicum (papulosquamous skin rash most commonly on soles of feet or palms of hands); Circinate balanitis; Hyperkeratotic nails; Painless oral ulceration

Ocular Involvement: Sterile conjuctivitis in 60% of patients; Acute anterior uveitis in 20% of patients. Uveitis tends to be unilateral.

Neurologic Involvement: Neuropathy, encephalopathy, and transverse myelitis

Cardiac Involvement: Aortitis with dilatation of the aortic ring and regurgitation in 1%

Gastrointestinal Involvement: Infectious ileitis/colitis or sterile ileitis/colitis

Renal Involvement: IgA nephropathy and amyloidosis

Genitourinary Involvement: Mild dysuria or mucopurulent discharge are typical symptoms more commonly in men and occasionally prostatitis or epididymitis are present; The pyuria, if present, is usually sterile

RISK FACTORS

(a) Enterogenic Infection: Salmonella, shigella, campylobacter, and yersinia; (b) Urogenital Infection: Chlamydia; HLA-B27 positive in 80%

FAMILY HISTORY

Likely an increased risk given the family passage of HLA-B27

RED FLAGS

Septic Arthritis - Non-gonococcal and gonococcal

DIFFERENTIAL DIAGNOSIS

(a) Infection: Septic arthritis: Non-gonococcal; Gonococcal arthritis; Viral arthritis; Spirochete - Lyme; (b) Crystalline arthritis (gout); (c) Another seronegative arthropathy - Enteropathic, psoriatic, ankylosing spondylitis; (d) Rheumatoid arthritis; (e) Rheumatic fever; (f) Connective tissue disease – Behcet's, SLE; (g) Sarcoidosis

PHYSICAL EXAMINATION

Vitals: Pulse: Normal; BP: Normal; RR: Normal; Temp: May have low-grade fever

Cutaneous: Nail changes such as hyperkeratosis or yellowing of the nails; Keratoderma blenorrhagicum on palms of hands and soles of tho feet

Head & Neck: Conjuctivitis; Oral ulceration; C-spine involvement with instability

Respiratory: No specific findings

Cardiovascular: Murmur of aortic regurgitation

Gastrointestinal: Circinate balanitis on the penis

Musculoskeletal: Involves joints of the lower extremity much more commonly but can have an inflammatory arthritis in the hands; Elbow and shoulder involvement; Costochondritis; Achilles tendonitis; Plantar fasciitis; Inflammatory arthritis affecting knees, ankles, MTPs and feet; Dactylitis of the toes; Tenosynovitis

Axial Examination: May have features to suggest an inflammatory arthritis such as: Flattening of the lumbar lordosis; Loss of lumbar extension and lateral flexion; Reduced lumbar forward flexion with increased finger tip to floor distance and abnormalities of the Modified Schober test and modified modified Schober test; Positive sacroiliac compression testing; Hip involvement with hip flexion; contractures found on the Thomas test; Red. chest expansion; Increased thoracic kyphosis with increased occiput to wall distance; Red. ROM of the cervical spine

Neurologic: Peripheral neuropathy

INVESTIGATIONS

CBC: Mild normochromic, normocytic anemia, leukocytosis is typical, reactive thrombocytosis

ESR/CRP: Elevated

HLA-B27: Occurs in 80% compared to 6% of general population

Immunoglobulins: Elevated IgA

Urinalysis: Pyuria

Urine Culture: Sterile

Radiology of Peripheral Joints: (a) Soft Tissue: Dactylitis; DIP swelling; Fusiform swelling around other joints; (b) Alignment: Malalignment secondary to deformities; (c) Bones: Evidence of new bone formation: Normal mineralization (lack of periarticular osteopenia); Periostitis (fluffy); Ankylosis of joints; Evidence of bone resorption: Acro-osteolysis (resorption of the distal tufts); Erosions – paramarginal

("Mickey Mouse Ears"); Osteolysis of bone (mutilans deformities); (c) Cartilage: Joint space may widen due to interposition of fibrous tissue as adjacent periarticular bone is resorbed; Narrowing of the joint space with progression; (d) Distribution: Bilateral but asymmetric; Distributed in a "ray-like" fashion; Oligoarticular

Radiology of Axial Joints: (a) Alignment: Loss of normal lumbar lordosis; Cervical spine abnormalities and subluxation; (b) Bones: Generalized osteoporosis of the spine; Fractures; Paravertebral ossification (thicker than syndesmophytes, runs from midbody to mid-body and may contain an unmineralized cleft between itself and the adjacent vertebral body; Whiskering of periosteum (Iliac crests, ischial tuberosities, greater trochanters); Squaring of vertebrae; Osteitis and erosion adjacent to the vertical endplate; Anterior longitudinal ligament mineralization may fill in the normal anterior concavity of the vertebral body; Syndesmophytes; Gracile ossification of the outer fibers of the annulus fibrosus; With maturation they create a bamboo spine; (c) Cartilage: Unilateral Sacroiliitis - Stage 1 – Pseudowidening of SI joints due to erosions of subchondral bone with loss of definition of joint margins, superficial erosions, and surrounding osteopenia; Stage 2 – Stage 1 & sclerosis; Stage 3 – Erosions of SI joints; Stage 4 – Ankylosis of SI joints; Apophyseal joint Involvement: Destruction then ankylosis; (d) Distribution: Segmental asymmetrical process; Patchy involvement of L, I, L, T, and C spines

Synovial Fluid: Gram stain & culture negative; Inflammatory infiltrate; Reiter's Cells – Large mononuclear cells containing many PMNs containing inclusion bodies

MANAGEMENT

General: Education; Vocational counseling; Arthritis self management programs

Physiotherapy: Pain relieving strategies and interventions; Mobility aids (canes & walkers) and braces; Exercise to improve ROM, muscle strength, aerobic conditioning; Weight loss; Manual therapy (manipulation) when appropriate

Occupational Therapy: Splints and orthotics; Joint protection measures and energy conservation; Assistive devices; Lifestyle management

Antibiotics: Should be given if an organism can be isolated; (a) Enterogenic infections: Controversy exists over the routine use of antibiotics in enterogenic reactive arthritis. Ciprofloxacin 500 mg PO BID has been given for a period of three months, in a few studies, with no significant improvement. However, when these patients were followed-up over a 2 year period there was some suggestion that those originally treated with ciprofloxacin tended to do better.   (b) Urogenital infections: Doxycycline 100 mg PO OD for chlamydia

NSAIDs: May dramatically reduce pain and spinal stiffness; Long-acting NSAIDs taken at night may reduce night discomfort and morning stiffness

Corticosteroids: Intra-articular corticosteroid injections may be of value for entheseal pain and peripheral synovitis; Local corticosteroid injection into the sacroiliac joints may be of benefit; Low doses of oral prednisone are NOT as effective as in RA

DMARDs: Sulfasalazine is the initial choice and may be used safely in patients with HIV – Doses of 2-3 grams per day. Can be discontinued if not effective after 4 months of use. Methotrexate & Azathioprine

Biologics: Etanercept & Infliximab – Case reports

PROGNOSIS

Risk Stratification for Chronic Arthritis: (a) Arthritis post-venereal disease – Worse than post-enterogenic disease; (b) HLA-B27; (c) Male gender

Prognosis: Self-limited disease course – Remission within 6 months (35%) to 2 years (70%); Intermittent recurrences – 15%; Chronic arthritis – 15%

RELAPSING POLYCHONDRITIS (RP)

DEFINITION & PATHOPHYSIOLOGY
Definition: A rare autoimmune disorder characterized by episodic widespread and progressive inflammation of cartilaginous structures leading to tissue destruction
Pathophysiology: Autoimmune disorder with evidence of cellular and humoral response to cartilaginous structures, including collagen II, IX, and XI

PRESENTATION
Identifying Data: All age groups, more common in age 40-50; Male: female ratio 1:1
Onset: Auricular chondritis is the most common initial symptom: Sudden onset of burning pain and swelling of the cartilaginous portion of the external ear with a purplish-red discoloration. The lobe of the ear is spared. May subside in a few days on its own or last several weeks often necessitating treatment. As the disease continues, progressive inflammation may result in deformities such as a soft and floppy ear (cauliflower ear); Migratory, asymmetric, episodic polyarthritis is the second most common initial symptom and is non-erosive and non-deforming; Other presenting features may include: Nasal chondritis which may progress to saddle-nose deformity; Ocular inflammation; Respiratory tract inflammation; Audiovestibular involvement with hearing loss and vertigo
Progression: The pattern of disease is highly individual but usually fits into one of the following categories: (a) Episodic disease activity, (b) Smoldering disease with ever-changing activity; (c) Fulminant downhill course; (d) Benign self-limited course
Constitutional Features: Fatigue & malaise prominent. Fever of unknown origin.
Functional Status: Red. functional status with difficulties in ADLs; Difficulty at work

RHEUMATOLOGIC REVIEW OF SYSTEMS
Mucocutaneous Involvement: A wide variety of skin abnormalities have been associated with relapsing polychondritis, however, none of them are specific for the condition; Abnormalities include alopecia, erythema nodosum, hyperpigmentation over involved cartilage, leukocytoclastic vasculitis, and pyoderma gangrenosum
Ear, Nose, & Throat Involvement: Inflammation of the cartilaginous nasal septa causing a saddle-nose deformity
Vascular Involvement: Ranges from leukocytoclasia to aortitis
Hematologic Involvement: Myelodysplasia
Ocular Involvement: Scleritis/episcleritis, conjunctivitis, iritis, and keratitis
Neurologic Involvement: Cranial neuropathies; Hearing loss; Vertigo; Headaches; Rare neurologic manifestations:hemiplegia, ataxia, seizures, confusion, & dementia
Cardiac Involvement: Aortic regurgitation, mitral regurgitation, AV block, pericarditis, and cardiac ischemia; Sudden heart valve rupture; Aortic aneurysms
Respiratory Involvement: Laryngeal involvement may lead to hoarseness, choking sensation, cough, & thyroid cartilage tenderness; Tracheobronchial involvement may lead to stridor, wheezing, wall thickening, stenosis, and major airway collapse.

RISK FACTORS
Unknown

FAMILY HISTORY
No known hereditary involvement

RED FLAGS
Look for ocular inflammation and inflammation of the respiratory tract

DIFFERENTIAL DIAGNOSIS
(a) Relapsing polychondritis; (b) Wegener's granulomatosis: saddle-nose deformity; (c) Syphilis; (d) Associated with another autoimmune disease: SLE; RA; Sjogren's syndrome; Behcet's (MAGIC – mucosal and genital ulceration with inflamed

cartilage); SSc; MCTD and overlap; Seronegatives (PsA, AS, ReA, IBD); (e) Thyroid; (f) Myelodysplastic syndrome; (g) Malignancy

PHYSICAL EXAMINATION

Vitals: Pulse: Normal; BP: Normal; RR: Elevations in RR may be an indicator of cardiac involvement, listen for stridor and wheezing; T: May have associated fever

Cutaneous: Vasculitic lesions on the finger tips; Livedo reticularis; Other skin rashes

Head & Neck: Alopecia; Auricular inflammation & cauliflower ear; Nasal inflammation and saddle nose; Ocular inflammation; Thyroid enlargement; Cranial nerve palsies

Respiratory: Wheezing and stridor; Hoarseness of the voice

Cardiovascular: Aortic or Mitral regurgitation; Pericardial friction rub with pericarditis

Gastrointestinal: Bruits if aortic involvement

Musculoskeletal: Inflammatory polyarthritis

Neurologic: Cranial neuropathies; Evidence of hearing loss

INVESTIGATIONS

CBC: Anemia of chronic disease, leukocytosis, and thrombocytosis. May also see a macrocytic anemia due to underlying myelodysplasia.

ESR: Elevated

Hypergammaglobulinemia

Rheumatoid Factor: Present in 20%

ANA: Present in 15 – 25%

ANCA: Has been reported in 25%

Radiology: A non-erosive, non-deforming polyarthritis with soft-tissue swelling

PFT's: Should be done in all patients to look for obstructive picture

CT Chest: To identify tracheobronchal narrowing or stricture

Echocardiogram: Routine test to look for cardiac involvement

MANAGEMENT

General: Education; Physiotherapy to improve ROM and functional abilities

Limited Disease: This includes active disease which does not compromise organ function such as auricular inflammation, nasal inflammation, and arthritis; (a) NSAIDs may be adequate; If NSAIDs fail, (b) Dapsone at doses of 50-100 mg PO OD may be used and titrated slowly (25 mg increments) to a maximum dose of 200 mg. Be aware of side effects of dapsone; (c) Corticosteroids are also useful with doses of 30-60 mg of prednisone per day in divided doses;

Organ Threatening Disease: Prednisone 60-100 mg in divided doses and slowly taper; 2nd Line agents for 3 reasons: (a) Significant organ-threatening disease; (b) Incomplete response to corticosteroids; (c) Unsatisfactory high-dose maintenance prednisone; 2nd Line agents include: Oral cyclophosphamide starting at 1-2 mg/kg and increasing to control disease activity and is the most common choice for significant organ-threatening disease. Continued for 6 months and then switched to azathioprine. Azathioprine at doses of 1-2 mg/kg. Methotrexate; Cyclosporine; IV Pulse Methylpred. – Used successfully for acute airway obstruction

Surgical: Sometimes required for acute airway obstruction

PROGNOSIS

Risk Stratification for Poor Progression: (a) Cardiac involvement is the 2nd most common cause of death; (b) Airway obstruction is a cause of death in 10% of cases and airway obstruction with infection in 28%; (c) Coexistent vasculitis; (d) Early saddle-nose deformity in a younger patient; (e) Anemia in an older patient (MDS)

Prognosis: The leading cause of death is infection due to airway obstruction and the use of immunosuppressive medication; Other causes of death include vasculitis; The survival rates are 74% at 5 years and 55% at 10 years

RHEUMATOID ARTHRITIS (RA)

DEFINITION & PATHOPHYSIOLOGY

Definition: Rheumatoid arthritis is a systemic inflammatory disease that predominantly manifests in the synovial membrane of diarthrodial joints; See the Classification Criteria for Rheumatoid Arthritis 245

Pathophysiology: The most widely accepted hypothesis is the disease is triggered in a genetically susceptible individual by an unknown antigen; The initial stages consist of T-cell infiltration into the synovial membrane. The T-cells are activated by an unknown antigen and subsequent clonal expansion ensues. The early inflammatory response results in recruitment of other cells to the synovium which is facilitated by upregulation of adhesion molecules and proliferation of new blood vessels. T-cells activate macrophages to secrete pro-inflammatory cytokines (TNF, IL-1, IFN). Tumor Necrosis Factor has the following actions: Activates neutrophils, macrophages, and synovial fibroblasts; Stimulates other cytokine production (IL-1), IL-6, GM-CSF etc; Upregulates adhesion molecules; Promotes the proliferation of synoviocytes and fibroblasts; Activates and induces differentiation of osteoclasts; Stimulates the release of matrix metalloproteinases (MMPs) resulting in proteolysis and tissue destruction. T-cells activate B-cells to produce rheumatoid factor. The natural anti-inflammatory and regulatory mechanisms are overwhelmed resulting in a runaway inflammatory process leading to the destruction of cartilage and bone

PRESENTATION

Identifying Data: Peak incidence between 30-50 years old (can occur at any age); Prevalence of 1% in general population; Female: Male = 2.5:1

Onset: Usually an insidious onset (70%) of joint pain and swelling in an oligoarticular pattern evolving to a polyarthritis; Occasionally can see a subacute presentation (20%), an acute presentation (10%), or a preceding palindromic presentation; Morning stiffness > 60 minutes, gelling phenomenon, decreased energy and poor sleep, occasionally appetite loss and weight loss although rare;

Progression: As the disease progresses more joints become continuously involved leading to the symmetrical polyarthritis. With continued inflammation damage to joints may result with the initial findings of erosions of plain radiographs. Almost 90% of the joints ultimately affected in a given patient are involved during the first year of disease. By 4 months of symptoms, 50% of patients will have erosions on MRI. By 3 years, 70-90% of patients demonstrate erosions on X-ray

Constitutional Features: Malaise, anorexia, and weight loss

Functional Status: Reduced functional status and difficulties with ADLs, Loss of employment

RHEUMATOLOGIC REVIEW OF SYSTEMS

Associated Conditions: Amyloidosis (rare)

Mucocutaneous Involvement: Rheumatoid nodules: Commonly found on pressure points along extensor surfaces; May become worse with methotrexate therapy; Secondary Sjogren's syndrome: Keratoconjuctivitis sicca; Raynaud's phenomenon

Hematologic Involvement: Anemia: Due to poor absorption, marrow suppression, GI loss secondary to NSAIDs; Felty's syndrome (RA, neutropenia, & splenomegaly): Seen in long-standing RA patients who are RF +ve, have subcutaneous nodules, and other extra-articular manifestations. The major complications include bacterial infections and chronic non-healing leg ulcers.

Ocular Involvement: Inflammation: Episcleritis, scleritis, & conjuctivitis; Corneal melt

Neurologic Involvement: C-spine instability with radiculopathy / myelopathy; Entrapment neuropathies; Peripheral neuropathy; Mononeuritis multiplex

Cardiac Involvement: Pericardial effusions; Valvular nodules

Respiratory Involvement: Cricoaretynoid inflammation – pain & dysphonia; Pulm. fibrosis; Pulmonary nodules; Bronchiolitis obliterans; Pleural inflammation

RISK FACTORS

(a) HLA DRB1 0401, 0404, & 0408 / HLA DRB1 0405 (Asian population). A genetic epitope which encodes for MHC structures codes for certain amino acids at the positions 67-74. Positively charged amino acids at positions 70, 71, and 74 related to the disease; (b) Smoking; (c) Age (increased risk within first 6 decades of life)

FAMILY HISTORY

15-30% concordance rate in monozygotic twins; RA does not frequently aggregate in families but familial cases are well reported

RED FLAGS

Cervical spine involvement

DIFFERENTIAL DIAGNOSIS

(a) Infection: Bacterial, viral; (b) Crystalline arthropathy: Polyarticular gout, CPPD; (c) Seronegative spondyloarthropathy: Psoriatic, reactive, IBD; (d) Connective tissue diseases: SLE, MCTD, vasculitis; (e) Inflammatory osteoarthritis; (f) Fibromyalgia

PHYSICAL EXAMINATION

Vitals: P: Usually normal (may see tachycardia with severe disease); BP: Usually normal; RR: May be an indicator of pulmonary/cardiac involvement; T: Normal

Cutaneous: Palmer erythema; Rheumatoid nodules on extensor surfaces of the hands, forearms

Head & Neck: Ocular involvement with scleritis, episcleritis, and conjuctivitis; Sicca features; C-spine instability

Respiratory: Crackles secondary to interstitial fibrosis; Diminished breath sounds and dullness on percussion due to pleural effusion; Pleural friction rub

Cardiovascular: Pericardial friction rub; Heart murmurs

Gastrointestinal: Splenomegaly if Felty's syndrome

Musculoskeletal: Sparing of the DIPs; PIPS – Fusiform swelling, pain, tenderness to palpate, flexion deformities, swan-neck deformities, boutonniere deformities, ligamentous instability, rheumatoid nodules; MCPs – Swelling, pain, tenderness to palpate, flexion deformities, ulnar drift, and subluxation; Thumbs - Z deformity; Wrists - Dorsal swelling, pain, tenderness, radial deviation, volar subluxation, carpal tunnel syndrome, and interosseus wasting; Flexor tendon thickening with nodules and trigger finger; Elbow and shoulder involvement; Knee and hip involvement; Foot - Hindfoot valgus deformity with forefoot varus deformity and forefoot abduction (pronated); MTP - Inflammation with loss visibility of the extensor tendons and splayed toes lifted off the ground. Subluxation of MTPs with distal migration of the fat pad and callous formation.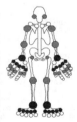

Neurologic: Neuropathy – Polyneuropathy or mononeuritis multiplex; Upper motor neuron signs with cervical spine involvement causing spinal cord compromise

INVESTIGATIONS

CBC: Anemia of chronic inflammation, anemia secondary to blood loss (NSAIDs), anemia secondary to bone marrow suppression, leukopenia with Felty's or secondary to medications, thrombocytosis with inflammation or thrombocytopenia secondary to Felty's or medications

ESR/CRP: Elevated
Rheumatoid Factor: Present in 70-85% of established cases
ANA: Present in 25% of patients
Plain Radiographs: *(a) Soft Tissue:* Periarticular swelling & evidence of joint effusions; ***(b) Alignment:*** Damage to joints results in malalignment: PIPs - Contractures, swan neck deformities, boutonniere deformities; MCPs - Subluxation and ulnar deviation; Thumbs - Z deformity; Wrists - Radial deviation and volar subluxation; C-Spine: A-A instability (vertical, horizontal, and lateral); MTPS: Subluxation, angulation deformities; ***(c) Bones:*** Periarticular osteopenia, periarticular cysts if rheumatoid robustus; ***(d) Joints:*** Uniform joint space narrowing and marginal erosions; Earliest Erosions: Second and third metacarpal heads; Ulnar styloid; Medial aspect of first metacarpal head
Synovial Fluid: Inflammatory cellular picture 5000 – 15,000 cells/mm3
Synovial Biopsy: (a) Hyperplasia of the synovial lining layer: Becomes 6-10 cells thick (normal 1-3); Cells hypertrophy; (b) Cellular infiltrate: Predominantly CD4 T-cells & macrophages; Also see B-cells, dendritic cells, PMNs, and activated fibroblasts; (c) Synovial neovascularization
Rheumatoid Nodule: Central area of fibrinoid necrosis; Surrounded by a layer of palisading histiocytes; Surrounded by a final layer of mononuclear cells

MANAGEMENT

Prior to Treatment: Prior to initiating therapy there are 4 (four) issues to consider: (a) Baseline disease activity and damage; (b) Prognostic factors; (c) Treatments (if any) have been used in the past; (d) Contra-indications to medications
Baseline Disease Activity & Impact: It is crucial to assess patients' disease activity and impact of the disease on their lives. This begins with features on **History** such as: (a) Duration of time with arthritis (early or long-standing); (b) Duration of morning stiffness; (c) Degree of pain; (d) Constitutional features such as energy loss, sleep disturbance, and weight loss; (e) Description of flares (duration & severity) and periods of quiescence; (f) Impact on activities of daily living (HAQ). The **Physical Examination** is then used to document: (a) number of swollen and tender joints; (b) damaged joints; (c) extra-articular features; (d) other co-morbidities. The **Laboratory** is used to document: (a) Evidence of inflammation (anemia, reactive thrombocytosis, elevated ESR/CRP); (b) Presence of a Rheumatoid Factor; (c) Other co-morbidities (liver function, renal function, hepatitis status); (d) Radiographic assessment of involved joints looking for sub-clinical damage.
Disease Classification and Prognostic Factors: Once the baseline disease activity and impact are established it becomes easier to classify the severity of the disease and prognosticate. RA can be classified as mild, moderate, or severe based on the ACR criteria. ***(a) Mild Disease:*** Less than 5 swollen joints, no extra-articular disease, RF –ve, no erosions; ***(b) Moderate Disease:*** 6-15 swollen joints, no extra-articular disease, RF +ve, no erosions; ***(c) Severe Disease:*** > 15 swollen joints, Reduced functional capacity, anemia, hypoalbuminemia, RF +ve, extra-articular disease, and erosions on radiographs.
General: It is essential to begin with education and other non-pharmacologic therapies as they for the support on which all other therapies are built.
Education: To understand the disease and the nature of the treatments
Physiotherapy: Pain relieving strategies and interventions, Mobility aids; Exercise to improve ROM, muscle strength, aerobic conditioning, and core stability training, Weight loss, Manual therapy (manipulation) when appropriate

Occupational Therapy: Splints and orthotics, Joint protection measures and energy conservation, Assistive devices, Lifestyle management

NSAIDs and COXIBs: Have analgesic and anti-inflammatory properties but do not alter the course of the disease or prevent joint destruction; Should not be used alone for the treatment of RA

DMARDs: All patients are candidates for DMARD therapy which have the potential to: (a) Reduce or prevent joint damage; (b) Preserve joint integrity and function; (c) Reduce health care costs; (d) Maintain economic productivity of the patient. Initial DMARD choice: What is the patient's severity of disease? ***(a) Mild:*** Hydroxychloroquine: Does not slow radiographic damage alone, early treatment has a significant impact on long-term function; Sulfasalazine: May act more quickly than hydroxychloroquine, has been shown to retard radiographic progression; ***(b) Moderate:*** Methotrexate: Standard of care due to its efficacy, low toxicity, low cost, and established track record. Patients are more likely to stay on MTX (50% at 3 years) and if they do discontinue it is usually due to adverse effects. Usual dose 15-15 mg per week; Sulfasalazine; Leflunomide: Similar efficacy to moderate doses of methotrexate; Gold; ***(c) Severe:*** Methotrexate; Leflunomide; ***Disease not controlled by initial DMARD (3-6 months):*** The options are as follows: (a) Maximize the dose of monotherapy; (b) Combination therapy: Combinations shown to be effective are: Methotrexate, Sulfasalazine, & Hydroxychloroquine; Methotrexate & Leflunomide; Methotrexate & Cyclosporine (rarely used); Methotrexate & Gold

Corticosteroids: Low dose corticosteroids (5 - 10 mg/day) are highly effective in controlling symptoms in patients with active RA; Recent evidence shows steroids to slow the rate of joint damage and therefore may have a disease modifying effect; The benefits of low-dose steroids should always be balanced against the risks; Options for Corticosteroid use include: Intra-articular corticosteroid injections into the most symptomatic joints; Intra-muscular injection of 80-120 mg depo-medrol: Has the benefit of lasting 2-3 weeks and can be used nicely as bridge therapy while waiting for a DMARD to work.

Biologics: When to Consider Biologic Therapy: In all patients with rheumatoid arthritis; Disease not controlled after trials of two (2) DMARDs; ***Adalimumab, Etanercept, & Infliximab:*** Effective in patients with early RA and those with active RA who have failed previous DMARD therapy. Effects include: Reduction in signs and symptoms; Reduction in disability; Reduction in radiographic progression; Seem to be more efficacious when used in combination with methotrexate; Anakinra: Does not appear to be as symptom controlling as TNF antagonists; Fair prevention of radiographic progression (35% reduction)

PROGNOSIS

Risk Stratification for Poor Prognosis: (a) High burden of inflammation (>15 swollen joints); (b) Reduced functional capacity (HAQ>1.0); (c) Persistently elevated ESR; (d) Rheumatoid factor positive; (e) Low education (< grade 11); (f) Presence of erosions on radiographs; (g) Presence of HLA DRB1 0401, 0404; (h) Smoker; (i) Extra-articular disease

Prognosis: Two general categories: 5-20% have intermittent disease with periods of exacerbation and a relatively good prognosis; 80-85% have progressive disease with either a slow or rapid course: 50% of patients will be functional class 3 or 4 within 10 yrs; 30% of patients will be unemployed at 5 yrs; Higher incidence of infections, cardiovascular disease, and lymphoma

SARCOIDOSIS

DEFINITION & PATHOPHYSIOLOGY

Definition: A multi-system granulomatous disorder characterized by the presence of non-caseating granulomas in involved organs.

Pathophysiology: The pathologic hallmark of sarcoidosis is the presence of T-lymphocytes, mono-nuclear phagocytes and non-caseating granulomas in the involved organs. Immunohistochemical staining reveals a predominance of CD-4 T-lymphocytes within the sarcoid granuloma. The exact pathophysiology of sarcoidosis is still unknown. The current theory is an unknown antigen (environmental trigger) stimulates the disease in a genetically susceptible host.

PRESENTATION

Identifying Data: Typically affects younger individuals with the onset between the ages of 10-40 in 70-90% of patients; It is more common in individuals of African-American descent being 3 to 4 times more common than in Caucasians; Affects women slightly more often than men

Onset: In 50% of cases the bilateral hilar adenopathy is found incidentally on a routine chest x-ray. Otherwise the lung is the most frequently involved organ with patients presenting with a cough, chest pain, or dyspnea. Sarcoid granuloma can affect any organ and therefore there is a vast array of initial presentations of sarcoidosis. Some of the more common musculoskeletal presentations include: *(a) Arthralgia:* The most common musculoskeletal manifestation of sarcoidosis which can be seen in up to 70% of patients with sarcoidosis; *(b) Acute Polyarthritis:* Usually presents as a non-migratory polyarthritis that has a predilection for joints of the lower extremity and can be confused with reactive arthritis; May present in isolation or as part of the triad of Lofgren's syndrome (arthritis, erythema nodosum, and hilar adenopathy); Associated periarticular swelling (periarthritis) may be dramatic; Erythema nodosum can be present in up to 75% of cases and hilar adenopathy is present in over 90%; The arthritis can occasionally present in an additive fashion resembling rheumatoid arthritis or it may present with a palindromic onset; *(c) Chronic Arthritis:* More often associated with a slower-onset more chronic form of sarcoidosis frequently associated with parenchymal lung disease and elevated ACE levels; It is most commonly a non-destructive mono or oligoarthritis involving the ankles, knees, and PIPs most commonly. Symmetric polyarthritis (like RA) has been described but it is rare; Dactylitic, tenosynovitic, or enthesitic manifestations may be associated with the presentation

Progression: The acute polyarthritis associated with sarcoidosis tends to be benign and self-limited (average 3 months) especially when the ACE level is not elevated at presentation. However, about 1/3 of patients will progress to have a more persistent arthritis.

Constitutional Features: The presentation with acute polyarthritis may be accompanied by fevers, chills, and general malaise. Fatigue may be prominent

Functional Status: Functional status is often severely impaired in the setting of acute polyarthritis, however, most patients follow a benign self-limited course and tend to recover completely; Otherwise functional status may be severely impaired with involvement of other organ systems

RHEUMATOLOGIC REVIEW OF SYSTEMS

Musculoskeletal Involvement: *(a) Joint Involvement:* Arthralgia; Acute Polyarthritis; Chronic Arthritis; *(b) Muscle Involvement:* Muscle biopsy reveals granulomas in up to 80% of individuals, however less than 5% will become symptomatic. Presentations for muscle involvement with sarcoidosis include:

Chronic Myopathy: Evolves over years resulting in symmetric proximal muscle weakness with wasting; Muscle enzymes are not usually elevated; Acute Myositis: Exceedingly rare; Symmetric proximal muscle weakness and elevated muscle enzymes similar to that seen with inflammatory myositis; Nodular Myositis: Single or multiple palpable granulomatous nodules. In one case a large palpable mass was present resembling a tumor; *(c) Bone Involvement:* Results from granulomatous invasion of bone; Radiographically, the lesions are usually cystic lesions but sclerotic lesions may occur (usually in the spine or pelvis). Lesions can involve the cortex and trabeculae resulting in a reticular or "lace-like" appearance on radiographs. Lesions have a predilection for the distal ends of the proximal and middle phalanges and tend to be bilateral; Commonly associated with chronic skin lesions

Mucocutaneous Involvement: (a) Erythema nodosum: The most common dermatologic abnormality; Sarcoid granulomas are usually not found on biopsy; Associated with surrounding arthritis; *(b) Lupus pernio:* Reflects "chronic" sarcoidosis; Violaceous indurated plaques on the ears, nose, cheeks, and lips which are non-painful and non-pruritic; May be associated with hypo/hyperpigmentation, alopecia, subcutaneous nodules, and maculopapular eruptions; Commonly associated with bone cysts and pulmonary fibrosis

Lymphatic & Glandular Involvement: Lymphadenopathy in up to 1/3 of patients; Unilateral or bilateral parotitis with swollen, painful, and enlarged glands; Heerfordt's syndrome - Fever, parotid enlargement, facial palsy, and uveitis

Vascular Involvement: Rare reports of vasculitic involvement in large, medium, and small sized vessels; Large vessel vasculitis resembles Takayasu Arteritis

Hematologic Involvement: Anemia in up to 20% of patients; Leukopenia which is usually mild and reflects either bone marrow involvement or redistribution of T-cells to sites of disease activity

Ocular Involvement: Anterior Uveitis: Most common ocular manifestation with blurred vision, photophobia, and excessive lacrimation. Frequently bilateral. Posterior Uveitis; Interstitial Keratitis; Keratoconjuctivitis; Lacrimal gland enlargement; Scleral plaques

Neurologic & Psychiatric Involvement: Neurosarcoidosis: Predilection for the base of the brain (basilar meningitis); Cranial neuropathies; Neuroendocrine dysfunction - central diabetes insipidus; Cognitive dysfunction; Seizures

Cardiac Involvement: Conduction disturbances; Papillary muscle dysfunction; Cardiomyopathy with CHF; Pericarditis

Respiratory Involvement: Five Radiographic Stages of Sarcoidosis as Follows: Stage 0: Normal; Stage 1: Bilateral hilar adenopathy; Stage 2: Bilateral hilar adenopathy plus pulmonary infiltrates; Stage 3: Pulmonary infiltrates alone; Stage 4: Pulmonary Fibrosis; Granulomatous endobronchial involvement of the airways may lead to stenosis, however, this is rare.

Gastrointestinal Involvement: Rare - Sarcoid lesions found in stomach; Hepatic Involvement: Granulomatous infiltration seen in up to 85%, however, only 20% will have clinical hepatomegaly or elevated liver enzymes; Splenomegaly

Renal Involvement: Hypercalciuria; Nephrolithiasis; Rare cases of granulomatous interstitial nephritis

Genitourinary Involvement: Ureteral obstruction from retroperitoneal lymph node involvement, retroperitoneal fibrosis, or ureteral involvement; Granulomas can be found in breast tissue, uterus, or testes

Endocrine Involvement: Hypercalcemia due to increased production of 1,25-(OH)2-VitaminD3 by activated macrophages and granulomas; Rarer endocrine abnormalities include hyper or hypothyroidism, adrenal suppression, or pituitary/hypothalamic involvement

RISK FACTORS
No known risk factors

FAMILY HISTORY
No association

RED FLAGS
None

DIFFERENTIAL DIAGNOSIS
Causes of Elevated ACE Levels include: (a) Sarcoidosis; (b) Hyperthyroidism; (c) Gaucher's disease; (d) Diabetes mellitus; (e) Leprosy; (f) Alpha-1 Anti-trypsin deficiency; (g) Other infections including miliary tuberculosis and histoplasmosis; (h) HIV infection; (i) Silicosis

Differential Diagnosis of Acute Arthritis with Erythema Nodosum: (a) Sarcoidosis; (b) Inflammatory bowel disease; (c) Histoplasmosis; (d) Coccidioidomycosis; (e) Psittacosis; (f) Hypersensitivity reaction to medications; (g) Behcet's disease

PHYSICAL EXAMINATION
Vitals: Pulse: May be elevated with respiratory or cardiac involvement; BP: Usually normal; RR: May be elevated with respiratory or cardiac involvement; Temp: May be slightly elevated

Cutaneous: Erythema nodosum; Lupus pernio

Head & Neck: Ocular involvement with glandular enlargement, conjunctivitis, photophobia, and excessive tearing; Tender, swollen parotid glands (can have associated facial nerve palsy); Cervical lymphadenopathy

Respiratory: Axillary adenopathy; May range from minimal findings to diffuse crackles secondary to interstitial involvement

Cardiovascular: Arrhythmias; Signs suggestive of congestive heart failure

Gastrointestinal: Hepatomegaly; Splenomegaly

Musculoskeletal: Arthralgia; Inflammatory oligoarthritis with a predilection for joints of the lower extremity; Proximal muscle weakness

Neurologic: Cranial neuropathies; Cognitive dysfunction; Peripheral neuropathy

INVESTIGATIONS
CBC: Anemia secondary to chronic inflammation, mild lymphopenia, mild eosinophilia. Otherwise, WBC & platelets usually normal except if significant bone marrow involvement.

Liver Enzymes: Elevated in 1/3 of patients with ALP and GGT more often elevated than ALT or AST.

Creatinine: Most common cause of elevation is pre-renal azotemia as a result of hypercalcemia, otherwise intra-renal (granulomatous interstitial nephritis) or post-renal (ureteral obstruction) may be the cause.

ESR: May be elevated during active disease

CRP: May be elevated during active disease

Serum Calcium: May be elevated

Urinary Calcium: Urinary calcium excretion may be elevated in the absence of hypercalcemia.

1,25 (OH)2 - Vitamin D3: Produced by macrophages and may be elevated

Hypergammaglobulinemia: Seen in active disease

Rheumatoid Factor: Can be seen in low titer in up to 40% of patients

ANA: A low titer, speckled pattern can be seen in up to 35% of patients

Angiotensin Converting Enzyme (ACE): This enzyme is produced by epithelioid cells and macrophages at the periphery of a granuloma in response to factors released by T-lymphocytes. Elevated in 40-90% of patients with sarcoidosis.

Other Screening Baseline Investigations for Sarcoidosis include: Two step tuberculin skin test; Ophthalmologic examination to rule out asymptomatic; abnormalities; Electrocardiogram

Chest X-Ray: Chest X-rays are abnormal in 90-95% of patients; Five Radiographic Stages of Sarcoidosis as follows: Stage 0: Normal; Stage 1: Bilateral hilar adenopathy; Stage 2: Bilateral hilar adenopathy plus pulmonary infiltrates; Stage 3: Pulmonary infiltrates alone; Stage 4: Pulmonary Fibrosis; HRCT scans are more sensitive that plain radiographs

Pulmonary Function Testing: Can range from normal to a restrictive pattern with preservation of flow rates and reduced diffusing capacity (DLCO)

Gallium-67 Citrate Scanning: Can reveal characteristic patterns of uptake including: The Panda sign - Produced by parotid and lacrimal uptake; The Lambda sign - Produced by paratracheal and bilateral hilar lymph nodes

Plain Radiographs: Osseous sarcoidosis may be seen as cystic lesions, a fine lattice, and diffuse osteoporosis on plain radiographs. Hand radiographs detect lesions at the heads of the proximal or middle phalanges. Osteopenia and osteoporosis can be seen due to dysregulation of calcium metabolism

Bone Scintigraphy: May be useful for evaluating osseous involvement with sarcoidosis

Biopsy: Tissue biopsy showing a non-caseating granuloma is the gold standard to confirm the diagnosis. Caseous necrosis is the destruction of cells which are converted to amorphous greyish debris located centrally in the granuloma. The center of the granuloma consists of a collection of epithelioid cells and giant-cells. Epithelioid cells are derived from macrophages. As macrophages mature to epithelioid cells they gain secretory and bactericidal activities but lose some phagocytic capability. Giant-cells are a conglomeration of epithelioid cells which share the same cytoplasm and have multiple nuclei. Cells where the nuclei are randomly arranged are called foreign body giant-cells whereas cells where the nuclei are located in the periphery are referred to as Langerhans giant-cells. The central collection of epithelioid and giant-cells is surrounded by a rim of T-lymphocytes - mainly CD4 - T-helper cells.

MANAGEMENT

General: Education; Physiotherapy; Occupational Therapy

Treatment of Arthritis: NSAIDs may be all that is necessary to treat the acute arthritis since it is often self limiting. Colchicine may be an alternative option. Low-dose corticosteroids may be useful for patients who fail NSAIDs. For more chronic arthritis, low-dose Corticosteroids or DMARDs (methotrexate, chloroquine, hydroxychloroquine, and azathioprine) have also been reported to be of benefit

Treatment of Bone Involvement: Unfortunately, bone involvement does not respond well to therapy; *Corticosteroids:* May improve swelling and pain but have no effect on the course; *DMARDs:* Methotrexate, hydroxychloroquine, and chloroquine have all been used anecdotally with variable success; *Bisphosphonates:* Useful to treat and prevent osteoporosis

Treatment of Muscle Involvement: Corticosteroids: Can be tried for symptomatic patients with acute sarcoid myositis using doses of 0.5 - 1 mg/kg/day are often used initially to control the disease followed by slow tapering. Chronic myopathy and mass lesions do not respond well to treatment

Treatment of Pulmonary Involvement: As pulmonary disease can remit spontaneously, it is recommended to initiate treatment with Corticosteroids under the following circumstances: (a) Patients with worsening pulmonary symptoms: cough, shortness of breath, hemoptysis; (b) Patients with deteriorating lung function; (c) Patients with progressive radiographic changes: Steroid sparing agents should be used in the following circumstances: (a) Patients unwilling to take corticosteroids; (b) Intolerable side effects to corticosteroids; (c) Progression of the disease despite adequate corticosteroid therapy; (d) Inability to taper patients to a maintenance dose of <15 mg/day of corticosteroids; ***Corticosteroids:*** Typically initiated at doses of 0.5-1 mg/kg/day for 4-6 weeks until disease is under control. If the patient is stable/ improved after 4-6 weeks the steroids can be tapered by 5-10 mg decrements every 4-8 weeks down to 15-30 mg/day. If the patient continues to be stable the dose can continued to be tapered until a maintenance dose is reached. If the disease reactivates while tapering, the corticosteroid dose should be increased to the last effective dose and held for 3-6 months. High-dose oral corticosteroids may be needed for patients with severe extra-pulmonary symptoms; ***Steroid Sparing Agents:*** The use of methotrexate, chloroquine, azathioprine, cyclophosphamide, chlorambucil, and cyclosporine in sarcoidosis is limited to small, uncontrolled trials and case reports.

PROGNOSIS

Risk Stratification for Poor Progression: In general, the more severe the disease and the more organ systems involved at presentation the worse the prognosis; (a) Stage 3 & 4 pulmonary involvement; (b) Cardiac involvement; (c) Neurologic involvement; (d) Cutaneous sarcoidosis; (e) Black race; (f) Onset > 40 years of age; (g) Symptoms present > 6 months

Prognosis: Patients presenting with Lofgren's syndrome have the best prognosis for full remission within 2 years. Isolated hilar adenopathy also has an excellent prognosis with 80% remitting spontaneously. Spontaneous Remission in 60% of patients with stage 2 radiographic disease and 30% with stage 3 disease. Chronic course in 10-30% of patients

SJOGREN'S SYNDROME (SS)

DEFINITION & PATHOPHYSIOLOGY

Definition: An autoimmune disorder characterized by ocular and oral dryness with glandular enlargement associated with polyarthritis. Please see the criteria for the classification of Sjogren's syndrome 247

Pathophysiology: An environmental agent triggers the condition in a genetically susceptible host (viral and hormonal factors theorized); Infiltration of CD4+ T helper cells in the periductal regions of exocrine tissues; B-cells become activated and produce increased quantities of autoantibody which are reactive towards IgG (RF), anti-Ro, and anti-La. B-cells also produce antibodies to the muscarinic M3 receptor which affect the neuromuscular junction akin to myasthenia gravis.

PRESENTATION

Identifying Data: Typical patient is a young female (30-50); Male: female ratio of about 1:9; Prevalence about 0.5-5% in the population

Onset: Patients typically present with one of the following: **Keratoconjunctivitis sicca or xerophthalmia:** These patients experience dry, gritty, painful eyes which usually worsen as the day progresses due to loss of moisture. Patients may be using artificial tear substitutes multiple times per day. **Xerostomia:** These patients may experience symptoms such as: (a) a sensation of decreased saliva with difficulty swallowing dry foods (bread) necessitating the use of water with meals (b) a burning sensation in the mouth with altered taste sensation (c) difficulty speaking (d) enlargement of the parotid gland, (e) gastroesophageal reflux, (f) sleep difficulty (dry mouth), (g) oral candidiasis & halitosis; **Vaginal dryness:** May be manifest as dyspareunia; **Dry skin**

Progression: As the disease progresses, symptoms of ocular and oral dryness typically worsen

Constitutional Features: Prominent fatigue

Functional Status: Reduced functional status and difficulties with ADLs if secondary Sjogren's or if associated with polyarthritis

RHEUMATOLOGIC REVIEW OF SYSTEMS

Musculoskeletal Involvement: Arthralgias and myalgias seen in up to 70% of patients; A rheumatoid-like non-erosive, non-deforming polyarthritis is occasionally seen; Inflammatory myositis

Lymphatic Involvement: Lymphadenopathy

Vascular Involvement: Raynaud's Phenomenon: Present in 20% of patients with Sjogren's syndrome at presentation and in 40% overall; Vasculitis: Palpable and non-palpable purpura on the lower extremities revealing a leukocytoclastic vasculitis. This is secondary to immune complex deposition.

Hematologic Involvement: There is a 44-fold greater risk of developing a B-cell lymphoma. About 5-8% of patients with SS will develop this. The earliest manifestation may be a monoclonal gammopathy.

Neurologic Involvement: Neuropathy: Sensorimotor glove and stocking symmetrical neuropathy in 10%. Cranial nerve neuropathies and autonomic neuropathies have been observed. CNS: Can range from discrete lesions on MRI to dementia and multiple sclerosis like symptoms

Respiratory Involvement: Chronic cough due to upper airway dryness; may be associated with reactive airway disease; Interstitial fibrosis may occur but is generally mild and seen in only 10% of cases

Gastrointestinal Involvement: Dysphagia due to dryness or esophageal dysmotility, like in scleroderma, can occur

Renal Involvement: Mild proteinuria and tubular dysfunction may result in RTA-1; Rare, but described, cases of glomerulonephritis

Endocrine Involvement: Hypothyroidism is common in primary SS

RISK FACTORS

Risk factors for reduced salivary gland function: (a) Medications (anticholinergics, anti-depressants, neuroleptics); (b) Viral infections (HIV (DILS), hepatitis C); (c) Malignancy (lymphoma); (d) Prior radiation therapy to the head and neck; (e) Trauma or surgery to the head and neck; (f) Presence of another systemic disease (sarcoidosis, RA, SLE)

FAMILY HISTORY

There is an increased risk of SS among family members

RED FLAGS

Think about malignancy and infectious etiologies

DIFFERENTIAL DIAGNOSIS

Differential Diagnosis of Decreased Salivary Secretion: (a) Primary Sjogren's syndrome; (b) Secondary Sjogren's syndrome: RA, SLE, and sarcoidosis; (c) Medications; (d) Infections: Hepatitis C, HIV (DILS), mumps; (e) Prior radiation or surgery to the head and neck; (f) Malignancy: Lymphoma

Differential Diagnosis of Bilateral Parotid Gland Enlargement: (a) Sjogren's syndrome; (b) Infection (bacterial, viral (mumps), HIV (DILS)); (c) Granulomatous disease (sarcoidosis); (d) Chronic alcohol abuse; (e) Others (cirrhosis, chronic pancreatitis, anorexia, diabetes mellitus, gonadal hypofunction, hyperlipoproteinemia)

PHYSICAL EXAMINATION

Vitals: Pulse: Normal; BP: Normal; RR: Elevations in RR may be an indicator of pulmonary involvement

Cutaneous: Raynaud's phenomenon; Dry skin; Vasculitic lesions; Livedo reticularis; Palpable purpura

Head & Neck: Alopecia; Ocular dryness – Lack of conjuctival pool, redness; Oral dryness – lack of salivary pooling, mucosal atrophy, mechanical irritation to the buccal mucosa due to dryness, poor dentition, halitosis, candidiasis; Parotid gland enlargement; Lymphadenopathy

Respiratory: Crackles secondary to interstitial fibrosis; Coughing

Cardiovascular: No specific findings

Gastrointestinal: No specific findings

Musculoskeletal: Inflammatory polyarthritis

Neurologic: Proximal myopathy secondary to inflammatory myositis; Cranial nerve palsies; Stocking paresthesia – peripheral neuropathy

INVESTIGATIONS

CBC: Anemia of chronic disease and leukopenia; thrombocytopenia is rare

SPEP: Polyclonal hypergammaglobulinemia

ESR: Usually elevated

Rheumatoid Factor (RF): Positive in 90% of cases

ANA: Positive in 80 - 90% of cases

Anti-Ro (SSA) Ab: Present in 70 - 90% of cases

Anti-La (SSB) Ab: Present in 40 - 50% of cases

Schirmer Test: Place a piece of filter paper under the inferior eyelid and measure the wetting of the paper over time. Wetting of < 5mm in 5 minutes is a strong indicator of reduced tear production. This test is not reliable in those >60 years of age.

Rose Bengal Staining: Taken up by damaged epithelium of the cornea and conjuctiva documenting the severity of dryness

Lashley cups: Measure the amount of oral saliva produced in 15 minutes (<1.5 mL) or 0.5 mL in 5 minutes

Parotid Sialography: Presence of diffuse sialectasias without evidence of obstruction of the major ducts

Salivary Scintigraphy: Measure the uptake of technetium-99 pertechnate during a 60 minute period showing delayed uptake, reduced concentration, or delayed excretion

Minor Salivary Gland Biopsy: Incisional biopsy through the lower labial mucosa containing 5-10 minor glands is adequate. Look for the # of lymphocytes found in 4 square mm of tissue (focus). If > 50 lymphocytes (focus) considered positive.

MANAGEMENT

General: Education about the disease; Vocational counseling; Arthritis self management programs

Physiotherapy: Pain relieving strategies and interventions; Mobility aids (canes & walkers) and braces; Exercise to improve ROM, muscle strength, aerobic conditioning, and core stability training; Weight loss; Manual therapy (manipulation) when appropriate

Occupational Therapy: Splints and orthotics; Joint protection measures and energy conservation; Assistive devices; Lifestyle management

Treatment of Xerophthalmia: (a) Tear substitutes: Preservative-free preparations; More concentrated hydroxypropylcellulose pellets inserted under the lower eyelids; Ointments may be used at night; (b) Glasses with shields; (c) Punctal occlusion: Collagen plugs initially (last for 2 days), if helpful permanent silicone plugs may be inserted; (d) Systemic Pilocarpine

Treatment of Xerostomia: Good oral hygiene & regular dental visits; Use of fluorinated toothpaste & regular use of anti-microbial mouthwash; Sugarless mints, candies, or gum; Oral lubricants (lacrilube); Systemic Pilocarpine or Cevimeline

Treatment of Systemic Manifestations: Hydroxychloroquine is often used for rashes and milder arthritis; Methotrexate and Azathioprine are used in patients with extra-glandular systemic involvement; Prednisone; NSAIDs for arthritis

Treatment of Raynaud's Phenomenon: Avoid cold and keep warm (socks, hat, scarf, gloves); Stop smoking; Avoid estrogen containing compounds; Calcium channel blockers – Nifedipine XL 30 – 60; Topical nitroglycerin paste; IV iloprost

PROGNOSIS

Survival is normal in most patients with the exception of those who develop lymphoproliferative disorders

SYSTEMIC LUPUS ERYTHEMATOSUS (SLE)

DEFINITION & PATHOPHYSIOLOGY

Definition: Systemic Lupus Erythematosus is an autoimmune disease characterized by the production of antibodies directed against nuclear constituents. See the Classification Criteria for SLE *(248)*

Pathophysiology: **(a) Genetic Component:** SLE occurs in genetically susceptible individuals, although the genes responsible have not been completely elucidated. Evidence for this comes from: High concordance rate in identical twins (up to 50%); Disease clustering within families (5-12%); **(b) Hormonal Component:** Increased estrogenic activity likely plays a role in the pathogenesis of SLE; **(c) Environmental Component:** Exposure to ultraviolet (UV) radiation; Viral exposure; **(d) Immunologic Component:** Garbage Disposal Theory of Auto-Antibody Generation: Step 1: Failure to clear autoantigens: May be a result of inherent complement deficiencies or dysfunction; Step 2: Uptake of autoantigen by immature dendritic cells: Occurs in the presence of inflammatory cytokines. Dendritic cells mature into antigen presenting cells. Step 3: Autoreactive B-cells take up autoantigen: B-cell acts as an antigen presenting cell. B-cell is stimulated through interaction with T-cells. B-Cell differentiates into a plasma cell and releases autoantibodies

PRESENTATION

Identifying Data: More common in women than men 6-10:1; Onset between the ages of 15-45, however, any age may be affected; Affects about 1 in 1000 individuals

Onset: SLE can present in many different ways (disease of 1000 faces); Common presentation would include: Constitutional features: Fatigue & low-grade fever; Arthritis/arthralgia; Rash; Abnormalities detected on bloodwork

Progression: Systemic lupus erythematosus is known as the disease of 1000 faces. As such, progression depends upon the severity of the disease and the organ systems involved.

Constitutional Features: Fever, chills, fatigue, sleep disturbance, anorexia, and weight loss. Lymphadenopathy can occur in up to 60% of patients.

Functional Status: Patients with SLE are often functionally impaired as a result of constitutional symptoms (fatigue) and musculoskeletal involvement; There is a higher incidence of depression in SLE contributing to functional impairment

RHEUMATOLOGIC REVIEW OF SYSTEMS

Musculoskeletal Involvement:

(1a) Arthralgia: Migratory, lasting 24-48 hours; joints are occasionally warm, although, there is little other objective evidence of inflammation; associated fatigue is a common debilitating symptom;

(1b) Inflammatory arthritis: Jacoud's arthropathy - A non-erosive, deforming, inflammatory polyarthritis with the same distribution as rheumatoid arthritis; occasionally can see an erosive arthritis which is commonly termed "Rupus" (overlap of Rheumatoid arthritis and lupus). It is often associated with a positive rheumatoid factor.

(1c) Muscle Involvement: Myalgias; inflammatory myositis; myositis related to medications (steroids & anti-malarials);

(1d) Fibromyalgia: Can occur in up to 30% of patients.

(1e) Avascular Necrosis: Occurs most commonly in the hips followed by knees and shoulders; can occur in up to 12% of patients; Risk factors include: High doses of prednisone (>20 mg/day); Raynaud's phenomenon; Vasculitis; African-American heritage; (h) Osteoporosis: Secondary to corticosteroid use

Mucocutaneous Involvement:

(2a) Chronic Cutaneous Lupus Erythematosus (CCLE): (a) Discoid Lupus: May be an isolated finding in otherwise healthy patients; Approximately 5-10% of these patients will go on to develop SLE; Otherwise it occurs in 15-30% of patients with SLE; Discrete, scaly, erythematous, slowly expanding plaques found on the head and neck which may have a central atrophic area; It is typically not photosensitive and heals with scarring; Lesions involving the scalp may result in alopecia due to hair follicle damage by inflammation (it is not reversible); Pathology shows a mononuclear cellular infiltrate around the dermal-epidermal junction, plugging of hair follicles, hyperkeratosis, and vacuolization of the basal layer; Immunofluorescence shows a banding at the dermal-epidermal junction consisting of immunoglobulins and complement; **(b) Lupus Panniculitis/Lupus Profundus:** Firm painful nodular lesions in the deep dermis and subcutaneous fat; With time the overlying skin becomes tethered to the nodules creating depressions; **(c) Lupus Tumidus:** Erythematous/violaceous plaques or nodules on sun exposed areas; Heal without scarring;

(2b) Subacute Cutaneous Lupus Erythematosus (SCLE): Seen in 10 - 25% of patients; Begins as erythematous papules or plaques in sun exposed areas such as the arms and upper torso; Progresses to widespread lesions which heal without scarring; The two variants of SCLE include: Annular - Erythematous rings with areas of central clearing; Papulosquamous - Plaques and papules with scale;

(2c) Acute Cutaneous Lupus Erythematosus (ACLE): (a) Malar Rash: Occurs in up to 60% of patients; Erythematous and slightly edematous; Photosensitive eruption which may persist for days; Classically located on the cheeks and over the bridge of the nose; May involve the forehead and chin; Spares the nasolabial folds; **(b) Diffuse Erythema; (c) Bullous Lupus Erythematosus; Vascular Lesions:** Livedo Reticularis; Palmar Erythema; Periungal Erythema - Due to dilated tortuous capillary loops; Can be seen on the upper eyelid as well; Raynaud's Phenomenon; Vasculitic Skin Lesions: Urticarial eruptions; Infarcts of the nailfolds and splinter hemorrhages; Palpable purpura; Telangiectasia: Appear commonly on the face and do not represent underlying disease activity; Seem to become worse with vasodilatation (blushing, heat, or alcohol);

(2d) Lupus Pernio (Chilblains): Localized inflammatory lesions of the skin as a result of exposure to the cold; Most common in young women, however, may occur in older patients with underlying vascular disease;

(2e) Mucous Membrane Lesions: Oral & nasal ulceration which are painless or painful; Found on the hard palate, buccal mucosa, and tongue; Secondary Sjogren's Syndrome;

(2f) Alopecia: (a) Telogen Effluvium - Transient diffuse shedding with flares of disease. Normal hair follicles are prematurely induced into a resting phase resulting in hair loss; (b) Lupus Hairs - Thin, weakened hairs that easily fragment causing diffuse alopecia most prominent along the periphery of the scalp and temples "lupus frizz"; (c) Permanent Hair Loss - Secondary to scarring discoid LE; (d) Secondary to medications

Renal Involvement: Renal involvement occurs in 75% of patients with SLE but is present in only 40% of patients at disease onset; Typically begins with proteinuria and/or hematuria; There are 5 World Health Organization (WHO) histologic categories of lupus nephritis: **(3a) WHO Class I:** Normal or Minimal Change Disease; **(3b) WHO Class II:** Mesangial (10-20%): Mildest form of involvement with normal or nearly normal renal function; Rarely require any treatment for their disease and prognosis is excellent; *(3c) WHO Class III:* Focal Proliferative (10-20%): Proteinuria and hematuria in almost all patients with some having nephrotic syndrome; May have associated renal failure and hypertension; By definition involves <50% of glomeruli with proliferation and necrosis; *(3d) WHO Class IV:* Diffuse Proliferative: Most common and most severe variant of lupus nephritis; All patients have proteinuria and hematuria; Involves >50% of the glomeruli with cellular hypertrophy proliferation, crescent formation, and areas of necrosis; Poor prognostic factors may include: (a) impaired renal function at presentation, (b) hypertension, (c) nephrotic range proteinuria, (d) older age, (e) anemia, (f) smoking, (g) diabetes, (h) elevated ds-DNA levels, (i) complement binding; *(3e) WHO Class V:* Membranous; Renal involvement is also scored with the activity and chronicity indices: *Activity Index:* Each parameter is graded from 0-3 depending on severity. Fibrinoid necrosis and cellular crescents are weighted twice. The maximum score is 24. Cellular proliferation (0-3); Fibrinoid necrosis (0-3) x 2; Cellular crescents (0-3) x 2; Hyaline thrombi (0-3); Leukocyte infiltration in glomerulus (0-3); Mononuclear cell infiltration in interstitium (0-3); *Chronicity Index:* Each parameter is graded 0-3 depending in severity. The maximal score is 12. Glomerular sclerosis (0-3); Fibrous crescents (0-3); Tubular atrophy (0-3); Interstitial fibrosis (0-3)

Hematologic Involvement:

(4a) Anemia: (a) Homolytic Anemia: Up to 10% of patients; Evidence of hemolysis (peripheral smear, LDH, haptoglobin, indirect bilirubin, Coomb's test); Compensatory reticulocytosis (Reticulocyte Production Index (RPI) = Reticulocytes (%) x (HCT/0.45) x (1/2)); (b) Anemia of Chronic Disease: Common (up to 80%) with a mild normocytic normochromic anemia; (c) Iron Deficiency Anemia: Microcytic, hypochromic anemia; (d) Blood Loss: Due to GI blood loss (medication related); (e) Bone Marrow Dysfunction: Pure red cell aplasia (PRCA); Medication related (immunosuppressants);

(4b) Leukopenia: (a) Neutropenia: Medications (immunosuppressants); Bone marrow dysfunction; Hypersplenism; Immune mechanisms; (b) Lymphopenia: Counts < 1500 cells/mm3; Seen in up to 75% of patient particularly with active disease; Associated with IgM, cold reactive, complement fixing, and presumably cytotoxic anti-lymphocyte antibodies; Increased apoptosis;

(4c) Thrombocytopenia: (a) Mild thrombocytopenia: 25-50% of patients will have mild thrombocytopenia (100-150,000 cells/mm3) which has no adverse effects; (b) Immune Thrombocytopenic Purpura: Profound thrombocytopenia is seen in the setting of immune thrombocytopenic purpura (ITP) where platelet destruction is mediated by anti-platelet antibodies; Antibodies directed against platelet glycoprotein IIb/IIIa have been detected; Presentations: > 50,000 - Asymptomatic; 30-50,000 - Increased bruising with minor trauma; 10-30,000 - Petechiae and purpura develop spontaneously; < 10,000 - High risk for internal bleeding, Medication related (Immunosuppressants); (c) Thrombotic thrombocytopenic purpura; (d) Anti-phospholipid antibodies

Pulmonary Involvement:

(5a) Airway & Alveoli: *(a) Infection:* Rates of infection appear increased in SLE due to underlying immune system dysfunction and immunosuppressive medications; *(b) Acute Lupus Pneumonitis:* Symptoms include dyspnea, cough, pleuritic chest pain, fever, hypoxemia, and rarely hemoptysis; CXR shows infiltrates in the lower lobes (may be bilateral); The pathology shows alveolar damage with alveolar wall injury, necrosis, edema, and hemorrhage *(c) Bronchiolitis Obliterans with or without Organizing Pneumonia (BOOP):* Symptoms include fever, cough, and

chest pain; Bronchiolitis obliterans (BO) is due to an organizing inflammatory exudate that occludes or obliterates bronchiolar lumens; Bronchiolitis obliterans organizing pneumonia (BOOP) is used when the inflammatory process extends into the alveolar spaces; CXR shows alveolar infiltrates with prominent air bronchograms (BO); Interestingly, PFTs show a restrictive pattern;

(5b) Interstitium: (a) Chronic Interstitial Lung Disease (Chronic pneumonitis): Rare in SLE (5%); May develop without any other pulmonary abnormalities or as a sequelae of acute lupus pneumonitis; Symptoms include progressive dyspnea and a chronic dry cough; CXR shows bibasilar interstitial or reticulonodular infiltrates with a restrictive pattern on PFTs; High Resolution Computed Tomography (HRCT); Ground glass opacities - Suggests active inflammation; Honey comb cysts - Suggests end-stage irreversible fibrosis;

(5c) Pleura: (a) Pleuritis: The most common abnormality of the respiratory system (45-60%); *(b) Pleural Effusion:* Think of other etiologies (PE, CHF, Infection, renal failure); Otherwise effusions in SLE predominantly exudative; Presence of LE cells is specific;

(5d) Diaphragm & Muscles: (a) Shrinking Lung Syndrome: Symptoms consist of dyspnea with or without chest pain; Reduced lung volumes on PFTs with elevated diaphragms on CXR; May be secondary to diaphragmatic muscle weakness;

(5e) Vasculature: (a) Pulmonary Hypertension: Symptoms consist of dyspnea, chest pain, palpitations, fatigue and a chronic dry cough with or without symptoms of right sided heart failure (orthopnea, PND, ascites, and peripheral edema); Rule out secondary causes of pulmonary hypertension (COPD, obstructive sleep apnea, Chronic pulmonary emboli, vasculitis, Cardiac valvular disease - mitral stenosis, mitral regurgitation, Pericarditis, Cardiac shunts - Left to right VSD/ASD, Pulmonary veno-occlusive disease); *(b) Pulmonary Hemorrhage:* Presenting symptoms include dyspnea, fever, cough, and hemoptysis; Hemoptysis does not have to be present; CXR shown bilateral infiltrates which may be confused with infection or pulmonary edema; Pathologic findings may include a capillaritis; *(c) Pulmonary Emboli*

Cardiac Involvement: (6a) Pericardial Disease: (a) Pericarditis: Most common form of cardiac involvement; Presents with retrosternal chest pain worse in the supine position and relieved by leaning forward; *(b) Pericardial Effusion:* Fibrinous exudative effusion; *(6b) Myocardial Disease:* Myocarditis; *Valvular Disease:* Libman Sacks endocarditis; *(6c) Arterial Disease: (a) Coronary Artery Disease:* SLE is an independent risk factor for accelerated atherosclerosis; *(b) Coronary Vasculitis;* Conduction System Disease

Neurologic & Psychiatric Involvement: Any patient with neurologic or psychiatric involvement should have a thorough work-up prior to attributing the cause to SLE. Considerations include: **Neurologic Causes (diffuse or focal):** Cerebrovascular insults; Infection - Focal (abscess) or diffuse (meningitis, encephalitis); Tumor - Primary or metastatic; Bleeding - Intracranial or subdural; Increased intracranial pressure; *Systemic Causes:* Impaired acid base balance (pH); Hypoxemia or hypercarbia; Hypo/hyperthermia; Dehydration; Hypo/hyperglycemia; Altered levels of electrolytes (Na, K, Cl, Mg, Ca, PO4); Altered levels of hormones (thyroid, steroids, parathyroid); Altered levels of vitamins (B12, thiamine, nicotinic acid); Systemic infection; Medications or toxins; Medication or toxin withdrawal; Organ failure (renal, hepatic, cardiac)

Common Neurologic Manifestations of SLE: (1) Headaches - common causes include: (a) Tension headaches; (b) Migraine headaches (up to 40%); (c) Cluster headaches; (d) Pseudotumor cerebri; (e) Aseptic meningitis / bacterial meningitis; *(2) Stroke* - common causes include: (a) Atherosclerotic disease; (b) Antiphospholipid antibody syndrome; (c) Vasculitis (rare); (d) Infection; *(3) Seizures; (4) Cognitive Dysfunction* - common causes include: (a) Active SLE; (b) Damage from previously active SLE; (c) Medications (corticosteroids); *(5) Peripheral Neuropathy* - common causes include: (a) Vasculitis; (b) Medications; (c) Associated diabetes;

(7a) Central Neurologic: Aseptic Meningitis: Fever, headache, meningeal irritation, CSF pleocytosis with negative cultures; Cerebrovascular Accidents: Neurologic deficits due to arterial insufficiency or occlusion, venous occlusive disease, or hemorrhage: Stroke, transient ischemic attack, chronic multifocal disease; Subarachnoid and intracranial hemorrhage; Sinus thrombosis; *Demyelinating Syndrome:* Acute or relapsing demyelinating encephalomyelitis with evidence of discrete neurologic lesions disseminated in space and time: Weakness of one or more limbs; Transverse myelopathy; Optic neuropathy; Diplopia due to isolated nerve palsies or internuclear ophthalmoplegia; Brain stem disease with vertigo, vomiting, ataxia, dysarthria, or dysphagia; *Headaches:* Migraine without aura; Migraine with aura; Tension headache; Cluster headache; Headache due to intracranial hypertension; *Movement Disorders:* Chorea: Irregular, involuntary, and jerky movements, that may involve any portion of the body in random sequence. Each movement is brief and unpredictable; *Seizure Disorders; Myelopathy:* Disorder of the spinal cord characterized by rapidly evolving parapesis and/or sensory loss, with a demonstrable motor and sensory cord level (may be transverse) and/or sphincter involvement; *Cognitive Disorders:* Implies a decline from a higher level of functioning and ranges from mild impairment to severe dementia. It may or may not impede social, educational, or occupational functioning, depending on the function(s) impaired and the severity of impairment. Significant deficits in any or all of the following cognitive functions: Simple or complex attention; Reasoning; Executive skills; Memory (learning/recall); Visual-spatial processing; Language (verbal fluency); Psychomotor speed; *Acute Confusional states:* Disturbance of consciousness or level or arousal characterized by reduced ability to focus, maintain, or shift attention, and accompanied by disturbances of cognition, mood, affect, and/or behavior. Typically develops over hours to days and fluctuates over the course of the day. Includes hypo and hyper aroused states and encompasses the spectrum from delirium to coma.

(7b) Peripheral Neurologic; Autonomic Neuropathy: Orthostatic hypotension, sphincteric erectile/ejaculatory dysfunction, anhidrosis, heat intolerance, constipation; *Demyelinating Neuropathy:* Symmetric, ascending, progressive polyradiculopathy, with motor predominance which peaks within 21 days; Loss of reflexes; CSF pleocytosis; *Myasthenia Gravis:* Neuromuscular transmission disorder characterized by fluctuating weakness and fatigability of bulbar and other voluntary muscles without loss of reflexes or impairment of sensation or other neurologic dysfunction: Diplopia, ptosis, dysarthria, weakness in chewing, swallowing difficulty, muscle weakness; Increased weakness with exercise; Dramatic improvement after administration of anticholinesterase medications; *Peripheral Neuropathy:* Mononeuropathy/Mononeuritis Multiplex: Disturbed function of one or more peripheral nerve(s) resulting in weakness/paralysis or sensory dysfunction due to either conduction block in motor nerve fibers or axonal loss; Plexopathy: Disorder of brachial or lumbosacral plexus producing muscle

weakness, sensory deficit, and/or reflex change not corresponding to the territory of single root or nerve; Polyneuropathy: Acute or chronic disorder or sensory and motor peripheral nerves with variable tempo characterized by symmetry of symptoms and physical findings in a distal distribution; *Sensorineural Hearing Loss; Cranial Neuropathy:* Disorder of sensory and/or motor function of a specific cranial nerve; *(c) Psychiatric: Anxiety Disorder:* Anticipation of danger or misfortune accompanied by apprehension, dysphoria, or tension. Includes generalized anxiety, panic disorder, panic attacks, and obsessive compulsive disorders; *Mood Disorders:* Prominent and persistent disturbance in mood characterized by: Depressed mood or markedly diminished interest or pleasure in almost all activities; Elevated, expansive, or irritable mood; *Psychosis:* Severed disturbance in the perception of reality characterized by delusions and/or hallucinations

Gastrointestinal Involvement: Esophageal: Esophageal hypomotility with dysphagia; GERD; Candidiasis; *Peritonitis:* Transudative effusions on paracentesis; *Mesenteric Vasculitis & Infarction:* Presents with abdominal pain (acute abdomen), nausea, vomiting, low-grade fever, and bloody diarrhea; Seen in patients with peripheral vasculitis; Can perforate; *Hepatitis:* (a) Lupoid hepatitis: Absence of anti-smooth muscle or antimitochondrial antibodies; Anti-ribosomal-P antibodies; (b) Medication associated hepatitis: NSAIDs; Methotrexate; Azathioprine; (c) Other causes of hepatitis: Hepatic congestion; Cholestasis; Arteritis; Non-alcoholic steatohepatitis (NASH); *Pancreatitis:* Can be secondary to vasculitis or thrombosis; Can be secondary to medications (azathioprine); *Protein Losing Enteropathy:* Profound hypoalbuminemia, edema, and diarrhea (in 50%); *Splenomegaly*

Infection: Patients with SLE are at increased risk for developing bacterial infections, which is the main reason for hospitalization; Risk factors for infection include: Active disease; Immunosuppressant medications (corticosteroids, azathioprine, cyclophosphamide); Renal failure with proteinuria and hypoalbuminemia

RISK FACTORS
No known risk factors for the development of SLE

FAMILY HISTORY
5-12% of relatives have SLE

RED FLAGS
Infection should always be ruled out in the presence of a fever

DIFFERENTIAL DIAGNOSIS
Lupus is known as the disease of 1000 faces as it can present in a multitude of ways; A separate differential diagnosis should be considered for each manifestation of the disease along with the organ systems involved

PHYSICAL EXAMINATION
Vitals: Pulse: May be elevated with active disease or with cardiac, pulmonary, or hematologic (anemia) involvement; *BP:* If elevated think renal disease and associated atherosclerosis; *RR:* May be elevated with cardiac, pulmonary, or hematologic (anemia) involvement; *Temperature:* May be elevated

Cutaneous: Splinter hemorrhages and nailfold infarcts; Rash across the knuckles (PIPs); Rashes specific to and associated with lupus; Livedo reticularis

Head & Neck: Alopecia and lupus hairs; Oral and nasal ulceration; Xerostomia and xerophthalmia; Malar rash; Discoid rash; Cervical adenopathy

Respiratory: Cough; Pleural friction rubs due to pleuritis; Pleural effusions secondary to pleuritis, infection, pulmonary hypertension, or cardiac failure; Diminished breath sounds due to infection, pulmonary hemorrhage, pneumonitis, or shrinking lung syndrome; Adventitious sounds (crackles) due to infection, edema, or pneumonitis; Axillary adenopathy

Cardiovascular: Abnormal rhythm secondary to conduction system disease; Pericardial friction rub secondary to pericarditis; Murmurs secondary to fever, hypoxia, anemia or valvular lesions associated with Libman-Sacks endocarditis; Congestive heart failure secondary to myocarditis or pericarditis; Pulmonary Hypertension: Loud P2, RV heave, pulmonary flow murmur, pulmonary regurgitation, tricuspid regurgitation, elevated JVP with prominent V waves due to TR

Gastrointestinal: May be normal

Musculoskeletal: Inflammatory arthritis

Neurologic: Peripheral neuropathy; Proximal myopathy

INVESTIGATIONS

CBC: Normochromic normocytic anemia is the most common finding, leukopenia with neutropenia and/or lymphopenia, and thrombocytopenia. (*see hematologic manifestations of SLE above*).

Creatinine: May be elevated with renal involvement. ALWAYS calculate the GFR.

Urinalysis: May show proteinuria, hematuria, or casts

Liver Enzymes: Usually normal

ESR/CRP: May be elevated with disease flare

ANA: Present in 99% of cases; Reasons for a negative ANA include: Anti-Ro/SSA antibody presence; Antiphospholipid antibodies; Hereditary compliment deficiencies

ds-DNA: Occur in 60-83% of patients. Highly specific (95%). In some patients, rising levels of ds-DNA may be associated with disease flare (renal disease).

Complement: C3 and C4 may be low. In some patients, falling levels of complement may herald the onset of disease flare.

ENA Panel: Anti-Sm antibodies: Insensitive but specific for SLE. Occur more commonly in African American and Asian patients. Generally not useful for following disease activity. Anti-RNP antibodies: Can occur in low titer in SLE; Anti-Ro/SSA antibodies: Found in 50% of patients with SLE. Associated with photosensitivity, subacute cutaneous lupus, cutaneous vasculitis, neonatal lupus, and congenital heart block. Anti-La/SSB antibodies: Found in 25% of patients with SLE usually associated with anti-Ro antibodies

Anti-Phospholipid Antibodies: Associated with stroke, seizures, depression, dementia, chorea, and transverse myelitis

Anti-Ribosomal-P Antibodies: Associated with psychosis and depression

Anti-Neuronal Antibodies: Associated with cognitive dysfunction

CT Imaging in NPSLE: Initial choice to identify tumors, bleeding, and cerebrovascular accidents

Magnetic Resonance Imaging in NPSLE: Usually normal in patients with psychiatric symptoms alone; Majority of lesions are small focal lesions concentrating in the periventricular and subcortical white matter; Focal NPSLE uniformly reveals large and small high-intensity MRI lesions in white and grey matter, which tend to persist despite treatment and correlate with antiphospholipid antibody production, livedo reticularis, and peripheral vasculitis

Electroencephalography (EEG) in NPSLE: 80% of patients with SLE will have abnormalities on routine EEG testing; Diffuse, slow wave activity is associated with organic brain syndromes; More useful for recording focal abnormalities due to seizures or other focal neurologic problems

Synovial Fluid: Clear to slightly cloudy fluid; Non-inflammatory cell counts (<2000/ mm3) with mononuclear cells; Low protein levels; ANA and LE cells can be found in synovial fluid

Cerebrospinal Fluid in NPSLE: Usually normal; CSF pleocytosis, elevated protein, and low glucose should increase suspicion of infection; Oligoclonal banding has been observed in patients with diffuse manifestations of NPSLE

Pleural Fluid: Exudative fluid with mild increase in LDH; Useful to rule out infection

MANAGEMENT

General: Education about the disease; Vocational counseling; Arthritis self management programs; Social support

Rest & Sleep Hygiene: No stressful activities at least one hour prior to bed (TV, work, exercise); Avoid caffeine; Go to bed at the same time each evening; Use the bedroom only for sleep, keep it dark, cool (65 degrees), and quiet; If not asleep after 30 minutes - get out of bed and leave the room; Try not to take worries to bed

Physiotherapy: Pain relieving strategies and interventions; Mobility aids (canes & walkers) and braces; Exercise program for: Corticosteroid induced weight gain, osteoporosis, and muscle weakness; Disease flares resulting in deconditioning. Manual therapy (manipulation) when appropriate

Occupational Therapy: Splints and orthotics; Joint protection measures and energy conservation; Assistive devices; Lifestyle management

Avoidance of the Sun: Can worsen photosensitive reactions and may activate systemic disease; Use a sunscreen with minimum SPF 30 (Recommend SPF 60) with an ingredient that will also block UVA (Parsol 1789); Long sleeves and broad rimmed hats; Review photosensitizing medications

Preventative Medicine: All patients with lupus should be followed closely by a specialist who has experience in managing lupus. Dimensions of preventative medicine include: Office evaluation every 3-6 months (more frequent for sicker patients) consisting of: Appropriate History; Physical Examination; Appropriate laboratory screening investigations which may include: CBC, Chemistry panel, Creatinine and urinalysis, ESR/CRP, Antibody profile - ds-DNA, anticardiolipin antibody titers, Complement - C3, C4, CH50

Cardiac Risk Assessment: Should be performed at least on a yearly basis and consist of: Evaluation of diet, weight control, and exercise status; Evaluation of smoking status; Blood pressure evaluation; Serum lipid profile; Fasting glucose; Homocysteine levels; Antiphospholipid antibody screening; Electrocardiogram; Chest X-ray

Osteoporosis: Bone mineral density testing should be performed every 1-2 years

(1) Treatment of Fatigue and Systemic Complaints: Non-pharmacologic based management is the cornerstone of therapy; Antimalarials may be beneficial and protective against major disease flares; NSAIDs and systemic corticosteroids may be useful; Some patients report benefit with Azathioprine

(2) Treatment of Musculoskeletal Involvement: (a) Analgesics; (b) NSAIDs (Be aware of associated renal and CNS disease); (c) Corticosteroids: Low-dose corticosteroids are often used for the treatment of musculoskeletal disease due to SLE. Must always be aware of the potential side-effects of long-term corticosteroids. Typical doses range from 5-10 mg/day; (d) Anti-Malarials: Hydroxychloroquine may protect against major disease flares; Beneficial for some patients with musculoskeletal complaints; (e) Methotrexate: Can be an effective steroid sparing agent for musculoskeletal involvement; (f) Azathioprine: Little evidence for the use of azathioprine for musculoskeletal complaints secondary to SLE. However, some patients report benefit with azathioprine.

(3) Treatment of Cutaneous Involvement: (a) Sun avoidance is the cornerstone of therapy *(see above)*. Referral to a dermatologist; (b) Topical Corticosteroids: Use low to medium potency non-fluorinated creams on facial lesions (hydrocortisone); Other lesions with medium potency fluorinated creams (betamethasone & triamcinolone) & lotions for scalp lesions; Can use short duration (< 2 weeks) of higher potency preparations in some cases (clobetasol, betamethasone dipropionate); (c) Intralesional Corticosteroids: Useful for discoid LE unresponsive to topical agents; Lidocaine 1% mixed in equal parts with triamcinolone acetonide (Kenalog®) 10 mg/mL. Use a 27 or 30 gauge needle and inject enough solution to blanch the lesion (about 0.1 cc for a 1.0 square cm lesion); (d) Antimalarials: Hydroxychloroquine is invaluable for the treatment of cutaneous LE with up to 70% of patients responding; Wait 6-8 weeks before considering alternative treatment. If monotherapy does not work, consider adding quinacrine 100 mg/day; do not use chloroquine and hydroxychloroquine together as the risk of retinal toxicity is very high. After a further 6-8 weeks, if the combination of hydroxychloroquine and quinacrine is still not working, consider replacing the hydroxychloroquine with chloroquine; (e) Retinoids: Isotretinoin and etretinate useful in a few cases of discoid LE; (f) Dapsone: Can be used in SCLE patients who fail antimalarials, works well in bullous LE, and is the treatment of choice in LE patients with vasculitis, Initial dose is 100 mg/day; Will produce dose related hemolysis, anemia, and methemoglobinemia in all patients. Follow CBC weekly for first month of treatment, monthly thereafter; Consider G6PD testing of patients at risk for deficiency; (g) Thalidomide: Useful in treatment resistant cases; (h) Oral Corticosteroids: Used for treatment resistant disease; Doses of 30 mg per day (15 mg PO BID) are used until disease is under control. The steroids are then tapered and patients are restarted on other therapy (i.e. antimalarials above); (i) Other Immunosuppressants: Methotrexate and Azathioprine have been used in treatment resistant cases

(4) Treatment of Renal Involvement: General supportive measures include: Nephrology referral; Low-protein diet; Low-salt diet if hypertensive; Treatment of hypertension and proteinuria with ACE-inhibitors; Treatment of hypercholesterolemia;

(4a) Treatment of Mesangial Glomerulonephritis (Class II): Does not require treatment if the patient has little proteinuria and an inactive urinary sediment (no hematuria or casts); If the patient has significant proteinuria (>1 gram/day), an active urinary sediment, or accompanied by elevated ds-DNA levels and hypocomplimentemia treatment should be considered with: Oral prednisone 0.5-1 mg/kg/day given from 4 to 12 weeks until disease activity is controlled. Prednisone is gradually tapered providing disease is adequately controlled;

(4b) Treatment of Proliferative Glomerulonephritis (Class III & IV): Treatment outcome parameters include: (a) Renal function - Creatinine clearance; (b) Proteinuria; (c) Hematuria; (d) Leukocyturia; (e) ds-DNA; (f) Complement levels. Treatment generally involves the use of corticosteroids plus a cytotoxic agent. Corticosteroids - 2 possible treatment approaches: Oral prednisone 1 mg/kg/day given for 4 - 12 weeks until disease activity is controlled and then tapered; IV methylprednisolone given as 1 gram pulses initially for 1 to 3 days and then 1 gram pulses monthly. This regimen is commonly used with rapidly progressive disease of recent onset. Cyclophosphamide: Considered to be the standard of care therapy for patients with proliferative glomerulonephritis (III/IV); Corticosteroids plus cyclophosphamide is effective in 60-90% of patients; The NIH regimen involves monthly intravenous pulses of cyclophosphamide for 6 months followed by pulses every 3 months thereafter, providing disease is adequately controlled. The total duration of treatment is 2 years. An example of treatment orders for a patient receiving IV cyclophosphamide and pulsed methylprednisolone is as follows: Initial pulses may vary from 0.25 to 2.5 grams at intervals of 1 week to 1 month. In Europe, mini-pulses given more frequently are routinely used. *Azathioprine:* Azathioprine may be used in the following circumstances: Patients intolerant to cyclophosphamide; After initial induction with cyclophosphamide, Azathioprine may work as a maintenance agent. This is typically done after 3-6 months of therapy with cyclophosphamide. There is some evidence to suggest that patients treated in this manner may have a slightly higher risk of renal relapse. *Mycophenolate Mofetil:* Initially used in a small trial (NEJM 2001) at doses of 1 gram BID and seemed to have similar efficacy to pulsed cyclophosphamide; However, on further analysis, there may be more relapses with use of mycophenolate; *Cyclosporine:* Shown to be effective in pure membranous nephritis; *Treatment of Membranous Nephritis (V):* Usually treated initially with 1mg/kg/day corticosteroids for 4-12 weeks and then tapered regardless of the response to treatment; Patients with associated proliferative component may be candidates for cytotoxic therapy

(5) Treatment of Hematologic Involvement

(5a) Autoimmune Hemolytic Anemia: Corticosteroids: Initial treatment with Prednisone 1.0 mg/kg/day; Splenectomy; Steroid Sparing Agents: Azathioprine; Cyclophosphamide; Plasmapheresis.

(5b) Immune Mediated Thrombocytopenia: Who should be treated: Hemorrhage - see *Urgent Treatment* below; Treat everyone with platelet counts < 30,000; 30-50,000 - No treatment or consider using prednisone; Corticosteroids: Initial treatment with Prednisone 1-1.5 mg/kg/day; Responses occur within 3 weeks; Response rates vary from 50-75%; Relapses are common with 5-30% achieving remission depending on the duration of the disorder; High-dose dexamethasone (40 mg/day) in primary ITP (NEJM 2003); Response rates of 85%; Remission of 50% at 6 months; Anti-D Immune Globulin: Initial dose is 75 mcg/kg/day; For Rh+ patients only; More expensive than corticosteroids but less toxic; Intravenous Immune Globulin (IVIG): Dose of 1 gram daily for 2-3 consecutive days for steroid refractory cases; Response rates of 80%, although remission is very rare; Used as acute intervention for severe thrombocytopenia; Splenectomy: The decision of when to undergo splenectomy is controversial; Consider splenectomy within 3 to 6 months if doses of 10-20 mg of prednisone are required to maintain a platelet count >30,000; Immunizations with Haemophilus influenzae type b, pneumococcal vaccines and meningococcal vaccines are mandatory 2 weeks prior to surgery; Medical alert bracelet; URGENT TREATMENT: Internal hemorrhage, neurologic symptoms, or emergency surgery are all indications for urgent treatment; Treatment consists of: IV Methylprednisolone 1 gram per day for 3 consecutive days; IVIG 1 gram daily for 3 consecutive days; Platelet infusions of 2-3 times the normal amounts usually required; Chronic ITP - Corticosteroid Sparing Agents: Danazol 10-15 mg/kg/day; Dapsone 75 mcg/day; Azathioprine; Cyclophosphamide

(6) Treatment of Pulmonary Involvement:

(6a) Pleuritis: NSAIDs - Often responsive to NSAIDs alone; Corticosteroids - Useful for NSAID refractory patients in moderate to high doses for short courses (i.e. 0.5-1 mg/kg/day);

(6b) Acute Pneumonitis: Treat as infection until proven otherwise - broad spectrum antibiotics; Corticosteroids: Prednisone 1-2 mg/kg/day is the mainstay of therapy; IV methylprednisolone for cases not responsive to oral prednisone or in cases with severe respiratory failure; Cyclophosphamide: Consider IV pulse cyclophosphamide for cases with severe respiratory failure or for those patients who have failed therapy with corticosteroids. See sample cyclophosphamide orders (119); Azathioprine: Consider oral Azathioprine for patients who have failed corticosteroids;

(6c) Chronic Interstitial Lung Disease: Treatment is aimed at reducing inflammation with the goal of preventing structural damage; Corticosteroids: Prednisone 1 mg/kg/day is the mainstay of therapy; However, response rate is quite low (30%); If no response after 3 months, withdraw the prednisone; Immunosuppressants: In patients with severe or progressive disease, a six month trial of IV pulse Cyclophosphamide or Azathioprine may be considered in patients who have failed corticosteroids. See sample cyclophosphamide orders above;

(6d) Pulmonary Hemorrhage: IV methylprednisolone 1 gram daily for 3 days followed by a dose of 80-120 mg of IV methylprednisolone daily thereafter; IV Cyclophosphamide for patients who are critically ill or are unresponsive to corticosteroids. See sample cyclophosphamide orders (119); Plasma exchange has been used with favorable responses;

(6e) Bronchiolitis Obliterans with or without Organizing Pneumonia (BOOP): Corticosteroids: Prednisone 1 mg/kg/day is the recommended as the initial therapy; Immunosuppressants: In patients with severe or progressive disease, a six month trial of IV pulse Cyclophosphamide or Azathioprine may be considered in patients who have failed or are intolerant to corticosteroids. See sample cyclophosphamide orders (119);

(6f) Pulmonary Hypertension: Oxygen (2 Lpm nasal cannulae); Warfarin - To reduce the formation of in-situ thrombosis; Diuretics & digoxin when appropriate; Calcium channel blockers; Bosentan – Endothelin receptor antagonist shown to increase exercise capacity and improve hemodynamics; IV-Epoprostenol – Flolan; Treprostinil; Sildenafil; ACE-Inhibitors; Lung and/or heart transplantation may be considered

(7) Treatment of Cardiac Involvement:

(7a) Pericarditis: NSAIDs; Prednisone 0.5 -1mg/kg/day in divided doses for NSAID failures;

(7b) Myocarditis: Prednisone 0.5-1 mg/kg/day; Resistant cases occasionally require the use of a cytotoxic agent such as cyclophosphamide or azathioprine;

(7c) Coronary Artery Disease: Imperative to periodically assess risk factors including: Smoking status; Diabetes screening; Hypertension; Cholesterol levels; Family history; Corticosteroid dose; Homocysteine levels; Anti-phospholipid antibody levels; Disease activity (ds-DNA, C3, & C4);

(7d) Libman-Sacks Endocarditis: Consider antibiotic prophylaxis for patients undergoing procedures with a higher risk of bacteremia (i.e. dental work); Consider anticoagulation therapy to reduce the risk of embolization

(8) Treatment of Neurologic Involvement: Consider other causes of neurologic involvement besides SLE *(see above)*; Due to the diffuse array of neuropsychiatric presentations the management differs depending upon the clinical presentation; Supportive: Serial neuropsychiatric testing to determine the presence, extent, and progression of cognitive dysfunction; Anti-epileptics in the face of seizure; Anti-psychotics; Anti-depressants; Anxiolytics; Contributing Factors: Withdraw offending

medications; Antibiotics for infection; Correct electrolyte and metabolic abnormalities; Replace hormones and vitamins; Immunosuppressive; ***Consider High Dose Corticosteroids for:*** Seizures in the setting of SLE; Cerebral vasculopathy; Any CNS manifestation in the setting of active SLE; ***Consider IV Pulse Cyclophosphamide for:*** Cerebral vasculopathy; Non-thrombotic focal neurologic defects; Transverse myelitis; ***Consider IVIG for:*** Any CNS manifestation unresponsive to steroids or cyclophosphamide; Concomitant thrombocytopenia; ***Consider Plasma Exchange for:*** Any CNS manifestation unresponsive to steroids, cyclophosphamide, or IVIG; ***Anti-Coagulation:*** ASA; Heparin; Warfarin

PROGNOSIS

Risk Stratification for Poor Progression: (a) Race: There may be racial differences in the expression of the disease and its outcome. Black patients are considered to have a poorer prognosis than Caucasians. (b) Age of Onset: Improved survival for patients who develop the disease at an older age; (c) Socioeconomic Status: Patients with higher education and better socioeconomic status seem to do better; (d) Disease Factors: A higher SLEDAI score at presentation has been found to adversely affect the disease outcome. Specific disease involvement which confer a worse prognosis include: CNS Involvement; Lupus Nephritis; Anemia; Thrombocytopenia; Pulmonary Involvement

Prognosis: Current survival rates are approximately 90% at 5 years and 70% at 20 years; Mortality rates are 3 fold higher than the general population; Mortality in SLE may result from: (a) Active disease (e.g. vasculitis resulting in CNS disease, pulmonary hemorrhage); (b) Damage from previously active disease; (c) Medication (e.g. infection while on immunosuppressants); (d) Associated coronary artery disease

SYSTEMIC SCLEROSIS (SSc)

DEFINITION & PATHOPHYSIOLOGY

Definition: A multi-systemic disease characterized by functional and structural abnormalities of small blood vessels, fibrosis of the skin and internal organs, immune system activation, and auto immunity. See the Classification Criteria for Systemic Sclerosis 249

Pathophysiology: The current theory is a susceptible host is exposed to an exogenous event which starts the process. The earliest findings are hypersensitive alpha-2 adrenergic receptors, endothelial damage and abnormal apoptosis. The subsequent smooth muscle hypertrophy creates luminal narrowing and thrombosis resulting in an obliterative arteriolopathy. Endothelial cell activation results in immune system activation and fibroblast activation. The primary profibrotic cytokines are IL-4 and TGF-Beta.

PRESENTATION

Identifying Data: Typical patient is a young female (35-65); Male: female ratio of about 1:7-12; Prevalence about 0.01% in the population

Onset: Initial symptoms are typically non-specific and include Raynaud's phenomenon, fatigue, and musculoskeletal complaints. The first specific clue is skin thickening that begins as swelling or puffiness of the fingers and hands. The patient feels a progressive tightening of the skin and decreased flexibility. In diffuse SSc various degrees of hypo or hyper pigmentation may occur giving the skin a tanned or "salt and pepper" appearance. ***Limited SSc (L-SSc):*** Usually have RP for 1-10 years prior to onset; skin involvement is distal to the elbows and knees but may involve the face. ***Diffuse SSc (d-SSc):*** Short interval between onset of RP and skin involvement which includes the trunk & extremities.

Progression: As SSc progresses the skin becomes progressively tighter and thicker. This stage may persist for one to three years, after which the skin tends to soften and either thins (becomes atrophic and thinned, with tethering to underlying structures) or returns toward normal texture. After this initial improvement the disease may be progressive.

Constitutional Features: Fatigue may be prominent, weight loss due to activity of the disease and GI involvement with anorexia.

Functional Status: Reduced functional status with difficulties with ADLs; Difficulty at work; Loss of libido – Erectile dysfunction in men is common; Depression in up to 50%

RHEUMATOLOGIC REVIEW OF SYSTEMS

Vascular Involvement: Raynaud's Phenomenon (RP): Present in 95% of patients with SSc vs 4% of general population; In SSC, RP is associated with tissue fibrosis of the fingers, loss of the digital pads, digital ulceration, and on occasion digital ischemia with amputation

Musculoskeletal Involvement: Arthralgias and myalgias are one of the earliest symptoms; A rheumatoid-like erosive polyarthritis is occasionally seen (<20%); Inflammation and fibrosis of the tendon sheaths also lead to pain and restriction of movement with accompanying tendon friction rubs; Muscle weakness and atrophy is a dominant problem in late SSc secondary to fibrosis, disuse, contractures of fibrotic skin, along with malnutrition

Mucocutaneous Involvement: Xerostomia and xerophthalmia

Neurologic Involvement: Trigeminal neuralgia; Other entrapment neuropathies such as carpal tunnel

Cardiac Involvement: Pericardial effusions; Myocardial fibrosis with diastolic dysfunction; Premature coronary artery disease

Respiratory Involvement: Leading cause of mortality in SSc; (a) Interstitial Fibrosis: Occurs with diffuse disease (30-60%), anti-topoisomerase-1 antibodies (Scl-70), and FVC<75 early in the course of disease; (b) Pulmonary hypertension without fibrosis occurs in 20-25% of limited SSc patients and less often in diffuse disease: Risk factors include long standing RP and limited SSc; Poor survival - 90% were dead at 5 years; Pulmonary arterial pressures (PAP) > 45 with right sided heart changes correlate with catheterization in 90% of cases. Right heart catheterization should be done in all cases to confirm the diagnosis.

Gastrointestinal Involvement: Small oral aperture; Dental disease and oral sicca features; Esophageal dysmotility with resulting GERD; Gastric ectasia (watermelon stomach); Pseudo obstruction secondary to small bowel involvement; Diminished peristalsis leading to bacterial overgrowth and malabsorption. Wide mouth diverticulae on barium enema; Loss of sphincter control

Renal Involvement: Scleroderma renal crisis is seen in about 10% of patients with systemic sclerosis and is characterized by: Abrupt onset of oliguric renal failure, abrupt onset of hypertension, bland urinary sediment (maybe a few RBCs or casts); Symptoms include fatigue, headaches, visual disturbances, encephalopathy and focal CNS events, seizures, congestive heart failure, and nausea and vomiting; Associated renal failure with fluid and electrolyte imbalance, consumptive thrombocytopenia, microangiopathic hemolysis, and elevated renin levels; Risk factors for renal crisis include: Diffuse SSc, early in the course of the disease, Medications (Corticosteroids and Cyclosporine)

RISK FACTORS

(a) Silica dust exposure and silicosis; (b) Exposure to organic solvents, (c) appetite suppressants (biogenic amines), and urea formaldehyde; (d) SSc like disorder with exposure to vinyl chloride, bleomycin, tainted rapeseed oil, L-tryptophan

FAMILY HISTORY

There are reported familial clusters of SSC but they are extremely rare.

RED FLAGS

Think about respiratory disease (pulmonary hypertension and fibrosis) and renal disease

DIFFERENTIAL DIAGNOSIS

(a) Systemic sclerosis; (b) Environmentally induced SSc - Chemicals; (c) Eosinophilic fasciitis; (d) Generalized morphea; (e) Scleredema – Seen in diabetics

PHYSICAL EXAMINATION

Vitals: Pulse: Normal; BP: Watch for elevations in BP as may be an indicator of renal crisis; RR: Elevations in RR may be an indicator of pulmonary/cardiac involvement

Cutaneous: Thickening of the skin (sclerodactyly) with a shiny appearance: L-SSc: Distal to the elbows and knees and may involve the face and neck; D-SSc: Involves proximal extremities and upper arms; Pigment changes in the skin – Hypo/hyper; Loss of skin appendages – Hair loss; Telangiectasia; Calcinosis; Finger tips: Loss of the finger pads and digital pulp with distal tuft resorption; Periungual capillary changes; Periungual infarcts; Digital pits/ulcerations from Raynaud's; Raynaud's phenomenon

Head & Neck: Skin thickening and tightness; Pigment changes; Telangiectasia; Alopecia; Ocular dryness; Cranial nerve abnormalities; Reduced oral aperture; Poor dentition with oral dryness

Respiratory: Crackles secondary to Interstitial fibrosis; Reduced chest expansion due to skin thickening and muscle fibrosis

Cardiovascular: Pulmonary hypertension – Loud P2, RV heave, pulmonary flow murmur, pulmonary regurgitation, tricuspid regurgitation, elevated JVP with prominent V waves due to TR; Diastolic dysfunction secondary to myocardial fibrosis; Congestive heart failure

Gastrointestinal: Weight loss, bloating

Musculoskeletal: Muscle atrophy, weakness; Flexion contractures of the digits; Decreased ROM secondary to fibrosis of the skin and joint capsules; Inflammatory arthritis; Tendon friction rubs

Neurologic: Cranial neuropathies (trigeminal); Carpal tunnel syndrome

INVESTIGATIONS

CBC: Thrombocytopenia and microangiopathic hemolysis (schistocytes) with renal crisis.

Urinalysis: Proteinuria with renal crisis

Creatinine: May be elevated with renal crisis

Elevated AST/ALT/ALP: Think PBC associated with L-SSc

ANA: In majority of cases

Anti-Topoisomerase-1 (Scl-70): Diffuse SSc associated with interstitial pulmonary fibrosis

Anti-centromere antibodies: Limited SSc

Anti-Polymerase-III: Diffuse SSc associated with cardiac or renal disease

Radiology: Soft-tissue calcification; Usually a non-erosive arthritis with deformities secondary to contraction of the overlying skin; Reported cases of erosive arthritis

Screening (yearly): Chest radiographs; ECG & echocardiogram; Pulmonary function tests

MANAGEMENT

General: Education

Physiotherapy: Reduce joint contractures; Improve ROM and functional abilities

Occupational Therapy

Disease Modifying Interventions: Methotrexate – Possible favorable outcome in skin; D-Penicillamine, chlorambucil, and interferon-alpha have not been fruitful

Treatment of Skin Disease: Topical moisturizers; Treat ulcers with anti-septic, antibiotic ointments, and analgesics; Calcinosis – Can try colchicine

Raynaud's Phenomenon: Avoid cold and keep warm (socks, hat, scarf, gloves); Stop smoking; Avoid estrogen containing compounds; Calcium channel blockers – Nifedipine XL 30 – 60 mg PO OD; Topical nitroglycerin paste; IV iloprost

Gastrointestinal: Reduce caffeine and alcohol, stop smoking, elevate head of the bed, avoid foods which precipitate GERD, eat frequent small meals; Oral antacids, H2 blockers, and proton pump inhibitors; Metoclopramide, erythromycin, or domperidone for dysmotility; Broad spectrum antibiotics; Supplemental vitamins

Cardiopulmonary: *(a) Interstitial Fibrosis:* Consider treatment if: Forced vital capacity (FVC) is reduced in early disease or it is steadily declining; Ground glass is seen on high resolution CT scan (HRCT); Polymorphonuclear cells or eosinophils on bronchoalveolar lavage; No significant pulmonary hypertension. Treat with IV cyclophosphamide and corticosteroids. *(b) Pulmonary Hypertension:* Oxygen (2 lpm nasal cannulae); Warfarin - To reduce the formation of in-situ thrombosis; Diuretics & digoxin when appropriate; Calcium channel blockers; Bosentan – Endothelin receptor antagonist shown to increase exercise capacity and improve hemodynamics; IV-Epoprostenol – Flolan; Treprostinil; Sildenafil; ACE-Inhibitors; Lung and/or heart transplantation may be considered.

Scleroderma Renal Crisis: Control blood pressure: Discontinue any medications which may worsen blood pressure; ACE-Inhibitors – Have improved survival from 10% in 1 year to 90% in 5 years. Captopril is most commonly used aiming to reduce blood pressure slowly. Dose 25 mg PO BID-TID increasing to max 150 mg TID; Angiotensin receptor blockers – Less effective than ACE (? Lack of bradykinin effect); Minoxidil start at 2.5 mg PO BID and gradually increase to 10 BID; Calcium channel blockers; Dialysis and renal care; Consult nephrology; Continue ACE during dialysis as persistent hyperreninemia may occur; Supportive Treatment: Consult cardiology if CHF is an issue; Oxygen; Careful use of diuretics; Nitrates; Statins; Neurology involvement if associated encephalopathy or seizures; Correct electrolyte abnormalities

Musculoskeletal: Physiotherapy – Early and aggressive to prevent joint contractures; Acetaminophen; NSAIDs and COXIBs; Methotrexate and corticosteroids for inflammatory myopathies

PROGNOSIS

Risk Stratification for Poor Progression: (a) Poor HAQ score; (b) Recent onset of Raynaud's phenomenon; (c) Acute onset of symptoms (fever, weight loss, polyarthritis); (d) Swelling of the extremities; (e) Carpal tunnel syndrome; (f) Tendon rubs; (g) Skin thickening proximal to the elbows and knees; (h) Anti-topoisomerase and/or anti-RNA polymerase III antibodies; (i) Elevated ESR, increased IgG (polyclonal), and reduced hemoglobin

Prognosis: The course of systemic sclerosis is highly variable; 10 year survival rates for limited & diffuse disease are 70% & 40-60% respectively; Cardiopulmonary disease is the leading cause of death in both variants of the disease

TAKAYASU ARTERITIS (TA)

DEFINITION & PATHOPHYSIOLOGY

Definition: A granulomatous vasculitis, occurring in younger individuals predominantly affecting the aorta and its main branches although coronary and pulmonary arterial involvement is seen. See the Classification Criteria for Takayasu Arteritis (250)

Pathophysiology: The etiology and pathogenesis of Takayasu arteritis is unknown. Current theories include: An infectious etiology playing a role in the pathogenesis, particularly tuberculosis; Autoimmune: These theories have been strengthened by a clear association with haplotypes such as HLAB52

PRESENTATION

Identifying Data: Female to male ratio is about 8-9:1; Usual age of onset is between 10 and 40; More common in Asians

Onset: The initial symptoms may be non-specific producing malaise, fatigue, fevers, night sweats, anorexia, weight loss, and myalgias; Often, patients are initially diagnosed as having a viral illness or other infection and delay to diagnosis has been reported between 2 - 11 years; Vascular symptoms are rarely present in the onset of disease

Progression: As the disease progresses, persistent vessel inflammation produces symptoms suggestive of vascular occlusion or dilatation. The particular symptom complex depends upon the vessel involved (see below). Symptoms may vary from asymptomatic pulseless disease to catastrophic neurologic impairment. Upper extremity vessels are usually involved with 85-95% of patients having diminished radial pulses with blood pressure discrepancies between the arms. Pulmonary arteries are involved in 50% of cases.

Constitutional Features: Fever, fatigue, myalgias, arthralgias, anorexia, weight loss, and night sweats

Functional Status: Patient may have considerable impairment in their functional status due to constitutional symptoms and symptoms from arterial occlusion

RHEUMATOLOGIC REVIEW OF SYSTEMS

Musculoskeletal Involvement: Arthralgias and myalgias, Rarely an inflammatory arthritis develops

Mucocutaneous Involvement: Skin rash resembling erythema nodosum or pyoderma gangrenosum. This rash may show vasculitis of small vessels on biopsy

Vascular Involvement: (a) Common carotid artery involvement: CVA and TIAs; Visual disturbances; Seizures; Headaches; Dementia; (b) Vertebral artery involvement: Vertigo; Visual disturbances (diplopia); Dysphagia; Dysarthria; Drop attacks; Headaches; Seizures; (c) Subclavian artery involvement (85-95%): Arm claudication; Pulseless arm; (d) Aortic arch involvement: Aortic valve regurgitation; Congestive heart failure; (e) Pulmonary artery involvement: Pulmonary hypertension; Hemoptysis; Chest pain; (f) Coronary artery involvement: Angina pectoris; (g) Mesenteric artery involvement: Abdominal pain; Diarrhea; Gastrointestinal hemorrhage; (h) Renal artery involvement: Hypertension (30-80% of patients); (i) Abdominal aortic involvement: Claudication of lower extremities; Hypertension; (k) Iliac artery involvement: Claudication of lower extremity

RISK FACTORS

Asian heritage; Age < 40

FAMILY HISTORY

Familial Takayasu arteritis has been reported

RED FLAGS

Look for complications of disease including cardiac and neurologic involvement

DIFFERENTIAL DIAGNOSIS

(a) Large Vessel Vasculitis: Takayasu arteritis; Giant-cell arteritis; Kawasaki disease (medium vessel); (b) Inflammatory Aortitis Related to Infection: Syphilis; Tuberculosis; (c) Inflammatory Aortitis Related to Other CTD: SLE; Rheumatoid arthritis; Ankylosing spondilitis; Behcet's disease; (d) Developmental Abnormalities: Marfan's syndrome; Congenital aortic coarctation

PHYSICAL EXAMINATION

Vitals: Pulse: Radial pulse may be absent; BP: Discrepancy between the arms & hypertension; RR: May be elevated if cardiac or pulmonary involvement; Temperature: May be elevated

Cutaneous: Cool cyanotic hands or arms suggestive of vascular occlusion; Cool, cyanotic feet

Head & Neck: Carotid and vertebral bruits

Respiratory: Subclavian bruits; Adventitious sounds due to CHF; Hemoptysis

Cardiovascular: Aortic regurgitation; Congestive heart failure (elevated JVP, edema, large heart, S3/S4); Pulmonary hypertension (elevated JVP, RV heave, pulmonic murmur, tricuspid regurgitation); Absent brachial pulse; Absent dorsalis pedis or posterior tibials; Absent femoral pulses or femoral bruits

Gastrointestinal: Aortic and renal bruits; Tenderness on palpation (mesenteric involvement)

Musculoskeletal: Arthralgia; arthritis is rare

Neurologic: Signs of CVA

INVESTIGATIONS

CBC: Normochromic normocytic anemia, reactive thrombocytosis, normal WBC

ESR/CRP: Usually elevated

Albumin: Low

Angiography is the Gold Standard: Complete aortic arteriography is useful for determining location and extent of disease; The lesions seen in TA are long, segmental stenoses with or without arterial occlusion; A classification system for angiographic findings is as follows: Type I - Branches of the aortic arch only; Type IIa - Ascending aorta, aortic arch and its branches; Type IIb - Ascending aorta, aortic arch and its branches, thoracic descending aorta; Type III - Thoracic descending aorta, abdominal aorta, and/or renal arteries; Type IV - Abdominal aorta and/or renal arteries; Type V - Combined features of type IIb and IV; Limitations of angiography include: Provides no information on the blood vessel wall; Invasive procedure associated with minimal risks

Computed Tomographic Angiography (CTA) and Magnetic Resonance Angiography (MRA): Advantages include visualization of the vessel wall and the non-invasive technique; Useful for following response to treatment

Pathology: Pathologic findings divided into inflammatory and fibrotic stages; (a) Inflammatory stage: Focal panarteritis with "skip lesions": Inflammation is localized to adventitia and outer parts of the media; Vasa vasoritis is seen in the adventitia; Infiltration of the media by lymphocytes and giant-cells (occasionally); Intimal thickening; (b) Fibrotic stage: Fibrosis with destruction of elastic tissue

MANAGEMENT

General: Education about the disease; Vocational counseling; Arthritis self management programs

Physiotherapy: Pain relieving strategies and interventions; Mobility aids (canes & walkers) and braces; Exercise to improve ROM, muscle strength, aerobic conditioning, and core stability training; Weight loss; Manual therapy (manipulation) when appropriate

Occupational Therapy: Splints and orthotics; Joint protection measures and energy conservation; Assistive devices; Lifestyle management

Corticosteroids: If patient has severe complications should consider IV Methylprednisolone; Otherwise, initiate Prednisone 1 mg/kg/day (40-60 mg) which can be given in divided doses (i.e. 20 mg PO TID); Increase the dose if the patient does not respond promptly; Continue the initial dose until all symptoms have disappeared and laboratory parameters have normalized (ESR/CRP); Slowly begin a tapering regimen such as: Reduce slowly by 5 mg every other week to 20 mg/day if the ESR remains normal; Below 20 mg reduce by 2.5 mg every 2-4 weeks as tolerated by symptoms and ESR; Below 10 mg reduce by 1 mg every 4 weeks as tolerated by symptoms and ESR

Repeat Vascular Imaging: Remember, about 50% of patients have active, progressive disease, despite normal ESR/CPR - therefore, repeat vascular imaging is important to guide immunosuppression

Osteoprotection: Given the dose and expected duration all patients should be placed on osteoprotective measures including: Education about glucocorticoid induced bone loss; Encouraged to exercise, stop smoking, and avoid excessive alcohol and caffeine; Calcium supplementation; Vitamin D; Bisphosphonates

Methotrexate: Methotrexate has been used with some success in an open label study of 18 patients; Doses of 20-25 mg are used for patients who relapse with corticosteroid treatment; Approximately 50% of patients treated with methotrexate will respond

Other Immunosuppressants: Cyclophosphamide, azathioprine, and mycophenolate mofetil have been helpful in some reported cases

Surgical: Indications for surgical or angioplastic management are as follows: Hypertension with critical renal artery stenosis; Extremity claudication limiting activities of daily living; Critical stenosis of three or more cerebral vessels; Moderate aortic regurgitation; Cardiac ischemia with confirmed coronary artery involvement; Surgery or angioplasty is best performed when disease is optimally controlled

PROGNOSIS

Risk Stratification for Poor Progression: Cardiac congestive heart failure associated with hypertension; Cerebrovascular disease

Prognosis: Overall 5 year survival rate ranges from 80-95% depending on severity of disease and aggressiveness of the intervention; Class IIb and III seem to have a worse prognosis; Prognosis depends upon complications of disease. No complications or a single mild complication has a much better prognosis than multiple complications.

VIRAL ARTHRITIS

DEFINITION & PATHOPHYSIOLOGY

Definition: An acute arthritis which develops during the prodromal phase of a viral infection, is usually symmetrical and polyarticular, and does not usually become chronic

Pathophysiology: Currently, no clear understanding of the mechanisms by which viruses induce arthritis. The following theories have been proposed: (a) Direct invasion of the joint; (b) Immune complex formation; (c) Dysregulation of the immune system; Viruses implicated with arthritic syndromes include: Hepatitis B & C; Rubella; Parvovirus B19; Human immunodeficiency virus (HIV); Alpha viruses; Adenovirus & coxsackieviruses; Mumps (paramyxoviridae)

PRESENTATION

Identifying Data: Age and patient sex is dependant upon the viral species: Hepatitis B & C: Risk factors for transmission; Rubella: Younger women; Parvo B19: More common in younger individuals. Arthritis is more common in adults and in women; HIV: Risk factors for transmission

Onset: Hepatitis B: Arthralgias most common; Can cause an immune complex mediated arthritis; Sudden and severe joint involvement which is limited to the prodromal phase of the hepatitis B infection; Involves small joints of the hands and the knees; Associated rash (urticarial, petechial, or maculopapular) in 40%; ***Hepatitis C:*** Arthritis & arthralgia independent of cryoglobulinemia; Mixed cryoglobulinemia type II (Raynaud's phenomenon, arthritis, & palpable purpura); ***Rubella:*** Arthritis may precede the maculopapular rash; Symmetric and migratory arthritis affecting the small joints of the hands, knees, wrists, ankles, and elbows; May have associated tenosynovitis and carpal tunnel syndrome; Arthritis is self-limited, resolving in days to weeks; ***Parvovirus B19:*** Rapid onset of symmetric polyarthritis; Primarily affects the hands and wrists; ***HIV:*** Arthralgias and myalgias; Acute onset of psoriatic arthritis; Vasculitis; Fibromyalgia; Diffuse infiltrative lymphocytosis syndrome (DILS)

Progression: Hepatitis B: Full recovery of arthritis with the onset of jaundice is the usual course; With chronic HBV, the most serious complication is the development of polyarteritis nodosa (10%); ***Hepatitis C:*** Mixed cryoglobulinemia type II (rash, arthritis, & palpable purpura); Development of fibromyalgia; ***Rubella:*** Usually self-limited, however, may become chronic in some cases; ***Parvovirus B19:*** Usually self-limited, however, may become chronic in 10% of cases

Constitutional Features: Fatigue, anorexia, weight loss, fevers, and general malaise may accompany viral arthritides

Functional Status: Patients may experience significant functional impairment during the acute inflammatory arthritis

RHEUMATOLOGIC REVIEW OF SYSTEMS

Hepatitis B: Acute and chronic hepatitis; Membranous or membranoproliferative; nephropathy, Polyarteritis nodosa

Hepatitis C: Mebranoproliferative glomerulonephritis; Thyroiditis; Porphyria cutanea tarda; Diabetes mellitus; Cryoglobulinemic vasculitis: Cryoglobulins consist of a monoclonal (type II) or polyclonal (type III) immunoglobulin directed against polyclonal IgG (hence the rheumatoid factor activity in 70-90%); HCV infection accounts for 90% of cases of mixed cryoglobulinemia; Develop a systemic small vessel vasculitis; Triad of palpable purpura, asthenia (weakness), and arthralgias begins the onset in most cases; Renal Involvement: Glomerulonephritis is the principal life-threatening complication; Nervous System Involvement: Mononeuritis multiplex; Corobral ischemia leading to stroke and TIA; Skin Involvement: Palpable purpura; Ulceration; Raynaud's phenomenon; Musculoskeletal Involvement: Arthritis & arthralgia; Sicca Features

Rubella: Maculopapular rash which usually starts on the face and spreads to involve the trunk and extremities; Lymphadenopathy

Parvovirus B19: Erythema infectiosum (slapped cheeks, reticular rash on the torso or extremities); Transient aplastic crisis

Human Immunodeficiency Virus (HIV): Articular: (a) Arthralgias (45%); (b) Reactive arthritis: Related to STDs acquired in high risk population, not HIV infection specifically; The incidence of HLA-B27 is the same in both HIV positive and HIV negative patients with reactive arthritis; May precede AIDS by several years; Oligoarthritis of lower extremities, urethritis common; conjunctivitis rare; Axial skeleton involvement rare; Can see severe erosive arthritis; (c) Psoriatic arthritis: Late in HIV infection; Significant clinical problem in patients not on anti-HIV treatment; (d) Undifferentiated spondyloarthropathy: Oligoarthritis, enthesitis, dactylitis, onycholysis, balanitis, uveitis or spondylitis but not enough to classify as Reiter's or psoriatic; (e) HIV-associated arthritis: Extreme disability & pain in knees and ankles lasting 1-6 weeks; No enthesopathy, mucocutaneous lesions, HLA-B27, and symptoms do not recur; (f) Painful articular syndrome (10%): Knees, shoulders, elbows - lasts 2 – 24 hrs; **Muscular:** (a) Myalgias; (b) Polymyositis: Clinically same as idiopathic polymyositis; Zidovudine-myopathy – after 11 months of treatment, clinically indistinguishable from polymyositis; (c) Myopathy (eg. HIV-wasting, zidovudine-induced, nemaline rod): Non-inflammatory, necrotizing myopathy & HIV-wasting syndrome in > 40% pts with myopathy (HIV); **Diffuse Infiltrative Lymphocytosis Syndrome (DILS) (5%):** Dx with HIV, bilateral salivary gland enlargement, and histological confirmation of salivary or lacrimal gland lymphocytic infiltration (no granulomas or neoplastic enlargement); Symptoms can start ~ 3 yrs pre-HIV diagnosis; Sicca, parotid gland enlargement, persistent circulating CD8 T cell lymphocytosis, diffuse visceral lymphocytic infiltration in HIV pt. Pulmonary involvement most serious with lymphocytic interstitial pneumonitis (decreased with protease inhibitors). Neurologic, hepatomegaly, transaminitis, renal insufficiency, interstitial nephritis, hyperkalemia, Type IV RTA, polymyositis, and lymphoma can all be seen. Rare to have autoantibodies with DILS; **Vasculitis:** PAN, GCA, Takayasu's, hypersensitivity angiitis, Henoch-Schonlein purpura, Wegener's granulomatosis, primary angiitis of CNS, Behcet's disease, and Kawasaki's disease; **Infection:** (a) Septic arthritis: Not common – no different than rest of population; Atypical mycobacterium consider in advanced HIV; Most common organism - Staphylococcus aureus; Fungal with severe immunosuppression; (b) Osteomyelitis - rare; (c) Pyomyositis: Seen in Africa & India; Fever, local muscle pain, erythema & swelling; Affects quads (single abscess in 75% cases); S. aureus – usually; Salmonella enteriditis, microsporidia, toxoplasmosis gondii have been seen; (d) Other: Soft tissue rheumatism (eg. tendonitis, bursitis); Fibromyalgia (30%); Avascular necrosis (related to protease-inhibitors); Gout

RISK FACTORS

HIV and Hepatitis B & C: Sexual transmission; Blood transfusions; Intravenous drug abuse; Organ transplantation; Tattoos; Nosocomial transmission (health care workers); Some cases have no obvious risk factors for transmission; **Rubella:** Wild-type rubella exposure; Some vaccines; **Parvovirus B19:** Exposure to parvovirus B19

FAMILY HISTORY

Vertical transmission with hepatitis B & C and HIV

RED FLAGS
Rule out other causes of acute arthritis; Consider HIV

DIFFERENTIAL DIAGNOSIS
(a) Infectious Arthritis: Viral arthritis; Subacute bacterial endocarditis; HIV; Gonococcal arthritis; Non-gonococcal bacterial arthritis; Lyme disease; *(b) Crystalline Arthropathies; (c) Rheumatoid Arthritis & Variants:* Rheumatoid arthritis; Adult onset Still's disease; Rheumatic fever; *(d) Seronegative Arthritides:* Psoriatic arthritis; Inflammatory bowel disease; Reactive arthritis; *(e) Connective Tissue Diseases:* Systemic lupus erythematosus; Inflammatory myositis; Sjogren's syndrome; *(f) Vasculitis:* (a) Large vessel vasculitis: Takayasu arteritis; Giant-cell arteritis; (b) Medium vessel vasculitis: Polyarteritis nodosa; Kawasaki disease; (b) Small vessel vasculitis: ANCA related - Wegener's granulomatosis; Churg-Strauss syndrome; Microscopic polyangiitis; Immune complex related: Hypersensitivity vasculitis - Cutaneous leukocytoclastic vasculitis; Cryoglobulinemic vasculitis; Connective tissue disease associated; Henoch-Schonlein purpura; Urticarial vasculitis; Miscellaneous: Malignancy related vasculitis; Behcet's Disease; Inflammatory bowel disease; *(g) Arthritis associated with Systemic Disease:* Thyroid disorders; Sarcoidosis

PHYSICAL EXAMINATION
Vitals: Pulse: Usually normal, elevated if unwell; BP: Normal; RR: Usually normal; Temperature: May have low-grade fever
Cutaneous: Erythema infectiosum rash with parvovirus B19; Rash & palpable purpura with cryoglobulinemia; Raynaud's phenomenon
Head & Neck: Lymphadenopathy
Respiratory: Axillary adenopathy
Cardiovascular: No Specific abnormalities
Gastrointestinal: Tender liver with hepatitis; Splenomegaly
Musculoskeletal: Inflammatory arthritis affecting the PIPs, MCPs, and wrists
Neurologic: Proximal myopathy with HIV

INVESTIGATIONS
CBC: Anemia (aplasia with parvovirus B19), reactive leukocytosis, reactive thrombocytosis. Lymphopenia with advanced HIV.
ESR/CRP: Elevated
Creatinine: Elevated with concomitant glomerulonephritis
Urinalysis: Concomitant glomerulonephritis
AST, ALT, LDH: May be elevated with hepatitis infection
Rheumatoid factor: Seen in high titers with cryoglobulinemia
Hepatitis B: Early phase of acute infection is characterized by the presence of HepBsAg, HepBeAg, IgM anti-HBc, and HBV DNA; HepBsAg and HepBeAg gradually disappear with IgM anti-HBC remaining during a "window" period. HBV DNA may or may not be found. Recovery of acute infection is seen with development of anti-HBs, anti-HBe, IgG anti-HBc, and the absence of HBV DNA; Chronic hepatitis B infection is seen with persistence of HepBsAg, HepBeAg, IgG anti-HBc, and the continued presence of HBV DNA
Hepatitis C: ELISA for anti-HCV; HCV RNA detection is the gold standard
Parvovirus B19: IgM antibodies to B19
Rubella: IgM antibodies to rubella
HIV: ELISA test for HIV; Confirmatory western blot
Radiology: In acute phases of viral related arthritis, soft-tissue swelling is the most common finding

MANAGEMENT
General: Education about the disease; Vocational counseling; Arthritis self management programs

Physiotherapy: Pain relieving strategies and interventions; Mobility aids (canes & walkers) and braces; Exercise to improve ROM, muscle strength, aerobic conditioning, and core stability training; Weight loss; Manual therapy (manipulation) when appropriate

Occupational Therapy: Splints and orthotics; Joint protection measures and energy conservation; Assistive devices; Lifestyle management

Hepatitis B: Symptomatic treatment with NSAIDs; Treatment of Hepatitis B associated PAN: Initial high dose Corticosteroids (see below) for the first few weeks of disease to control severe life-threatening manifestations; Conventional immunosuppression treatment enhances the viruses ability to replicate and may jeopardize the patients outcome. Instead a combination of plasma exchange and anti-viral agents seems to be effective. Plasma Exchange: To remove circulating immune complexes (9-12 exchanges over 3 weeks); Anti-Viral Agents: Interferon-alpha-2b or lamivudine; A good prognostic sign is conversion from HBeAg to HBeAb

Hepatitis C: Symptomatic treatment with NSAIDs; Interferon-alpha and ribavirin therapy for HCV infection; Corticosteroids and cyclophosphamide are often required for cryoglobulinemic vasculitis

Rubella: Symptomatic treatment with NSAIDs

Parvovirus B19: Symptomatic treatment with NSAIDs

Human Immunodeficiency Virus (HIV): Symptomatic treatment with NSAIDs; Intra-articular corticosteroid injections for localized involvement; Low-dose prednisone may be beneficial in some cases; Sulfasalazine; Hydroxychloroquine; Methotrexate and other immunosuppressants should be used with care

PROGNOSIS
Generally, viral related arthritides are self-limited processes that improve after a two week course. It is rare for chronic arthritis to develop.

HIV and hepatitis B & C may have a worse prognosis due to the chronic nature of these infections.

WEGENER'S GRANULOMATOSIS (WG)

DEFINITION & PATHOPHYSIOLOGY

Definition: A multi-systemic disease characterized by a necrotizing granulomatous vasculitis affecting small blood vessels. Extra-vascular granulomatous inflammation may also occur.

Pathophysiology: The initiating factor(s) responsible for the development of vasculitis is/are unknown; Endothelial cells are quickly activated and upregulate adhesion molecules, cytokines, growth factors, and receptors recruiting and activating components of the innate and adaptive immune systems; PMNs express antigens (MPO, PR3) on their surface and are activated through ANCA binding to these antigens; Activated PMNs release MPO, PR3, & reactive oxygen species further upregulating the immune response, which may result in significant damage to endothelial cells

PRESENTATION

Identifying Data: Majority of patients are adults; Male to female ratio is equal; Prevalence is about 1 in 20,000 - 30,000 people

Onset: Essentially, all patients seek medical attention because of upper or lower airway symptoms with 30% having both. *(a) Upper Airway* - Due to chronic inflammation, vasculitis, and tissue necrosis: Chronic sinusitis is a presenting feature in 50% of cases - may have purulent discharge; Epistaxis; Oral & nasal mucosal inflammation & ulceration; Otitis media due to inflammation of the naso-pharyngeal mucosa obstructing the auditory canal; Laryngeal inflammation results in hoarseness of the voice; Tracheal inflammation leads to subglottic stenosis causing stridor and respiratory difficulty; *(b) Lower Airway* - Characteristically due to chronic granulomatous inflammation; acute inflammation may result in neutrophilic infiltration: Chronic cough; Dyspnea with pneumonitis; Hemoptysis with alveolar hemorrhage; *(c) Musculoskeletal:* Arthralgias/myalgias; Inflammatory arthritis; *(d) Renal:* Present in 15-50%; Rapidly progressive glomerulonephritis

Progression: The course of the disease may be indolent or progressive. As the disease progresses, inflammation in organs may result in permanent damage and/ or deformity and new organs may become involved. Untreated WG affecting the kidneys and lower respiratory tract is uniformly fatal and prior to the 1970s 50% of patients survived five months and 80% dead at one year.

Constitutional Features: Fever, night sweats, anorexia, malaise, weight loss, and fatigue may be prominent features

Functional Status: Functional status may be considerably reduced with severe disease

RHEUMATOLOGIC REVIEW OF SYSTEMS

Musculoskeletal Involvement: Arthralgias and myalgias are common; Inflammatory arthritis is much less common and when present does not result in destruction

Mucocutaneous Involvement: Palpable purpura; Subcutaneous nodules; Ulcers, vesicles, and papules

Ocular Involvement: Conjuctivitis; Dacrocystitis; Proptosis due to retro-orbital pseudotumor; Uveitis; Scleritis / episcleritis; Corneal ulceration; Optic neuritis

Neurologic Involvement: Mononeuritis multiplex is the most frequent peripheral neurologic abnormality; Cranial neuropathies; CVA, seizures, and cerebritis

Cardiac Involvement: Pericarditis

Respiratory Involvement: Chronic inflammation with granuloma formation leads to the characteristic typical findings of multiple, bilateral nodal infiltrates that tend to cavitate and/or are associated with fixed focal alveolar infiltrates; Acute inflammation is seen as acute pneumonitis and is thought secondary to necrotizing vasculitis with neutrophilic infiltration; Pleural effusions are seen in 20%

Renal Involvement: 75% of patients will eventually develop glomerulonephritis; The typical lesion is pauci-immune, focal and segmental, necrotizing glomerulonephritis; In more severe cases a diffuse proliferative and crescentic GN occurs; Renal disease is usually asymptomatic

RISK FACTORS
No known risk factors

FAMILY HISTORY
No known family history

RED FLAGS
Must always rule out sepsis as it can present as multi-organ failure and can mimic vasculitis; Refractory vasculitis is an infection until proven otherwise (it may also be damage)

DIFFERENTIAL DIAGNOSIS
Small Vessel Vasculitis: (a) ANCA Related (Wegener's granulomatosis; Churg-Strauss syndrome; Microscopic polyangiitis); (b) Immune Complex Related (Hypersensitivity vasculitis - Cutaneous leukocytoclastic vasculitis; Cryoglobulinemic vasculitis; Connective tissue disease associated vasculitis; Henoch-Schonlein purpura; Urticarial vasculitis); (c) Miscellaneous (Malignancy related vasculitis; Behcet's Disease; Inflammatory bowel disease); (d) Granulomatous Infections: Tuberculosis; Syphilis; Fungi; (e) Pseudo-vasculitis syndromes: SBE & atrial myxoma

PHYSICAL EXAMINATION
Vitals: Pulse: Elevated if unwell; BP: HTN if concomitant renal disease; RR: Elevated RR may be an indicator of underlying pulmonary disease. Listen for stridor. Temperature: Fever is not uncommon

Cutaneous: Splinter hemorrhages and nailfold infarcts; Other skin lesions (palpable purpura, nodules, ulceration, vesicles)

Head & Neck: Ocular involvement; Nasal mucosal inflammation & ulceration, saddle-nose deformity; Oral mucosal inflammation & ulceration; Hoarse voice; Serous otitis media; Lymphadenopathy

Respiratory: Stridor and wheezing; Adventitous sounds; Reduced breath sounds due to hemorrhage, edema, or pleural effusion

Cardiovascular: Pericardial friction rub

Gastrointestinal: No specific findings

Musculoskeletal: Inflammatory arthritis

Neurologic: Neuropathy - polyneuropathy or mononeuritis multiplex

INVESTIGATIONS
CBC: Normochromic normocytic anemia, leukocytosis - Can see eosinophilia, and reactive thrombocytosis

Albumin: low

Complement: Normal or elevated C3, C4

Creatinine: Elevated

ESR/CRP: Elevated

Urinalysis: Hematuria and proteinuria

ANCA: c-ANCA - The presence of a c-ANCA represents antibodies to proteinase-3 and is highly specific (98%) for the diagnosis of WG. The sensitivity varies from 30-90% which is due to fluctuating levels of c-ANCA based on disease severity and extent. Some studies suggest a rising c-ANCA may be indicative of disease activity.
p-ANCA - Seen in 10% of cases

Tissue Pathology: The highest yield for tissue pathology comes from open lung biopsies followed by renal biopsies. Three major pathologic findings in the lung include: (a) Parenchymal necrosis; (b) Vasculitis in arteries, veins, and capillaries; (c) Granulomatous inflammation with a mixed cellular infiltrate. The minor features include: (d) Tissue eosinophilia; (e) Alveolar hemorrhage; (f) Interstitial fibrosis; (g) Lipoid pneumonia; (h) Bronchial lesions

MANAGEMENT

General: Education about the disease; Vocational counseling; Arthritis self management programs

Physiotherapy: Pain relieving strategies and interventions; Mobility aids (canes & walkers) and braces; Exercise to improve ROM, muscle strength, aerobic conditioning, and core stability training; Weight loss; Manual therapy (manipulation) when appropriate

Occupational Therapy: Splints and orthotics; Joint protection measures and energy conservation; Assistive devices; Lifestyle management

Supportive: Treatment of pulmonary-renal syndrome usually requires fluid resuscitation with hemodynamic and ventilatory support; Renal failure requires nephrology consultation as may require dialysis

High-Dose Corticosteroids: Pulsed IV Methylprednisolone 1 gram over 60 minutes daily for 3-5 days; After 3 days give Prednisone 1 mg/kg PO OD - This can be given in 3 - 4 divided daily doses for 7 - 10 days consolidating to a single morning dose by 2-3 weeks. As the patient improves clinically and the ESR normalizes the Prednisone can be slowly tapered. *Example Tapering Regimens:* Taper to 50% original dose by decreasing by 2.5 mg q10days; Maintain at this dose for 3 weeks; Taper to 20 mg by decreasing by 2.5 mg qweekly; Taper to 10 mg by decreasing by 1 mg q2weeks; Maintain at 10 mg for 3 weeks; Taper to 0 by decreasing by 1 mg qmonthly OR Taper by 5 mg on alternate days qweekly gradually converting the treatment regimen to alternate daily Prednisone; Thereby the Prednisone is tapered by 2.5-5 mg each week until it is discontinued

Cyclophosphamide: Indications for Cyclophosphamide are as follows: (a) Severe pulmonary-renal disease; (b) Mononeuritis multiplex; (c) CNS disease; (d) RPGN; (e) Mesenteric vasculitis; (f) Cardiac involvement; (g) Alveolar hemorrhage

Pulsed IV Cyclophosphamide: Initial pulses may vary from 0.25 to 2.5 grams at intervals of 1 week to 1 month. In Europe, mini-pulses given more frequently are routinely used. Example orders for Cyclophosphamide see page 166.

Oral Cyclophosphamide: More effective (less relapses) and used second line when IV fails; Given as 1-2 mg/kg/day orally for a maximum of one year. Use cyclophosphamide as the induction agent aiming to stop it at 3-6 months and continue with one of the maintenance agents. The initial NIH regimen states to continue cyclophosphamide for one year after remission then taper by 25 mg every 2-3 months, however, they do state that the "necessary duration of treatment is open to question and our views have changed over the years". REMEMBER TO PROPHYLAX WITH SEPTRA

Remission with Azathioprine: European Union Vasculitis Study Group used the CYCAZAREM regimen (2 studies one in abstract form in *A&R, 1999* and the other in *NEJM 349:1, 2003*). *Induction:* Oral Cyclophosphamide **2 mg/kg/day for 3 months**; *Remission:* Oral Cyclophosphamide 1.5 mg/kg/day OR Azathioprine 2 mg/kg/day; *Results:* 93% remission rate with cyclophosphamide & prednisone; Mortality at 18 months ~ 5%; Relapse rate 14-15% (same in both CYC and AZA groups); Adverse events 21-26%

Remission with Methotrexate: Has been used for maintenance of remission in patients with Wegener's Granulomatosis; Oral Cyclophosphamide was used to initiate disease remission and weekly Methotrexate was substituted given 1-2 days after the last dose of CYC. An open labeled trial showed equal efficacy in maintaining remission between MTX and CYC (*A&R 1999*). Extended follow-up showed a higher rate of renal relapse (*A&R June, 2002, Am J Med, April, 2003*).

Mycophenolate Mofetil: Also under investigation as a maintenance agent

Trimethoprim/Sulfamethoxazole (Septra): 1 DS PO 3x per week is used as prophylaxis for Pneumocystis carinii in patients taking Cyclophosphamide; Not used for induction but may be useful for remission in a patient with localized upper airway WG; In very mild disease (nasal only) TMP/SMX may be used alone (1 DS PO BID)

Chlorambucil, Cyclosporine, and Tacrolimus: Have been successfully used as second line agents in cyclophosphamide failures

IVIG: Conflicting results

Plasmapheresis/Plasma Exchange: Uncertain benefit & undeniable risks

Treatment of Localized Disease: Nasal Perforation & Saddle Nose Deformity: Do not repair perforated nasal septae; Correct saddle nose deformities once the inflammation has subsided; ***Subglottic Stenosis:*** Intralesional corticosteroids and mechanical dilatation is the most effective therapy; Carbon dioxide laser treatments are contraindicated because they may exacerbate the condition; Systemic therapy with Corticosteroids or Cyclophosphamide is usually not effective; Tracheostomy is sometimes required; ***Orbital Inflammation:*** Results from extension of inflammation from the sinuses or from retro-orbital pseudotumor; Systemic therapy should be instituted; Pulsed IV Methylprednisolone is sometimes helpful in those resistant to oral therapy.

PROGNOSIS

Risk Stratification for Poor Progression: Rapid onset with rapid progression; Generalized involvement

Prognosis: Historically, mortality figures from early trials (prior to 1970) show a 5 month survival of 50%; Aggressive treatment with Corticosteroids and Cyclophosphamide has: Shown marked improvement in 90%; Achieved clinical remission in 75%; Reduced the 8 year mortality to 13%

ANALGESICS

ACETAMINOPHEN (TYLENOL, PANADOL, TEMPRA, ✚ABENOL, ATASOL, FROSST 222 AF)

INDICATIONS
Approved: Treatment of mild to moderate pain and fever
DOSE & DRUG ADMINISTRATION
Dose: 650-1000 mg PO q4-6h (10-15 mg/kg/day); *Max Dose:* 4 g/day; *Supplied:* Tablets: 160 ✚, 325, & 500 mg; Del. release tablets: 650 mg; Soft-chew tablets: 80 & 160 mg; Gelcaps: 325 ✚ & 500 mg; Liquid: 80 mg/2.5 mL, 80, 120mL, & 160 mg/5mL, 500 mg/15 mL; Suppositories: 80, 120, 125, 300, 325, 650 mg;
DOSE ADJUSTMENT
Hepatic Failure: Acetaminophen undergoes primary hepatic metabolism; use with caution in patients with severe hepatic impairment or a history of excessive alcohol use (> 3 drinks/day). Recommend < 2 g per day with severe hepatic impairment.
Renal Failure: CrCl > 50 ml/min: No initial dose adjustment; *CrCl 10-50 ml/min:* Dose initially at q6h intervals; *CrCl < 10 ml/min:* Dose initially at q8h intervals.
ONSET OF ACTION
Initial Response: 30 minutes
MONITORING
No specific laboratory monitoring is necessary
CONTRAINDICATIONS & PRECAUTIONS
(a) Hypersensitivity to acetaminophen; (b) Excessive alcohol use (> 3 drinks/day)
TOXICITY
When used as directed, acetaminophen is virtually free of side effects
PREGNANCY & LACTATION
Pregnancy: Considered to be a safe medication to use during pregnancy, although, no formal studies have been conducted. (**CATEGORY NOT LISTED**)
Lactation: Although small amounts of acetaminophen are excreted in breast milk; it is generally considered a safe medication to use while breast feeding.
DRUG INTERACTIONS
Acetaminophen may ↑ toxicity of: Warfarin (occasional elevations in INR)
Drugs which may ↓ acetaminophen levels: St. Johns wort
MECHANISM OF ACTION
Acetaminophen is the active metabolite. The site and mechanism of action of acetaminophen is unclear but is believed to be related to the inhibition of prostaglandin synthetase. It is postulated that the analgesic effect is produced by an elevation of the pain threshold and fever reduction is mediated by direct action on the hypothalamic heat regulating center that dissipates body heat via vasodilatation and sweating.
PHARMACOKINETICS
Bioavail: 80%; *1/2 Life:* 1-4 hours; *Metab:* Metabolized in the liver via glucuronidation, sulfation, and by the mixed function oxidase system; *Prot Bind:* Low – mainly exists in the free form; *Excret:* Metabolites in the urine

AMITRIPTYLINE (ELAVIL, VANATRIP)

INDICATIONS
Approved: Management of depressive illness; *Off-Label Uses:* Chronic pain, fibromyalgia, neuropathic pain

DOSE & DRUG ADMINISTRATION
Initial Dose: 10-25 mg PO qhs for fibro, 25 mg PO TID for depression; *Max Dose:* 300 mg/day; *Supplied:* Tablets: 10,25,50,75,100,150 mg

DOSE ADJUSTMENT
Hepatic Failure: Amitriptyline undergoes primary hepatic metabolism; use with caution in patients with severe hepatic impairment.
Renal Failure: No specific dosage reduction recommended.

ONSET OF ACTION
Initial Response: A sedative effect can be observed within an hour which is useful to aid in restoration of sleep in fibromyalgia patients. It may take up to 30 days before an adequate anti-depressant effect is seen.

MONITORING
No specific laboratory monitoring is necessary

CONTRAINDICATIONS & PRECAUTIONS
(a) Known hypersensitivity to amitriptyline; (b) Current MAO inhibitor use or use within the past 14 days; (c) Acute myocardial infarction or congestive heart failure and other cardiovascular disorders including arrhythmias; (d) History of seizures; (e) Impaired hepatic function or hepatic damage; (f) Narrow angle glaucoma; (g) Hyperthyroidism or thyroid replacement medication

TOXICITY
Reversible: (a) Gen: Diaphoresis, weight gain, taste disturbances; *(b) GI:* Nausea, vomiting, constipation, dry mouth; *(c) CNS:* Drowsiness, fatigue, dizziness, headache, akathisia; *(d) GU:* Urinary retention
Potentially Serious: (a) CNS: Seizures in overdose, hallucinations, delusions, confusional states; *(b) CVS:* Unexplained death, arrhythmias, myocardial infarction, orthostatic hypotension; *(c) Hem:* Anemia, thrombocytopenia, leukopenia, agranulocytosis, eosinophilia; *(d) Optho:* Acute angle glaucoma

PREGNANCY & LACTATION
Pregnancy: **RISK CANNOT BE RULED OUT. (CATEGORY C)**
Lactation: Amitriptyline is detected in breast milk, nursing is generally not recommended.

DRUG INTERACTIONS
Amitriptyline may ↑ toxicity of: MAO-I inhibitors (do not use together or within 14 days of each other), anticholinergic agents, sympathomimetics, alcohol, carbamazepine, Warfarin (↑ INR).
Drugs which may ↑ toxicity of amitriptyline: CNS sedating drugs, cimetidine, other tricyclic antidepressants (respiratory), SSRI, ketoconazole, quinidine. Amitriptyline may prolong the QT interval; do not combine two or more agents capable of prolonging the QT interval since additive effects on cardiac conduction are possible. The sedative effects of amitriptyline are additive with alcohol, other tricyclic antidepressants, barbiturates, and benzodiazepines.

MECHANISM OF ACTION
Amitriptyline is a dibenzocycloheptadiene derivative. Amitriptyline is the active form. Amitriptyline inhibits the membrane pump responsible for the uptake of norepinephrine and serotonin in adrenergic and serotonergic neurons. This effect may potentiate or prolong neuronal activity since reuptake of these biogenic amines is important in terminating transmitting activity. Interference with the reuptake of norepinephrine and/or serotonin may be responsible for the antidepressant effects. Other mechanisms of action include potentiation of the descending analgesic pathways, upregulating CNS endorphins, & effect on peripheral pain receptors.

PHARMACOKINETICS
Bioavail: Moderate (60% absorption); *1/2 Life:* 31 - 46 hours; *Metab:* Cytochrome P450 2D6, 2C9, & 3A4 pathways. Metabolized in the liver via glucuronidation & sulfation; *Prot Bind:* High (99%); *Excret:* Glucuronide and sulfide metabs in the urine

CYCLOBENZAPRINE (FLEXERIL)

INDICATIONS
Approved: Muscle spasm associated with acute, painful musculoskeletal conditions;
Off-Label Uses: Fibromyalgia

DOSE & DRUG ADMINISTRATION
Initial Dose: 10 mg PO TID for muscle spasm, 5 - 40 mg PO qhs for fibromyalgia;
Max Dose: 60 mg/day; *Supplied:* Tablets: 5 & 10 mg

DOSE ADJUSTMENT
Hepatic Failure: Cyclobenzaprine undergoes primary hepatic metabolism; use 5 mg/day in mild hepatic impairment and avoid use with severe hepatic impairment.
Renal Failure: No specific dosage reduction is recommended.

ONSET OF ACTION
Initial Response: Clinical improvement has been observed as early as the first day of therapy, however, may take 1-2 weeks for peak effect.

MONITORING
No specific laboratory monitoring is necessary

CONTRAINDICATIONS & PRECAUTIONS
(a) Known hypersensitivity to cyclobenzaprine; (b) Current MAO inhibitor use or use within 14 days; (c) Acute recovery phase of myocardial infarction; (d) Arrhythmias, conduction disturbances, or heart block; (e) Hyperthyroidism and thyroid replacement medications; (f) History of seizures

TOXICITY
Reversible: (a) Gen: Taste disturbances, fatigue, dizziness; *(b) GI:* Nausea, vomiting, constipation, dry mouth; *(c) CNS:* Drowsiness, headache, blurred vision, confusion, tinnitus
Potentially Serious: (a) CNS: Extra-pyramidal symptoms; *(b) CVS:* Unexplained death, arrhythmias, myocardial infarction; *(c) GI:* Abnormal liver function; *(d) Endo:* SIADH, gynecomastia, galactorrhea; *(e) Hem:* Bone marrow depression

PREGNANCY & LACTATION
Pregnancy: NO EVIDENCE OF RISK IN HUMANS. (CATEGORY B)
Lactation: Unknown whether cyclobenzaprine is excreted in breast milk. Since cyclobenzaprine is closely related to the tricyclic antidepressants, caution should be used when given to a nursing mother.

DRUG INTERACTIONS
Cyclobenzaprine may ↑ toxicity of: Alcohol, barbiturates, & other CNS sedatives

MECHANISM OF ACTION
Cyclobenzaprine is the active form. Cyclobenzaprine is structurally similar to tricyclic antidepressants and acts in the CNS to reduce skeletal muscle activity. The net effect of cyclobenzaprine is a reduction in tonic somatic motor activity, influencing both gamma and alpha motor systems.

PHARMACOKINETICS
Bioavail: Oral absorption is almost complete; *1/2 Life:* 24 - 72 hours; *Metab:* Metabolized in the liver via glucuronidation; *Prot Bind:* High (99%); *Excret:* Glucuronide metabolites in the urine

GABAPENTIN (NEURONTIN)

INDICATIONS
Approved: Epilepsy, post-herpetic neuralgia; *Off-Label Uses:* Neuropathic pain
DOSE & DRUG ADMINISTRATION
Initial Dose: Day 1 - 300 mg, Day 2: 300 mg BID, Day 3: 300 mg TID; *Dose Increments:* Dose may be increased up to 1800 mg/day titrating to pain. In general, doses > 1800 mg have little increased effect; *Max Dose:* 3600 mg/day; *Supplied:* Capsules: 100, 300, & 400 mg; Tablets: 600 & 800 mg; Liquid: 250 mg/5mL
DOSE ADJUSTMENT
Hepatic Failure: None, gabapentin is not metabolized.
Renal Failure: CrCl > 60 ml/min: 900-3600 mg/d (300 tid, 400 tid, 600 tid, 800 tid,1200 tid); *CrCl 30-59 ml/min:* 400-1400 mg /d (200 bid, 300 bid, 400 bid, 500 bid, 700 bid); *CrCl 15-29 ml/min:* 200-700 mg/d (200 qd, 300 qd, 400 qd, 500 qd, 700 qd); *CrCl <15 ml/min:* 100-300 mg/d (100 qd, 125 qd, 150 qd, 200 qd, 300 qd).
ONSET OF ACTION
Initial Response: Clinical improvement has been observed as early as the first day of therapy, however, may take greater than 6 weeks for peak effect.
MONITORING
No specific laboratory monitoring is necessary
CONTRAINDICATIONS & PRECAUTIONS
(a) Known hypersensitivity to gabapentin; (b) Use with caution in patients with impaired renal function; (c) Withdraw slowly as may precipitate a seizure; (d) Use with caution in the elderly (sedation)
TOXICITY
Reversible: (a) CVS: Peripheral edema; *(b) CNS:* Somnolence, dizziness, ataxia, fatigue, depression, tremor, dysarthria, nervousness; *(d) Mucocut:* Pruritis; *(e) GI:* Weight gain, nausea, vomiting, dyspepsia; *(f) Optho:* Blurred vision, diplopia
Potentially Serious: (a) Hem: Leukopenia
PREGNANCY & LACTATION
Pregnancy: RISK CANNOT BE RULED OUT. (CATEGORY C)
Lactation: Unknown whether gabapentin is excreted in breast milk, therefore, nursing is generally not recommended.
DRUG INTERACTIONS
Drugs which may ↓ gabapentin levels: Antacids (reduce bioavailability); *Drugs which may ↑ gabapentin levels:* Cimetidine, morphine; *Drugs which may ↑ toxicity of gabapentin:* Alcohol (sedation)
MECHANISM OF ACTION
Gabapentin is the active form. The mechanism of action of gabapentin is unknown. Gabapentin is structurally related to the neurotransmitter GABA, although it does not interact with GABA receptors, is not converted to GABA, and is not an inhibitor of GABA uptake or degradation.
PHARMACOKINETICS
Bioavailability: Oral absorption is 50 - 60%; *Half Life:* 5 - 6 hours; *Metabolism:* No appreciable metabolism in humans; *Protein Binding:* None; *Excretion:* Excreted as unchanged drug in the urine 56 - 80%

OPIOID ANALGESICS – GENERAL INFORMATION

INDICATIONS
Approved: Relief of mild, moderate, and severe pain.

EQUIANALGESIC DOSE INFORMATION

Generic Name	Trade Name	★PO Dose	★IM Dose	Freq
Codeine	Tylenol® #1, #2, #3, #4, Codeine-Contin®	200 mg	130 mg	q4h
Fentanyl	Sublimaze®	---	0.05 mg	-
Hydromorphone	Dilaudid®, Hydromorph-Contin®	7.5 mg	1.5 mg	q6h
Meperidine	Demerol®	300 mg	75 mg	q4h
Morphine	Morphine®	30-60 mg	10 mg	q4h
LA Morphine	M-Eslon®, MS-Contin®	90 mg	-	q12h
Oxycodone	Supeudol®, Percocet®, Percodan®	30 mg	15 mg	q6h
Propoxyphene	Darvon®	195 mg	---	q4h

DOSE ADJUSTMENT
Hepatic Failure: Use with caution since the opioid analgesics may have a prolonged duration and cumulative effect in patients with hepatic impairment. Use the lowest dose whenever possible.

Renal Failure: Use with caution since the opioid analgesics may have a prolonged duration and cumulative effect in patients with renal impairment. Use the lowest dose whenever possible.

MONITORING
No specific laboratory monitoring is necessary

CONTRAINDICATIONS & PRECAUTIONS
(a) Known hypersensitivity to opioid analgesics; (b) Diarrhea caused by poisoning; (c) Current MAO inhibitor use or use within the past 14 days; (d) Acute respiratory depression, acute asthma attack, or upper airway obstruction; (e) Use with care in the elderly; (f) Cardiac arrhythmias

TOXICITY
Reversible: (a) Gen: Diaphoresis, weakness; ***(b) GI:*** Nausea, vomiting, constipation, dry mouth; ***(c) CNS:*** Drowsiness, sedation, euphoria, dysphoria, headache, agitation, seizures, mood alterations, dreams, hallucinations & disorientation; ***(d) Genitourinary:*** Urinary retention; ***(e) Mucocut:*** Rash

Potentially Serious: (a) Abuse: Psychological or physical dependence; ***(b) CNS:*** Severe CNS depression, hallucinations & disorientation; ***(c) CVS:*** Hypotension; ***(d) Resp:*** Severe respiratory depression & respiratory arrest; ***(e) Other:*** Withdrawal syndrome

DRUG INTERACTIONS
Opioids may ↑ toxicity of: MAO-inhibitors (do not use together or within 14 days of each other), warfarin (monitor INR closely), neuromuscular blocking agents; ***Drugs which may ↑ toxicity of opioids:*** CNS sedating drugs, drugs with anti-muscarinic activity, cimetidine, tricyclic antidepressants (respiratory)

MECHANISM OF ACTION
Opioids produce their effect by interacting with specific receptors distributed throughout the central nervous system, peripheral nervous system, and the

gastrointestinal tract. Opioid-receptor activation results in inhibition of adenyl cyclase activity, activation of receptor-operated K^+ currents, and suppression of voltage-gated Ca^{2+} currents. These effects cause hyperpolarization of the cell membrane, which decreases neurotransmitter release, resulting in less pain transmission. Patients still perceive some pain, but it does not bother them.

There are 5 opioid receptors – mu, kappa, sigma, delta, and epsilon. Opioid analgesia occurs at the mu, kappa, and sigma receptors. Most analgesia is mediated through mu-1 receptors located within the brain which is also primarily responsible for the euphoric effects of the opioids.

CODEINE PHOSPHATE (TYLENOL 2, 3, 4, ♣CODEINE CONTIN®, ♣EMTEC, ♣EMPRACET, FIORINAL WITH CODEINE, ♣FIORINAL C1/4 & C1/ 2, FIORICET WITH CODEINE, ♣LENOLTEC, ♣FROSST 292, ♣TECNAL C1/ 4 & C1/2)

INDICATIONS
Approved: Pain, cough, & ♣ diarrhea.
DOSE & DRUG ADMINISTRATION
Initial Dose: Start with a low dose 15 - 60 mg PO q4-6h; *Max Dose:* The most common codeine preparation is Tylenol #3®. The dose of acetaminophen must not exceed the recommended dose (<4g/day).
Supplied: Reg Tablets. 15, 30, & 60 mg; *Liquid:* 15mg/5ml ; *Injectable Sol'n:* 30 & 60 mg/mL. *Acetaminophen with Codeine (#2, #3, #4):* 300 mg Acetaminophen/ 15, 30, & 60 mg codeine (♣Tylenol and Lenoltec include 15 mg of caffeine while Emtec and Empracet do not contain caffeine). *ASA with Codeine:* 300 mg ASA/15 & 30 mg codeine (♣*Frosst 292* tablets contain 15 mg of caffeine and 30 mg of codeine). *Fiorinal with Codeine:* 330 mg ASA/ 50 mg butalbital/ 40 mg caffeine/ 30 mg codeine (♣*Fiorinal C1/4, C1/2 & Tecnal C1/4, C1/2* contain 15 & 30 mg of codeine). *Fioricet with Codeine:* 330 mg Acetaminophen/ 50 mg butalbital/ 40 mg caffeine/ 30 mg codeine. ♣*Codeine-Contin®* tablets: 50, 100, 150, 200 mg.
DOSE ADJUSTMENT
Hepatic Failure: May have a prolonged or cumulative effect in patients with hepatic impairment. Use the lowest dose possible and use with caution.
Renal Failure: CrCl > 50 ml/min: No initial dose adjustment; *CrCl 10-50 ml/min:* Reduce initial dose by 25%; *CrCl < 10 ml/min:* Reduce initial dose by 50%
ONSET OF ACTION
Initial Response: 30 - 45 min; *Peak Effect:* 60 - 90 min, 4 hours for codeine contin
PREGNANCY & LACTATION
Pregnancy: RISK CANNOT BE RULED OUT. (CATEGORY C)
Lactation: Codeine is detected in breast milk; nursing is generally not recommended, however, it is reasonably safe if used for short periods of time.
MECHANISM OF ACTION
Approximately 10% of a dose of codeine is demethylated to morphine by the CYP4502D6 enzyme system in the liver. Conversion to morphine and morphine-6-glucuronide accounts for the opioid effects of codeine. *About 5 - 10% of the Caucasian population, 1 - 2% of Asians, and 1% of the Arabic population lack the CYP4502D6 enzyme and thus receive no effect from codeine*
PHARMACOKINETICS
Bioavail: Unknown; *1/2 Life:* 3-4 hours; *Metab:* In the liver mainly by glucuronidation. 10% is demethylated in the liver to morphine; *Excret:* Metabs in urine

FENTANYL (DURAGESIC, ACTIQ)

INDICATIONS
Approved: Sedation, relief of pain, preoperative medication, adjunct to general or regional anesthesia, management of chronic pain (transdermal product); ♣Severe chronic pain.

DOSE & DRUG ADMINISTRATION
Initial Dose: Calculate the previous 24 hour analgesic requirement; Convert this amount to the equianalgesic dose of morphine (*Use the table in Opioids – General Information to do this – 142*). *Morphine < 134 mg/d:* Fentanyl 25 ug/hr; *Morphine 135-224 mg/d:* Fentanyl 50 ug/hr; *Morphine 225-314 mg/d:* Fentanyl 75 ug/hr; *Morphine 315-404 mg/d:* Fentanyl 100 ug/hr; *Morphine 405-494 mg/d:* Fentanyl 125 ug/hr; *Morphine 495-584 mg/d:* Fentanyl 150 ug/hr. 5 mcg/kg of Transmucosal form is equivalent to 0.75-1.25 mcg/kg IM fentanyl.

Max Dose: Should be adjusted to severity of pain and the response of the patient;
Supplied: 25, 50, 75, &100 ug/hr sustained release patches, raspberry flavored lozenges (transmucosal form) on a stick 200, 400, 600, 800, 1200, 1600 ugs.

DOSE ADJUSTMENT
Hepatic Failure: May have a prolonged or cumulative effect in patients with hepatic impairment. Use the lowest dose possible and use with caution.
Renal Failure: CrCl > 50 ml/min: No initial dose adjustment; *CrCl 10-50 ml/min:* Reduce initial dose by 25%; *CrCl < 10 ml/min:* Reduce initial dose by 50%.

ONSET OF ACTION
Initial Onset: 6 - 8 hrs; *Peak Effect:* 24 hrs; *Duration:* 72 hrs

PREGNANCY & LACTATION
Pregnancy: RISK CANNOT BE RULED OUT. (CATEGORY C)
Lactation: Use of fentanyl patches is not advisable.

MECHANISM OF ACTION
Fentanyl is a semi-synthetic narcotic analgesic.

PHARMACOKINETICS
Bioavail: Unknown; *1/2 Life:* 17-22 hours; *Metab:* Metabolized by CYP4503A4 system by oxidative N-dealkylation to norfentanyl and other inactive metabolites; *Excret:* Conjugated metabolites (75%) & unchanged drug (10%) in the urine. Metabolites in the faeces (10%)

HYDROMORPHONE (DILAUDID, DILAUDID-5, ♣HYDROMORPH-CONTIN)

INDICATIONS
Approved: Pain & cough

DOSE & DRUG ADMINISTRATION
Initial Dose: Start with a low dose 2 - 4 mg PO q3-6h ;
Max Dose: Should be adjusted to severity of pain and the response of the patient;
Supplied: Regular Tablets: 1, 2, 4, 8 mg dosed q4-6h; *Suppositories:* 3 mg dosed q6-8h; ♣*Controlled Release Capsules (Hydromorph-Contin):* 2, 6, 12, 18, 24, & 30 ug dosed q12h; Oral Liquid: 1 mg/ml dosed q4-5h.

DOSE ADJUSTMENT
Hepatic Failure: May have a prolonged or cumulative effect in patients with hepatic impairment. Use the lowest dose possible and use with caution.
Renal Failure: Metabolites of hydromorphone are inactive; therefore no dose adjustment in renal failure is necessary.

PREGNANCY & LACTATION
Pregnancy: RISK CANNOT BE RULED OUT. (CATEGORY C)

Lactation: It is unknown if hydromorphone is excreted in breast milk, therefore, nursing is generally not recommended.

MECHANISM OF ACTION

Hydromorphone is a semi-synthetic narcotic analgesic. Hydromorphone is the active compound.

PHARMACOKINETICS

Bioavail: 25%; *1/2 Life:* 2 - 3 hours; *Metab:* Conjugated in the liver ; *Excret:* Conjugated metabolites & unchanged drug in the urine

MEPERIDINE (DEMEROL, PETHIDINE)

INDICATIONS

Approved: Relief of moderate to severe pain; ♣ cough.

DOSE & DRUG ADMINISTRATION

Initial Dose: Start with a low dose 50 mg PO/SC/IM q3-6h; *Max Dose:* Should be adjusted to severity of pain and the response of the patient;

Supplied: Regular Tablets: 50 & 100 mg; *Syrup:* 50 mg/5ml banana flavored.

DOSE ADJUSTMENT

Hepatic Failure: May have a prolonged or cumulative effect in patients with hepatic impairment. Use the lowest dose possible and use with caution.

Renal Failure: Meperidine is generally avoided in renal failure. Normeperidine, an active metabolite, is about one-half as potent as meperidine but it has twice the CNS stimulatory effects. The normal half-life of normeperidine is about 15 hours which is increased to 30 hours in patients with renal impairment. In renal failure, normeperidine can accumulate leading to worsening CNS toxicity such as seizures.

PREGNANCY & LACTATION

Pregnancy: RISK CANNOT BE RULED OUT. (CATEGORY C)

Lactation: Meperidine is excreted in breast milk, therefore, nursing is generally not recommended. However, use for short periods is likely safe.

MECHANISM OF ACTION

Meperidine is a semi-synthetic narcotic analgesic. Meperidine and its metabolite normeperidine are the active compounds.

PHARMACOKINETICS

Bioavail: 25%; *1/2 Life:* 3 - 5 hours; *Metab:* Hydrolyzed in the liver to meperidinic acid followed by partial glucuronidation. Meperidine also undergoes N-demethylation to normeperidine; *Excret:* Conjugated metabolites & unchanged drug in the urine

MORPHINE SULFATE (AVINZA, KADIAN, ♣M-ESLON, MS-CONTIN, ♣M.O.S., MSIR, ORAMORPH-SR, ROXANOL, ♣STATEX)

INDICATIONS

Approved: Severe pain

DOSE & DRUG ADMINISTRATION

Initial Dose: Start with a low dose 5 - 7.5 mg PO q4-6h; *Max Dose:* Should be adjusted to severity of pain and the response of the patient;

Supplied: Regular Tablets: 15 & 30 mg (♣ 5, 10, 20, 25, 30, 40, 50, & 60 mg); *Controlled Release Tablets (MS-Contin, Oramorph-SR):* 15, 30, 60, 10 mg (200 mg MS-Contin only); *Controlled Release Capsules (Kadian):* 20, 30, 50, 60, & 100 mg; *Extended Release Capsules (Avinza):* 30, 60, 90, & 120 mg; *Suppositories:* 5, 10, 20, & 30 mg; *Oral Liquid:* 10 mg/5ml, 10 mg/2.5 ml, 20 mg/5 ml, 20 mg/ml (concentrate), 100 mg/5ml (concentrate).

DOSE ADJUSTMENT
Hepatic Failure: May have a prolonged or cumulative effect in patients with hepatic impairment. Use the lowest dose possible and use with caution.
Renal Failure: CrCl > 50 ml/min: No initial dose adjustment; *CrCl 10-50 ml/min:* Reduce initial dose by 25%; *CrCl < 10 ml/min:* Reduce initial dose by 50%.

PREGNANCY & LACTATION
Pregnancy: RISK CANNOT BE RULED OUT. (CATEGORY C)
Lactation: Morphine is detected in breast milk, nursing is generally not recommended. However, it is reasonably safe if used for short periods of time.

MECHANISM OF ACTION
Morphine is the active compound

PHARMACOKINETICS
Bioavail: Unknown; *1/2 Life:* 2 - 3 hours; *Metab:* Metabolized in the liver mainly by glucuronidation; *Excret:* Glucuronide metabolites in the urine

OXYCODONE (✿ENDOCODONE, SUPEUDOL, ✿OXYCOCET, ✿OXYCODAN, OXY LR, OXYFAST, PERCOCET, ✿PERCOCET-DEMI, PERCODAN, ✿PERCODAN-DEMI, OXYCONTIN, PERCOLONE, ROXICET, ROXICODONE, TYLOX)

INDICATIONS
Approved: Moderate to severe pain.

DOSE & DRUG ADMINISTRATION
Initial Dose: Start with a low dose 5 – 10 mg PO q3-6h; *Max Dose:* Should be adjusted to severity of pain and the response of the patient;
Supplied: Regular Tablets: 5, 15, & 30 mg; *Regular Capsules:* 5 mg; *Controlled Release Tablets (Oxycontin):* 10, 20, 40, 80, & 160 mg, *Oral Liquid:* 5 mg/5 ml & 20mg/ml; ✿*Suppositories:* 10 & 20 mg; *Acetaminophen/Oxycodone:* Generic: 5/325, 5/500, Percocet 2.5/325, 7.5/500, 7.5/500, 10/325, 10/650, Roxicocet 5/325, Caplet 5/500, ✿Percocet-Demi: 325/2.5; *ASA/ Oxycodone:* Percodan, Oxycodan: 5/325, ✿Percodan-Demi: 2.5/325.

DOSE ADJUSTMENT
Hepatic Failure: May have a prolonged or cumulative effect in patients with hepatic impairment. Use the lowest dose possible and use with caution.
Renal Failure: CrCl > 50 ml/min: No initial dose adjustment; *CrCl 10-50 ml/min:* Reduce initial dose by 25%; *CrCl < 10 ml/min:* Reduce initial dose by 50%.

PREGNANCY & LACTATION
Pregnancy: RISK CANNOT BE RULED OUT. (CATEGORY C)
Lactation: It is unknown if oxycodone is excreted in breast milk, therefore, nursing is generally not recommended.

MECHANISM OF ACTION
Oxycodone is a semi-synthetic narcotic analgesic. Oxycodone is the active compound.

PHARMACOKINETICS
Bioavail: 60%; *1/2 Life:* 3 hours; *Metab:* Metabolized to noroxycodone in the liver; Conjugated in the liver; *Excret:* Conjugated metabolites & noroxycodone in the urine

PENTAZOCINE (TALWIN, TALWIN-NX)

INDICATIONS
Approved: Moderate to severe pain.

DOSE & DRUG ADMINISTRATION
Initial Dose: 50 mg q3-4h, may increase to 100 mg q3-4h; *Max Dose:* 600 mg/day;
Supplied: 50 mg tablets with 0.5 mg naloxone per tablet

DOSE ADJUSTMENT
Hepatic Failure: May have a prolonged or cumulative effect in patients with hepatic impairment. Use the lowest dose possible and use with caution.
Renal Failure: CrCl > 50 ml/min: No initial dose adjustment; *CrCl 10-50 ml/min:* Reduce initial dose by 25%; *CrCl < 10 ml/min:* Reduce initial dose by 50%.

ONSET OF ACTION
Initial Onset: 15 - 30 min; *Duration:* 4 - 5 hrs

PREGNANCY & LACTATION
Pregnancy: RISK CANNOT BE RULED OUT. (CATEGORY C)
Lactation: Pentazocine is excreted in breast milk, use with caution.

MECHANISM OF ACTION
Pentazocine is a mixed agonist / antagonist at the opioid receptor. It is a member of the benzazocine series of synthetic benzomorphans.

PHARMACOKINETICS
Oral Bioavail: 20% due to extensive first pass metabolism; *1/2 Life:* 2-3 hours; *Metab:* Oxidative and glucuronide conjugation in the liver; *Excret.* Metabolites in the urine, small amount of unchanged drug

PROPOXYPHENE (DARVON, DARVON-N)

INDICATIONS
Approved: Mild to moderate pain, (❦Moderate to severe pain)

DOSE & DRUG ADMINISTRATION
Initial Dose: Start with a low dose 65 mg PO q4h; *Max Dose:* 390 mg/day;
Supplied: Darvon 65 mg capsules & *Darvon-N* 100 mg tablets

DOSE ADJUSTMENT
Hepatic Failure: May have a prolonged or cumulative effect in patients with hepatic impairment. Use the lowest dose possible and use with caution.
Renal Failure: CrCl > 50 ml/min: No initial dose adjustment; *CrCl 10-50 ml/min:* Reduce initial dose by 25%; *CrCl < 10 ml/min:* Reduce initial dose by 50%.

ONSET OF ACTION
Initial Onset: 15 - 60 min; *Peak Effect:* 2 hrs; *Duration:* 4 - 6 hrs

PREGNANCY & LACTATION
Pregnancy: RISK CANNOT BE RULED OUT. (CATEGORY C)
Lactation: Low levels of propoxyphene have been detected in human milk. In postpartum studies involving nursing mothers who were given propoxyphene, no adverse effects were noted in infants receiving mother's milk.

MECHANISM OF ACTION
Propoxyphene is a centrally acting narcotic analgesic agent structurally related to methadone. It is metabolized in the liver to norpropoxyphene which has a substantially lower CNS effect but greater local anesthetic effect.

PHARMACOKINETICS
Oral Bioavail: 60% due to first pass metabolism; *1/2 Life:* 6 - 12 hours; *Metab:* Metabolized in the liver to yield norpropoxyphene; *Excret:* Metabolites in the urine

TRAMADOL (✤Tramacet, Ultracet, Ultram)

INDICATIONS
Approved: Moderate to moderate severe pain. (✤Short term for acute pain)

DOSE & DRUG ADMINISTRATION
Initial Dose: Tramacet or *Ultracet* 1-2 tabs q4-6h, *Ultram* 50-100 mg PO q4-6h; *Max Dose: Tramacet* or *Ultracet* 8 tabs/day, *Ultram*® 400 mg/day;
Supplied: Ultracet, ✤*Tramacet:* 37.5mg tramadol/325mg acetaminophen; *Ultram:* 50 mg tabs

DOSE ADJUSTMENT
Hepatic Failure: Not studied in hepatic impairment, avoid with severe hepatic impairment.
Renal Failure: Not extensively studied. Recommended to increase dosing interval to q12h for patients with CrCl< 30 mL/min with a maximum daily dose of 200 mg of tramadol.

ONSET OF ACTION
Initial Onset: 30 - 60 min; *Peak Effect:* 2 hrs; *Duration:* 4 - 6 hrs

PREGNANCY & LACTATION
Pregnancy: RISK CANNOT BE RULED OUT. (CATEGORY C)
Lactation: Low levels of tramadol have been detected in human milk. It is not advisable to use tramadol while nursing.

DRUG INTERACTIONS
Carbamazepine may significantly reduce the analgesic effect of tramadol. Concomitant administration with carbamazepine is not recommended.

MECHANISM OF ACTION
Tramadol is a centrally acting synthetic opioid analgesic. It works through two complementary mechanisms: (a) binding to the mu opioid receptors; (b) through a weak inhibition of the re-uptake of norepinephrine and serotonin.

PHARMACOKINETICS
Oral Bioavail: 75%; *1/2 Life:* 5 hours; *Metab:* Metabolized in the liver by N- and O-demethylation and glucuronidation or sulfation; *Excret:* 30% unchanged in the urine and 60% metabolites in the urine

BIOLOGICS
ADALIMUMAB (HUMIRA)

INDICATIONS
Approved: Moderate to severe rheumatoid arthritis (can be used with methotrexate or other DMARDs); Psoriatic arthritis *Off-Label Uses:* Seronegative spondyloarthropathies (ankylosing spondylitis, etc.); juvenile rheumatoid arthritis

DOSE & DRUG ADMINISTRATION
Initial Dose: 40 mg sc injection every other week; *Dose Increase:* Can be increased to 40 mg sc injection every week.
Supplied: Pre-loaded 1 mL syringes containing 40 mg of adalimumab.

DOSE ADJUSTMENT
Hepatic Failure: No pharmacokinetic data is available
Renal Failure: No pharmacokinetic data is available

ONSET OF ACTION
Initial Response: 2 - 4 weeks; *Maximal Response:* 2 - 4 months

MONITORING
The American College of Rheumatology does not recommend any routine laboratory monitoring, but patients should be alerted to report any signs or symptoms of infection. *Baseline:* AST, ALT, ALP, albumin, bilirubin, CBC, serum creatinine, PPD skin testing and CXR

CONTRAINDICATIONS & PRECAUTIONS
(a) Known hypersensitivity to adalimumab; (b) Active infections chronic and localized; (c) History of recurring infections or conditions which may predispose to infections (i.e. diabetes); (d) Use with extreme caution concomitantly with other TNF blocking agents; (e) Do not administer live vaccines to any patient receiving adalimumab; (f) History of malignancy or family history of a first degree relative with malignancy; (g) Multiple sclerosis or family history of multiple sclerosis; (h) Concomitant connective tissue disease such as systemic lupus erythematosus

TOXICITY
Reversible: *(a) Mucocut:* Injection site reactions (20%, mild to moderate), rash; *(b) CNS:* Headache; *(c) GI:* Nausea, abdominal pain; *(d) MSK:* Back pain; *(e) Gen:* Flu-like symptoms
Potentially Serious: *(a) Infection:* Serious infections and sepsis, including fatalities, have been reported with the use of adalimumab, with common infections including URTI, sinusitis, and UTI; reactivation of tuberculosis; *(b) Malignancy:* Increased risk of lymphoma (a concern, however, no conclusive evidence to quantify the magnitude of this risk versus patients with RA; *(c) Hematologic:* Agranulocytosis, granulocytopenia, leukopenia, pancytopenia, polycythemia; *(d) CNS:* New onset or exacerbation of CNS demyelinating disorders (rare); *(e) Autoantibody formation:* Increased ANA positivity with a lupus-like syndrome

PREGNANCY & LACTATION
Pregnancy: NO EVIDENCE OF RISK IN HUMANS. (CATEGORY B) There is very little pregnancy experience with adalimumab. It should be used in pregnancy only if benefits clearly outweigh potential risks.
Lactation: Unknown whether adalimumab is excreted in breast milk. Because many drugs are excreted in breast milk, caution should be used if adalimumab is given to a nursing mother.

DRUG INTERACTIONS
Use caution when combining adalimumab with anakinra as the combination may increase the risk of serious infections and neutropenia. Methotrexate reduced

adalimumab apparent clearance by up to 44% after multiple doses, however, no dose modification is required. Adalimumab can be used safely with other DMARDs.

MECHANISM OF ACTION

Adalimumab is a recombinant human IgG1 monoclonal antibody specific for human Tumor Necrosis Factor (TNF). Adalimumab is the active compound with no initial metabolism. Adalimumab binds specifically to TNF-alpha and blocks its interaction with the p55 and p75 cell surface receptors. Adalimumab also lyses surface TNF expressing cells in-vitro in the presence of complement. This inhibits TNF from binding to cell surface TNF-receptors which results in: ↓ Levels of other pro-inflammatory cytokines (IL-1, IL-6, Gm-CSF); ↓ Production of matrix metalloproteinases (MMP-3 and stromelysin); ↓ Osteoprotegrin ligand ==> decreased osteoclast activation; Down-regulation of the expression of adhesion molecules (ICAM).

PHARMACOKINETICS

Parenteral Bioavail: 64%; *Max Plasma Concentration:* 131 56 hours; *1/2 Life:* 10-20 days; *Metab:* Proteolysis; *Prot Bind:* None; *Excret:* Protein is lysed

ANAKINRA (KINERET)

INDICATIONS

Approved: Rheumatoid arthritis. *Off-Label Uses:* Seronegative spondyloarthropathies (psoriatic arthritis, ankylosing spondylitis, etc.)

DOSE & DRUG ADMINISTRATION

Dose: 100 mg sc injection per day. *Supplied:* Pre-loaded 1 mL syringes containing 100 mg of anakinra.

DOSE ADJUSTMENT

Hepatic Failure: No dosage adjustment recommended, however, no formal pharmacokinetic studies have been conducted in patients with hepatic impairment.

Renal Failure: CrCl < 30mL/minute 70-75% reduction in mean plasma clearance of anakinra; however, no formal pharmacokinetic studies have been conducted in patients with renal impairment.

ONSET OF ACTION

Initial Response: 2 - 4 weeks; *Maximal Response:* 6 months

MONITORING

Baseline: AST, ALT, ALP, albumin, bilirubin, CBC, serum creatinine, PPD skin testing and CXR

Monthly: CBC, creatinine, AST, ALT, ALP, albumin

CONTRAINDICATIONS & PRECAUTIONS

(a) Known hypersensitivity to anakinra or E. coli derived products; (b) Active infections – chronic and localized; (c) History of recurring infections or conditions which may predispose to infections (i.e. diabetes); (d) Use with extreme caution concomitantly with other TNF blocking agents; (e) Do not administer live vaccines

TOXICITY

Reversible: (a) Mucocut: Injection site reactions (70%), mild to moderate and tend to improve with time; *(b) CNS:* Headache; *(c) GI:* Nausea, diarrhea, abdominal pain; *(d) Gen:* Flu-like symptoms

Potentially Serious: (a) Infection: Serious infections and sepsis, including fatalities, have been reported with the use of anakinra; *(b) Malignancy:* A concern, however, currently no evidence to suggest increased incidence; *(c) Hem:* Leukopenia; Neutropenia

PREGNANCY & LACTATION
Pregnancy: NO EVIDENCE OF RISK IN HUMANS. (CATEGORY B) There is very little pregnancy experience with anakinra. It should be used in pregnancy only if benefits clearly outweigh potential risks.

Lactation: Unknown whether anakinra is excreted in breast milk. Because many drugs are excreted in breast milk, caution should be used if anakinra is given to a nursing mother.

DRUG INTERACTIONS
Use caution when combining a TNF blocking agent (adalimumab; etanercept; infliximab) with anakinra as the combination may increase the risk of serious infections and neutropenia. Otherwise no drug-drug interaction studies have been performed in human subjects. Anakinra can be used safely in combination with other DMARDs

MECHANISM OF ACTION
Anakinra is a recombinant, non-glycosylated form of human interleukin-1(IL-1) receptor antagonist (IL-1Ra). Anakinra is the active compound with no initial metabolism. Interleukin-1 is induced in response to inflammatory stimuli and mediates various physiological inflammatory and immunological responses. Anakinra blocks the binding of interleukin-1 to its receptor by competitive inhibition. This inhibits the effects of IL-1 resulting in: ↓ Levels of other pro-inflammatory cytokines (TNF, IL 6); ↓ Expression of COX-2 and PGE2; ↓ Production of collagenases; ↓ Angiogenic factors; ↓ Osteoclast activation, chondrocyte activation, and fibroblast proliferation; ↓ Expression of adhesion molecules (ICAM)

PHARMACOKINETICS
Parenteral Bioavail: 95%; *Max Plasma Concentration:* 3 - 7 hours; *1/2 Life:* 4 - 6 hours; *Metab:* None; *Prot Bind:* None; *Excret:* Renal

ETANERCEPT (ENBREL)

INDICATIONS
Approved: Rheumatoid arthritis; juvenile rheumatoid arthritis; psoriatic arthritis; ankylosing spondylitis; psoriasis (US only). *Off-Label Uses:* Vasculitis (Wegener's Granulomatosis) & autoimmune eye disease.

DOSE & DRUG ADMINISTRATION
Initial dose: 50 mg sc per week given as a single dose or two 25 mg injections at 72 - 96 hours apart; Max dose: 100 mg per week.

Supplied: Cartons with four dose trays each containing a 25 mg vial of etanercept, a syringe with 1mL bacteriostatic water for injection, and two alcohol swabs. A 50 mg prefilled syringe is now available.

DOSE ADJUSTMENT
Hepatic Failure: No dosage adjustment recommended, however, no formal pharmacokinetic studies have been conducted in patients with hepatic impairment.

Renal Failure: No dosage adjustment recommended, however, no formal pharmacokinetic studies have been conducted in patients with renal impairment.

ONSET OF ACTION
Response: 2 weeks to 3 months

MONITORING
The American College of Rheumatology does not recommend any routine laboratory monitoring, but patients should be alerted to report any signs or symptoms of infection. *Baseline:* AST, ALT, ALP, albumin, bilirubin, CBC, serum creatinine, PPD skin testing and CXR

CONTRAINDICATIONS & PRECAUTIONS

(a) Hypersensitivity to etanercept; (b) Active infections – chronic and localized; (c) Congestive heart failure; (d) History of recurring infections or conditions which may predispose to infections (i.e. diabetes); (e) Patients receiving etanercept should not be given live vaccines; (f) History of malignancy or family history of a first degree relative with malignancy; (g) Multiple sclerosis or family history of multiple sclerosis; (h) Concomitant connective tissue diseases such as systemic lupus erythematosus

TOXICITY

Reversible: (a) Mucocut: Injection site reactions (37%), mild to moderate and tend to improve with time, rash; ***(b) CNS:*** Headache, dizziness; ***(c) GI:*** Nausea, vomiting, abdominal pain, dyspepsia; ***(d) MSK:*** Weakness

Potentially Serious: (a) Infection: Serious infections and sepsis, including fatalities, have been reported with the use of etanercept; with common infections including URTI, sinusitis, and UTI; reactivation of tuberculosis; ***(b) Malignancy:*** Increased risk of lymphoma is a concern, however, no conclusive evidence to quantify the magnitude of this risk versus patients with RA; ***(c) Autoantibody formation:*** Increased ANA positivity with a lupus-like syndrome; ***(d) Cardiac:*** Worsening congestive heart failure; ***(e) Hem:*** Pancytopenia including aplastic anemia (rare); ***(f) CNS:*** New onset or exacerbation of CNS demyelinating disorders (rare)

PREGNANCY & LACTATION

Pregnancy: **NO EVIDENCE OF RISK IN HUMANS. (CATEGORY B).** There is very little pregnancy experience with etanercept. It should be used in pregnancy only if benefits clearly outweigh potential risks.

Lactation: Unknown whether etanercept is excreted in breast milk. Because many drugs are excreted in breast milk, caution should be used if etanercept is given to a nursing mother.

DRUG INTERACTIONS

Use caution when combining etanercept with anakinra as the combination may increase the risk of serious infections and neutropenia. Otherwise no drug-drug interaction studies have been performed in human subjects. Etanercept can be used safely in combination with other DMARDs.

MECHANISM OF ACTION

Etanercept is a dimeric fusion protein of the extracellular ligand-binding portion of the human p75 TNF receptor linked to the Fc portion of human IgG1. Etanercept is the active compound with no initial metabolism. Etanercept serves as a p75 TNF decoy receptor, competitively binding to TNF molecules (both TNF & TNF) specifically. This inhibits TNF from binding to cell surface TNF-receptors which results in: ↓ Levels of other pro-inflammatory cytokines (IL-1, IL-6, Gm-CSF); ↓ Production of matrix metalloproteinases (MMP-3 and stromelysin); ↓ Osteoprotegrin ligand → decreased osteoclast activation; Down-regulation of the expression of adhesion molecules (ICAM)

PHARMACOKINETICS

Maximum serum concentration: 72 hours (48 - 96); ***Half Life:*** 115 hours; ***Metabolism:*** Proteolysis; ***Protein Binding:*** None; ***Excretion:*** Protein is lysed

INFLIXIMAB (REMICADE)

INDICATIONS
Approved: Used in combination with methotrexate for rheumatoid arthritis; ankylosing spondylitis; psoriatic arthritis. *Off-Label Uses:* Vasculitis (Wegener's Granulomatosis); Sjogren's syndrome; inflammatory myopathies; juvenile rheumatoid arthritis.

DOSE & DRUG ADMINISTRATION
Infliximab is administered concomitantly with oral or subcutaneous *methotrexate* to help prevent the formation of human anti-chimeric antibodies (HACA) which may neutralize infliximab. *Initial Dose:* 3 mg/kg infusion at week zero followed by doses at 2 and 6 weeks; *Maintenance Dose:* 3 mg/kg every 8 weeks; *Dose Adjustments:* For improved clinical efficacy, the interval between infusions can be decreased to every 6 weeks or the infusion dose can be increased; *Maximum Dose:* 10 mg/kg. *Supplied:* Vials of 20 mL containing 100 mg of infliximab. *METHOTREXATE:* At least 7.5 mg/week

DOSE ADJUSTMENT
Hepatic Failure: No dosage adjustment recommended, however, no formal pharmacokinetic studies have been conducted in patients with hepatic impairment.
Renal Failure: No dosage adjustment recommended, however, no formal pharmacokinetic studies have been conducted in patients with renal impairment.

ONSET OF ACTION
Initial Response: hours to days; *Maximal Response:* 4 – 6 weeks

MONITORING
The American College of Rheumatology does not recommend any routine laboratory monitoring, but patients should be alerted to report any signs or symptoms of infection. *Baseline:* AST, ALT, ALP, albumin, bilirubin, CBC, serum creatinine, PPD skin testing and CXR

CONTRAINDICATIONS & PRECAUTIONS
(a) Hypersensitivity to infliximab or murine proteins; (b) Active infections – chronic and localized; (c) History of tuberculosis; (d) Congestive heart failure; (e) History of recurring infections or conditions which may predispose to infections (i.e. diabetes); (f) History of malignancy or family history of a first degree relative with malignancy; (g) Multiple sclerosis or family history of multiple sclerosis; (h) Live vaccines should not be administered to patients receiving infliximab

TOXICITY
Reversible: (a) Acute Infusion Reactions (17%): During or 1-2 hours after infusion – fever or chills, pruritis or urticaria, and cardiopulmonary reactions (chest pain, hypotension, hypertension or dyspnea) ➔ stop infusion, administer benadryl and/ or corticosteroids. If reaction clears, restart infusion at a slower rate. *(b) CNS:* Headache; *(c) GI:* Abdominal pain, nausea, vomiting, diarrhea; *(d) Mucocut:* Rash, transient increase in joint pain and/or swelling; *(e) MSK:* Back pain; arthralgia; *(f) Gen:* Fever; fatigue
Potentially Serious: (a) Hypersensitivity: Urticaria, dyspnea, & hypotension within 2 hours of infusion; *(b) Infection:* Serious infections and sepsis, including fatalities, have been reported with the use of infliximab with common infections including URTI, sinusitis, and UTI; Reactivation of Tuberculosis; *(c) Malignancy:* Increased risk of lymphoma is a concern, however, no conclusive evidence to quantify the magnitude of this risk versus patients with RA. *(d) Autoantibody formation/ Lupus-like syndrome:* ANA & ds-DNA; *(e) Cardiac:* Worsening congestive heart failure; *(f) CNS:* New onset or exacerbation of CNS demyelinating disorders (rare)

PREGNANCY & LACTATION

Pregnancy: NO EVIDENCE OF RISK IN HUMANS. (CATEGORY B). There is very little pregnancy experience with infliximab. It should be used in pregnancy only if benefits clearly outweigh potential risks.

Lactation: Unknown whether infliximab is excreted in breast milk. Because many drugs are excreted in breast milk, caution should be used if infliximab is given to a nursing mother.

DRUG INTERACTIONS

Use caution when combining infliximab with anakinra as the combination may increase the risk of serious infections and neutropenia. Otherwise no drug-drug interaction studies have been performed in human subjects. Infliximab can be used safely in combination with other DMARDs

MECHANISM OF ACTION

Infliximab is a chimeric (mouse-human) IgG1 monoclonal antibody. Infliximab is the active compound with no initial metabolism. Infliximab binds to the soluble and trans-membrane forms of TNF- molecules. This inhibits TNF- from binding to cell surface TNF-receptors which results in: ↓ Levels of other pro-inflammatory cytokines (IL-1 & IL-6); ↓ Production of matrix metalloproteinases (MMP-3 and stromelysin); ↓ Osteoprotegrin ligand → decreased osteoclast activation; ↓ Regulation of the expression of adhesion molecules (ICAM) and ↓ in lymphocyte migration

PHARMACOKINETICS

1/2 Life: 8 - 10 days; *Metab:* Proteolysis; *Prot Bind:* None; *Excret:* Protein is lysed

CORTICOSTEROIDS

SYSTEMIC CORTICOSTEROID PREPARATIONS

INDICATIONS

Approved: As adjunctive therapy for short-term administration (to tide the patient over an acute episode or exacerbation) in: Psoriatic arthritis; Rheumatoid arthritis, including juvenile rheumatoid arthritis (selected cases may require low-dose maintenance therapy); Ankylosing spondylitis; Acute and subacute bursitis; Acute nonspecific tenosynovitis; Acute gouty arthritis; Post-traumatic osteoarthritis; Synovitis of osteoarthritis. Epicondylitis; Collagen Diseases: During an exacerbation or as maintenance therapy in selected cases of: Systemic lupus erythematosus; Systemic dermatomyositis (polymyositis); Acute rheumatic carditis.

DOSE & DRUG ADMINISTRATION

Biologic Half-Life (hrs): Hydrocortisone (Solu-Cortef®) 8-12 hours, Prednisone 18-36 hours, Methylprednisolone (Solu-Medrol®) 18-36 hours, Dexamethasone (Decadron®) 36-54 hours

Equivalent Dose: Hydrocortisone (Solu-Cortef®) 20 mg = Prednisone 5 mg = Methylprednisolone (Solu-Medrol®) 1 mg = Dexamethasone (Decadron®) 0.75 mg

Relative Mineralocorticoid Potency: Hydrocortisone (Solu-Cortef®) 2, Prednisone 1, Methylprednisolone (Solu-Medrol®) 0, Dexamethasone (Decadron®) 0

DOSE ADJUSTMENT

Hepatic Failure: No specific dosage adjustment is recommended.

Renal Failure: No specific dosage adjustment is recommended, however, use with caution as may exacerbate hypertension & edema in the setting of renal impairment.

MONITORING

Baseline: Blood pressure, CBC, electrolytes, BUN, Cr, glucose, urinalysis, consider bone mineral densitometry (BMD) testing for high-risk patients or patients in whom prolonged use of corticosteroids is anticipated, weight, consider Tb skin testing and CXR for those who may be at increased risk; *At Each Visit:* Blood pressure, weight; *Yearly:* Serum glucose, lipid levels (TG, HDL, LDL), electrolytes (especially potassium), BMD

CONTRAINDICATIONS & PRECAUTIONS

(a) Known hypersensitivity to corticosteroids; (b) Current active infection or history of frequent recurrent infections; (c) History of untreated tuberculosis or histoplasmosis; (d) Hypertension, edema, hypokalemia; (e) Diabetes (worsen blood sugar control); (f) Osteoporosis; (g) Active peptic ulcer or previous history of peptic ulcer disease or concomitant use of NSAIDs; (h) Glaucoma; (i) Diverticulosis; (j) Hyperlipidemia; (k) atherosclerosis and risk factors; (l) Children still growing

TOXICITY

Reversible: (a) Gen: Hypertension, peripheral edema, hypokalemia; *(b) GI:* Nausea, vomiting, dyspepsia, diarrhea, hyperphagia, weight gain (truncal obesity & moon face), abdominal distension; *(c) CNS:* Euphoria, insomnia, mood swings, agitation, anxiety, personality changes; *(d) Mucocut:* Acne, hirsutism; *(e) Hem:* Neutrophilia, lymphopenia, monocytopenia

Potentially Serious: (a) Infection: Serious infections and sepsis, including fatalities, have been reported with the use of corticosteroids; *(b) Ocular:* Posterior subcapsular cataracts & glaucoma; *(c) Lytes:* Hypokalemia, sodium retention; *(d) Endo:* Hypoadrenalism if abruptly withdrawn, iatrogenic Cushing's syndrome, diabetes mellitus, menstrual irregularities; *(e) Psychiatric:* Major depression, psychosis; *(f) CVS:* Congestive heart failure, atherosclerosis, hyperlipidemia; *(g)*

MSK: Myopathy, aseptic necrosis (especially of femoral and humeral heads), osteoporosis, stunt growth in children; *(h) GI:* Peptic ulcer disease, pancreatitis, esophageal ulceration, inc. LFTs, fatty liver, silent intestinal perforation; *(i) Mucocut:* Impaired wound healing, thin fragile skin, petechiae and ecchymoses, facial erythema, increased sweating, hirsutism, acne, and striae, and may suppress reactions to skin tests; *(j) CNS:* Pseudotumor cerebri; *(k) Sudden death with rapid administration of high dose pulse*

PREGNANCY & LACTATION

Pregnancy: **RISK CANNOT BE RULED OUT. (CATEGORY C)**

Conception & Fertility: The use of corticosteroids prior to pregnancy does not seem to adversely impact fertility. *Maternal Effects:* Premature rupture of membranes and exacerbation of gestational diabetes and hypertension. *Fetal Effects:* Monitor for adrenal suppression and infection, may increase the risk of cleft lip and palate. Prednisone can cross the placenta and umbilical cord concentrations are about 10% of maternal serum concentrations. Dexamethasone easily crosses the placenta and is used to treat congenital heart block in patients who are anti-Ro positive.

Lactation: Small amounts of corticosteroids can be found in the breast milk; however, the American Academy of Pediatrics considers prednisone and prednisolone safe and compatible with breast feeding.

Recommendations: Use the lowest possible dose of corticosteroids needed to control disease activity. In women treated with corticosteroids during pregnancy, "stress doses" of hydrocortisone may be required for cesarean sections or prolonged labor and delivery. Women who choose to breast feed may wish to wait 4 hours after ingesting a dose; this may minimize the amount of glucocorticoid found in the milk. Corticosteroids may be considered safer than NSAIDs or DMARDs to manage inflammatory disease during pre-pregnancy and pregnancy.

DRUG INTERACTIONS

Drugs which may ↑ *efficacy/toxicity of corticosteroids:* Cyclosporine, erythromycin & ketoconazole (inhibit metabolism), estrogens, potassium depleting diuretics; *Drugs which may* ↓ *efficacy of corticosteroids:* Phenobarbital, phenytoin, rifampin; *Corticosteroids may* ↑ *efficacy/toxicity of:* Ketoconazole (inhibit metabolism), cyclosporine, digoxin, NSAIDS (gastrointestinal toxicity); *Corticosteroids may* ↓ *efficacy of:* Anticholinesterase agents (neostigmine), isoniazid; Variable effects on anticoagulation - monitor coagulation indices closely

MECHANISM OF ACTION

Glucocorticoids circulate as free glucocorticoid or bound to cortisol-binding globulin. Free glucocorticoid diffuses into the cytoplasm and attaches to the glucocorticoid receptor (GR). Binding of the glucocorticoid to the GR results in an activated GR-glucocorticoid complex which can then translocate into the nucleus. Glucocorticoids then have the ability to enhance or inhibit gene expression. Glucocorticoids enhance gene expression by binding to specific short sequences of DNA called glucocorticoid responsive elements (GRE) which results in the induction of gene transcription. Glucocorticoids inhibit gene expression by binding to transcription factors such as activated protein-1 (AP-1) or nuclear factor (NF-) preventing their interaction with DNA and inhibiting protein synthesis. Glucocorticoids inhibit inflammation through multiple effects on immune response cells, cytokines, and other mediators which are capable of producing tissue injury: ↑ Production of anti-inflammatory cytokines such as IL-10, IL-1Ra, & annexin-1; ↓ Production of adhesion molecules (E-selectin, ICAM-1); ↓ Production of inflammatory cytokines including TNF-, IL-2, and IL-6; Glucocorticoids also have cellular effects including: ↓ Processing of antigens by monocytes for presentation to lymphocytes; ↓ Activation and proliferation of immature T lymphocytes, T-effector lymphocytes, natural killer cells and immature B cells; ↓ Expression of proinflammatory cytokines such as TNF-, IL-1, IL-2, and IFN by numerous cells, including fibroblasts, macrophages, and endothelial cells; ↓ Generation of other mediators of inflammation such as prostaglandins and nitric oxide by inhibiting COX-2 and iNOS; Stabilize lysosomal membranes on neutrophils and retard neutrophil apoptosis

DEXAMETHASONE SODIUM PHOSPHATE (DECADRON)
INDICATIONS
Approved: As adjunctive therapy for short-term administration (to tide the patient over an acute episode or exacerbation) in: Psoriatic arthritis; Rheumatoid arthritis, including juvenile rheumatoid arthritis (selected cases may require low-dose maintenance therapy); Ankylosing spondylitis; Acute and subacute bursitis; Acute nonspecific tenosynovitis; Acute gouty arthritis; Post-traumatic osteoarthritis; Synovitis of osteoarthritis. Epicondylitis; Collagen Diseases: During an exacerbation or as maintenance therapy in selected cases of: Systemic lupus erythematosus; Systemic dermatomyositis (polymyositis); Acute rheumatic carditis.
DOSE & DRUG ADMINISTRATION
Initial Dose: 0.5 - 100 mg with dosage requirements being variable and dependant upon the disease being treated and the response of the patient; *Maintenance Dose:* High-dose corticosteroid therapy should be continued only until the patient's condition has stabilized – usually not beyond 48 - 72 hours.
Supplied: 0.25, 0.5, 0.75, 1, 1.5, 2, 4, & 6 mg tablets; 4 mg/mL (vials of 1, 5, 10, 25, & 30 mL), 10mg/mL (vials of 1 & 10 mL), & 24 mg/mL (vials of 5 mL).
PHARMACOKINETICS
Active Form & Initial Metabolism: Dexamethasone is a potent anti-inflammatory steroid. It has a greater anti-inflammatory potency than prednisolone and has less tendency than prednisolone to induce sodium and water retention; *Bioavail:* 100%; *1/2 Life:* 2 - 3 hours; *Biologic 1/2 Life:* 36 - 54 hours; *Metab:* Hepatic; *Prot Bind:* Highly bound to cortisol binding globulin or albumin; *Excret:* Glucuronide and sulfide metabolites in the urine

HYDROCORTISONE SODIUM SUCCINATE (SOLU-CORTEF)
INDICATIONS
Approved: As adjunctive therapy for short-term administration (to tide the patient over an acute episode or exacerbation) in: Psoriatic arthritis; Rheumatoid arthritis, including juvenile rheumatoid arthritis (selected cases may require low-dose maintenance therapy); Ankylosing spondylitis; Acute and subacute bursitis; Acute nonspecific tenosynovitis; Acute gouty arthritis; Post-traumatic osteoarthritis; Synovitis of osteoarthritis. Epicondylitis; Collagen Diseases: During an exacerbation or as maintenance therapy in selected cases of: Systemic lupus erythematosus; Systemic dermatomyositis (polymyositis); Acute rheumatic carditis.
DOSE & DRUG ADMINISTRATION
May be administered by IV infusion or IM injection. *Initial Dose:* 50 mg to 1000 mg IV and may be repeated at intervals of 2, 4, or 6 hours; *Maintenance Dose:* High-dose corticosteroid therapy should be continued only until the patient's condition has stabilized – usually not beyond 48-72 hours;
Supplied: 100, 250, 500, & 1000 mg powder for reconstitution.

PHARMACOKINETICS

Active Form & Initial Metab: Solu-Cortef® is the highly water soluble sodium succinate ester of hydrocortisone; ***Bioavail:*** 100%; ***Plasma 1/2 Life:*** 1 - 2 hours; ***Biologic 1/2 Life:*** 8 - 12 hours; ***Metab:*** Hepatic; ***Prot Bind:*** Highly bound to cortisol binding globulin or albumin; ***Excret:*** Glucuronide and sulfide metabolites in the urine

METHYLPREDNISOLONE SODIUM SUCCINATE (SOLU-MEDROL)

INDICATIONS

Approved: As adjunctive therapy for short-term administration (to tide the patient over an acute episode or exacerbation) in: Psoriatic arthritis; Rheumatoid arthritis, including juvenile rheumatoid arthritis (selected cases may require low-dose maintenance therapy); Ankylosing spondylitis; Acute and subacute bursitis; Acute nonspecific tenosynovitis; Acute gouty arthritis; Post-traumatic osteoarthritis; Synovitis of osteoarthritis.   Epicondylitis; Collagen Diseases: During an exacerbation or as maintenance therapy in selected cases of: Systemic lupus erythematosus; Systemic dermatomyositis (polymyositis); Acute rheumatic carditis.

DOSE & DRUG ADMINISTRATION

May be administered by IV infusion or IM injection. ***Initial Dose:*** 50 mg to 1000 mg IV and may be repeated at intervals dictated by the patients response to treatment; ***Maintenance Dose:*** High-dose corticosteroid therapy should be continued only until the patient's condition has stabilized – usually not beyond 48 - 72 hours; ***Supplied:*** 40, 125, 500, & 1000 mg powder for reconstitution.

PHARMACOKINETICS

Active Form & Initial Metab: Methylprednisolone is a potent anti-inflammatory steroid. It has a greater anti-inflammatory potency than prednisolone and has less tendency than prednisolone to induce sodium and water retention. ***Bioavail:*** 100%; ***Plasma 1/2 Life:*** 1 - 3 hours; ***Biologic 1/2 Life:*** 18 - 36 hours; ***Metab:*** Hepatic; ***Prot Bind:*** Highly bound to cortisol binding globulin or albumin; ***Excret:*** Glucuronide and sulfide metabolites in the urine

PREDNISONE

INDICATIONS

Approved: As adjunctive therapy for short-term administration (to tide the patient over an acute episode or exacerbation) in: Psoriatic arthritis; Rheumatoid arthritis, including juvenile rheumatoid arthritis (selected cases may require low-dose maintenance therapy); Ankylosing spondylitis; Acute and subacute bursitis; Acute nonspecific tenosynovitis; Acute gouty arthritis; Post-traumatic osteoarthritis; Synovitis of osteoarthritis.   Epicondylitis; Collagen Diseases: During an exacerbation or as maintenance therapy in selected cases of: Systemic lupus erythematosus; Systemic dermatomyositis (polymyositis); Acute rheumatic carditis.

DOSE & DRUG ADMINISTRATION

Dose: May vary from 5 to 100+ mg/day depending on the specific disease entity being treated. The initial dose should be maintained or adjusted until a satisfactory response is obtained. After a favorable response is noted, the proper maintenance dosage should be determined by decreasing the initial drug dosage in small decrements at appropriate time intervals until the lowest dosage that will maintain an adequate clinical response is reached. If after long-term therapy the drug is to be stopped, it is recommended that it be withdrawn gradually rather than abruptly. If prednisone therapy is anticipated for long periods (>5 mg/day for > 3 months) administration of an osteoprotective agent is mandatory (i.e. bisphosphonate);

Supplied: 1, 5, 10, 20 & 50 mg tablets; Sterapred (5 mg tablets tapering 30 mg to 5 mg over 6 days or 30 mg to 10 mg over 10 days); Sterapred DS (10 mg tablets tapering from 60 mg to 10 mg over 6 days or 60 mg to 20 mg over 12 days)

PHARMACOKINETICS

Initial Metab: Prednisone itself is biologically inactive and must be converted to prednisolone in the liver. Prednisolone is the biologically active form; **Bioavail:** 90%; **Plasma 1/2 Life:** 2 - 4 hours; **Biologic 1/2 Life:** 18 - 36 hours; **Metab:** Hepatic; **Prot Bind:** Highly bound to cortisol binding globulin or albumin; **Excret:** Glucuronide and sulfide metabolites in the urine

INTRA-ARTICULAR CORTICOSTEROIDS

INDICATIONS

Approved: Adjunctive therapy for short-term administration in synovitis of osteoarthritis, acute and subacute bursitis, epicondylitis, post-traumatic osteoarthritis, rheumatoid arthritis, acute gouty arthritis, acute nonspecific tenosynovitis. **Rheumatologists use these corticosteroid preparations to inject joints, tendon sheaths, trigger points, and peri-articular structures.**

DOSAGE & DRUG ADMINISTRATION

Methylprednisolone Acetate (Depo-Medrol): 40 mg/mL (1,2,5 mL vials); Lg Joint: 40-80 mg, Med Joint: 20-40 mg, Sm Joint: 10 mg

Triamcinolone Acetonide(Kenalog): 40 mg/mL (1, 5 mL vials); Lg Joint:40-80 mg, Med Joint: 20-40 mg, Sm Joint: 10 mg

Triamcinolone Hexacetonide (Aristospan): 20 mg/mL (5 mL vials); Large Joint: 40-80 mg, Med Joint: 20-40 mg, Sm Joint: 10 mg

Betamethasone Sodium Phosphate / Acetate (Celestone, Soluspan): 3 mg/mL (1, 5 mL vials) Large Joint: 6-12 mg, Med Joint: 3-6 mg, Sm Joint: 3 mg

Which Preparation to Choose: There are no large, randomized controlled trials comparing various intra-articular corticosteroid preparations as to efficacy or toxicity. Methylprednisolone acetate and triamcinolone acetonide seem to cause less post-injection flares than other long acting agents. The triamcinolone compounds are less water soluble and therefore may be longer acting

Should Lidocaine be Used: Possible effects of mixing lidocaine include: (a) Reduced propensity to cause steroid atrophy; (b) Reduced propensity of steroid crystals to cause a post-injection flare; (c) Immediate relief from the injection

How Frequently Should Injections be Given: Controversy exists regarding the maximal safe frequency of intra-articular corticosteroid injections. Some evidence to suggest that frequent intra-articular corticosteroid injections may accelerate osteoarthritic changes. However, corticosteroids inhibit mediators of cartilage destruction (metalloproteinases and collagenases), in rheumatoid and osteoarthritis, which may slow cartilage loss. In general a conservative approach is currently recommended. As an example, some physicians inject joints affected by RA every month and joints affected by OA every 3 months. The duration of such therapy is still unknown. For increased efficacy of the injection, it is advisable to limit weight bearing activity for 24 hours after a lower extremity joint is injected.

DOSE ADJUSTMENT

Hepatic Failure: No specific dosage adjustment is recommended.

Renal Failure: No specific dosage adjustment is recommended.

MONITORING

No recommended laboratory monitoring for intra-articular corticosteroid injections

CONTRAINDICATIONS & PRECAUTIONS
(a) Hypersensitivity to corticosteroids; (b) Septic arthritis of the joint to be injected; (c) Cellulitis overlying the joint to be injected; (d) Anticoagulation

TOXICITY
Intra-articular corticosteroid injection does result in some systemic absorption; therefore, toxicity can be systemic. Please see general information on corticosteroids to review other systemic toxicities.

Minor: (a) Articular: Post-injection flare usually occurring within 24 hours and thought to be induced by the steroid crystals. Will resolve usually within 48 hours; *(b) Other:* Facial flushing, uterine bleeding

Major: (a) MSK: Septic arthritis (iatrogenic infection - rare), tendon rupture; *(b) Radiologic Deterioration of Joints:* "Steroid arthropathy"; Charcot like arthropathy; osteonecrosis; *(c) Mucocut:* Fat necrosis or calcification at the injection site; *(d) Neuro:* Inadvertent injection of a nerve (median, sciatic) resulting in a peripheral neuropathy; *(e) Ophtho:* Cataracts

PREGNANCY & LACTATION
Pregnancy: **RISK CANNOT BE RULED OUT. (CATEGORY C)**
Lactation: Small amounts of corticosteroids can be found in breast milk, however, thought to be safe.

MECHANISM OF ACTION OF CORTICOSTEROIDS
See Systemic Corticosteroid Preparations – Mechanism of Action

COXIBs

CELECOXIB (CELEBREX)

INDICATIONS
Approved: Osteoarthritis; rheumatoid arthritis; colorectal cancer prevention (familial adenomatous polyposis), dysmenorrhea. *Off-Label Uses:* Acute and chronic pain

DOSE & DRUG ADMINISTRATION
Dose: Osteoarthritis 100 mg PO BID; rheumatoid arthritis 200 mg PO BID; familial adenomatous polyposis 400 mg PO BID. *Supplied:* 100, 200, & 400 mg capsules.

DOSE ADJUSTMENT
Hepatic Failure: Dosage reduction of 50% in moderate hepatic impairment. Not recommended in severe hepatic impairment.
Renal Failure: Use with caution as celecoxib may worsen existing renal impairment.

ONSET OF ACTION
Initial Response: 60 min (dental pain model)

MONITORING
Baseline: CBC, creatinine, AST, ALT, ALP, albumin; *Every 3 months:* Consider creatinine & blood pressure in patients with pre-existing hypertension or those who are elderly; *Yearly:* CBC, creatinine, AST, ALT, ALP, albumin

CONTRAINDICATIONS & PRECAUTIONS
(a) Known hypersensitivity to celecoxib; (b) Allergic-type reactions to sulfonamides; (c) Asthma, urticaria, or allergic-type reactions after ASA or other NSAIDs; (d) Active peptic ulcer disease, active GI bleeding, or active inflammatory disease of the bowel; (e) Use with caution in patients with a past history of peptic ulcer disease; (f) Significant hepatic impairment or active liver disease; (g) Severe renal impairment (CrCl < 30 mL/min) or deteriorating renal disease ; (h) Avoid in patients who have recently had a CABG, myocardial infarction, cerebrovascular accident, or experienced significant chest pain related to heart disease; (i) Use with caution in patients at high risk for cardiovascular disease (MI & CVA) and those with angina, fluid retention, hypertension, or heart failure; (j) Concomitant use with other NSAIDs

TOXICITY
Reversible: (a) CVS: Hypertension, fluid retention, and edema; *(b) GI:* Dyspepsia, abdominal pain, diarrhea
Potentially Serious: (a) Resp: Worsening of ASA sensitive asthma; *(b) Hepatic:* 15% of patients experience borderline ↑ in liver enzymes with rare cases of associated fulminant hepatitis, liver necrosis, and fatal hepatic failure; *(c) Renal:* Worsening of renal function; *(d) Hem:* Anemia; *(e) GI:* Complicated GI ulceration with perforation, obstruction, and bleeding; *(f) CNS:* Aseptic meningitis; *(g) CVS:* Worsening angina, myocardial infarction

PREGNANCY & LACTATION
Pregnancy: RISK CANNOT BE RULED OUT. (CATEGORY C). Celecoxib should be avoided in the 3rd trimester due to a risk of premature closure of ductus arteriosus.
Lactation: Unknown whether celecoxib is excreted in breast milk. Celecoxib should not be used by women who are breastfeeding or plan to breastfeed
Recommendations: (a) Coxibs should be given in the lowest effective dose, intermittently if possible, and discontinued at least 6 to 8 weeks prior to delivery. (b) Coxibs should not be used by nursing mothers. (c) Acetaminophen should be considered as an alternative analgesic. (d) If an NSAID is required, consider switching to older NSAIDs such as ibuprofen or naproxen which have been used

more frequently in pregnancy. Consider using a short acting NSAID to help minimize the concentration found in the breast milk.

DRUG INTERACTIONS

Coadministration of celecoxib with drugs that inhibit cytochrome P450 2C9 should be done with caution. ***Drugs which may ↑ toxicity of celecoxib:*** Corticosteroids (GI side effects), fluconazole, other NSAIDs; ***Celecoxib may ↑ toxicity of:*** Anticoagulants (monitor INR closely); ***Celecoxib may ↑ levels of:*** Lithium

MECHANISM OF ACTION

Celecoxib is a cyclooxygenase-2 selective, non-steroidal, anti-inflammatory drug that exhibits anti-inflammatory, analgesic, and anti-pyretic activities. Celecoxib is the active compound with no initial metabolism. Inhibition of prostaglandin synthesis, primarily via inhibition of cyclooxygenase-2 (COX-2). At therapeutic levels there is no inhibition of cyclooxygenase-1 (COX-1)

PHARMACOKINETICS

Bioavail: Unknown; ***Max Plasma Concentration:*** 2.8 hours; ***1/2 Life:*** 11 hours. ***Metab:*** Hepatic via cytochrome P450 2C9 to carboxylic acid, a primary alcohol, & its glucuronide conjugate; ***Prot Bind:*** High (97%); ***Excret:*** Faeces (57%) & urine (27%)

DISEASE MODIFYING ANTI-RHEUMATIC DRUGS (DMARDs)

AZATHIOPRINE (IMURAN, AZASAN)

INDICATIONS
Approved: Rheumatoid arthritis. ***Off-Label Uses:*** Systemic lupus erythematosus and other collagen vascular diseases; vasculitis; Sjogren's syndrome; inflammatory myopathies

DOSE & DRUG ADMINISTRATION
Initial Dose: 1 - 2 mg/kg per day (~ 50 - 100 mg per day); ***Increase:*** 0.5 – 1.0 mg/kg every 4 - 8 weeks until reach 2.5 mg/kg per day; ***Maximum Dose:*** 4 mg/kg per day
Supplied: 50 mg tablets, Azasan® 25, 75, & 100 mg tablets;

DOSE ADJUSTMENT
Hepatic Failure: No dosage adjustment recommended; however, use with caution as the metabolism of azathioprine may be impaired.
Renal Failure: Azathioprine and its metabolites are excreted by the kidneys. Use the lowest possible dose in the setting of renal impairment. ***CrCl > 50 ml/min:*** No initial dose adjustment; ***CrCl 10-50 ml/min:*** 50% initial dose reduction; ***CrCl < 10 ml/min:*** 75% initial dose reduction; ***Dialysis:*** 0.25 mg/kg after dialysis.

ONSET OF ACTION
Initial Response: 2-4 months; ***Maximal Response:*** 4 months

MONITORING
Baseline: CBC, platelets, creatinine, AST, ALT, ALP; ***Weekly during first month or dose adjustments:*** CBC, platelets; ***Twice monthly for second and third months:*** CBC, platelets; ***Then monthly:*** CBC, platelets, creatinine, AST, ALT, ALP

CONTRAINDICATIONS & PRECAUTIONS
(a) Hypersensitivity to azathioprine or 6-mercaptopurine: Severe nausea & vomiting which may be accompanied by diarrhea, rash, fever, malaise, myalgias, ↑ LFTs, and rarely hypotension; (b) Patients previously treated with alkylating agents may have a risk of neoplasia; (c) History of recurring infections or conditions which may predispose to infections; (d) Reduced activity of thiopurine methyltransferase (TPMT) can result in increased hematologic toxicity. May occur in up to 10-15% of patients.

TOXICITY
Reversible: **(a) GI:** Nausea & vomiting (may be ↓ by dividing the daily dose), diarrhea; **(b) Mucocut:** Skin rash, alopecia; **(c) Gen:** Fevers, malaise (common reason for discontinuation); **(d) MSK:** Arthralgias
Potentially Serious: **(a) Infection:** Serious infections and sepsis have been reported with the use of azathioprine; **(b) Hematologic:** Reversible myelosuppression, leukopenia and/or thrombocytopenia, macrocytic anemia and severe bone marrow depression; **(c) Malignancy:** May ↑ risk of lymphoproliferative disease. AML and solid tumors have been reported in patients with RA receiving azathioprine; **(d) Fertility:** May cause a temporary ↓ in spermatogenesis; **(e) GI:** Hepatotoxicity (rare), veno-occlusive disease (rare), pancreatitis

PREGNANCY & LACTATION
Pregnancy: POSITIVE EVIDENCE OF RISK. (CATEGORY D)
Conception & Fertility: Azathioprine does not appear to be teratogenic in humans. There appears to be no effect on fertility and no increase in the abortion rate. Azathioprine appears to be safe for men who are attempting to father children.
Fetal Effects: Azathioprine crosses the placenta but the fetal liver lacks the enzyme to convert it to 6-mercaptopurine, the active metabolite. A variety of adverse effects

have been reported throughout pregnancy; however, normal pregnancies have been reported in patients who were treated with azathioprine and prednisone.
Lactation: Low concentrations of azathioprine are found in breast milk. Breast feeding is generally not recommended.
Recommendations: Use of azathioprine should be reserved for pregnant women whose rheumatic diseases are severe or life-threatening.

DRUG INTERACTIONS
Azathioprine may ↓ *efficacy of:* Warfarin, non-depolarizing muscle relaxants;
Drugs which may ↑ *toxicity of azathioprine:* Allopurinol (patients receiving azathioprine and allopurinol concomitantly should have a dose reduction of azathioprine of approximately ½ to ¼), sulfasalazine (increased myelosuppression), ACE inhibitors (anemia & leukopenia), other bm suppressing meds, zidovudine

MECHANISM OF ACTION
Azathioprine is rapidly converted to 6-mercaptopurine (6-MP) enzymatically by glutathione S-transferase on first pass through the liver. 6-Mercaptopurine (6-MP) is the biologically active form which is converted to cytotoxic thioguanine nucleotides (6-thioguanine) by hypoxanthine-guanine phosphoribosyltransferase (HGPRT). Azathioprine is a purine analogue which hinders the synthesis of adenosine & guanine. The exact mechanism of action is not known - possible mechanisms include: ↓ Circulating lymphocyte count and proliferation by cytotoxicity through incorporation into nucleic acids or by ↓ cellular proliferation by inhibiting purine synthesis; ↓ Antibody production, ↓ Monocyte production; Suppression of natural killer cell activity; ↓ Cell-mediated and humoral immunity

PHARMACOKINETICS
Bioavail: 47% (27 - 83); *Max Plasma Concn:* 1- 3 hours; *1/2 Life:* 6-MP (1 - 2 hours), thioguanine nucleotides (1 - 2 weeks); *Metab:* 6-MP is inactivated to 6-methylthiouric acid by xanthine oxidase. 6-MP is inactivated to 6-methylmercaptopurine by thiopurine methyltransferase (TPMT); *Prot Bind:* 30%; *Excret:* Renal

CHLORAMBUCIL (LEUKERAN)

INDICATIONS
Approved: No approved rheumatologic indications.   *Off-Label Uses:* Vasculitides (WG; PAN; MPA; CSS; Takayasu's arteritis; GCA); SLE; uveitis; Behcet's disease

DOSE & DRUG ADMINISTRATION
Initial Dose: 2 - 4 mg PO OD; *Increase:* 1 - 2 mg per day at 1 to 2 month intervals;
Maximum Dose: None specified (titrate to bone marrow effects);
Supplied: 2 mg tablets.

DOSE ADJUSTMENT
Hepatic Failure: increases 1/2-life;Dose modifications are generally not required;
Renal Failure: CrCl > 50 ml/min: No initial dose adjustment; *CrCl 10-50 ml/min:* Reduce initial dose by 50-70%; *CrCl < 10 ml/min:* Reduce initial dose by 75%

ONSET OF ACTION
Initial Response: 4 - 8 weeks; *Maximal Response:* Months

MONITORING
Baseline: CBC, Cr, AST, ALT, ALP; *Every one to two weeks for initial 2 months or with dosage change:* CBC; *Monthly thereafter:* CBC, Cr, AST, ALT, ALP

CONTRAINDICATIONS & PRECAUTIONS
(a) Known hypersensitivity to chlorambucil; (b) Active infection – chronic and localized; (c) History of recurring infections or conditions which may predispose to infections (i.e. diabetes); (d) Previous malignancy

TOXICITY
Reversible: *(a) GI:* Nausea, vomiting, abdominal pain, diarrhea, anorexia; *(b) Mucocut:* Oral ulceration, skin rash; *(c) CNS:* Reversible tremors, muscle twitching, confusion, agitation, ataxia, flaccid paresis, and hallucinations

Potentially Serious: *(a) Hem:* Reversible myelosuppression is common but may be severe; *(b) Reproductive:* Azospermia and amenorrhea which are usually reversible; *(c) Infection:* Serious infections and sepsis, including fatality, have been reported with the use of chlorambucil; *(d) Mucocut:* Severe skin reactions progressing to erythema multiforme, toxic epidermal necrolysis, or Stevens-Johnson syndrome; *(e) Malignancy:* ↑ Risk of leukemia and lymphoma

PREGNANCY & LACTATION
Pregnancy: POSITIVE EVIDENCE OF RISK. (CATEGORY D)

Conception & Fertility: Limited evidence that chlorambucil impairs fertility.

Fetal Effects: Chlorambucil has been associated with significant congenital abnormalities.

Lactation: There is very limited information on the safety of chlorambucil during lactation. Breast feeding should likely be avoided by patients receiving chlorambucil.

Recommendations: Chlorambucil is generally contraindicated during pregnancy and lactation; It should be discontinued at least 3 months before the patient tries to conceive; Consideration should be given to preserving ovarian function.

DRUG INTERACTIONS
Drugs which may ↑ toxicity of chlorambucil: Other bone marrow suppressing medications

ACTIVE FORM & INITIAL METABOLISM
Chlorambucil is a bifunctional alkylating agent of the nitrogen mustard type which is extensively metabolized in the liver to phenylacetic acid mustard. Both chlorambucil and phenylacetic acid mustard are biologically active

MECHANISM OF ACTION
Chlorambucil works by alkylation of DNA by the active metabolites, such as phosphoramide mustard. Alkylation results in cross-linking of DNA, breaks in DNA, ↓ DNA synthesis, and apoptosis. The resulting effects include a reduction in numbers of T and B lymphocytes, ↓ lymphocyte proliferation, ↓ antibody production, and suppression of delayed hypersensitivity. Effects are not limited to any particular cell type, however, effects are more marked with rapidly dividing cells.

PHARMACOKINETICS
Bioavail: >70%; *Max Plasma Concn:* 40 - 70 minutes; *Elim 1/2 Life:* 1.5 hrs; *Metab:* Cytochrome P450 enzyme system in liver; *Prot Bind:* 99%; *Excret:* Metabs in urine

CHLOROQUINE PHOSPHATE (ARALEN)

INDICATIONS
Approved: No approved rheumatologic indications. *Off-Label Uses:* Rheumatoid arthritis & other inflammatory arthritides; systemic lupus erythematosus

DOSE & DRUG ADMINISTRATION
Dose: 125 - 250 mg PO OD (must be < 3 mg/kg/day of lean body weight);
Supplied: 250 & 500 mg tablets

DOSE ADJUSTMENT
Hepatic Failure: Use with caution, drug is known to concentrate in the liver.

Renal Failure: CrCl > 10 ml/min: No initial dose adjustment; *CrCl < 10 ml/min:* Reduce initial dose by 50%; *Dialysis:* No dose adjustment

ONSET OF ACTION
Initial Response: 8 - 12 weeks; *Maximal Response:* Several months

MONITORING
Baseline: Ophthalmologic monitoring (central visual fields (one eye only) and color vision); *Every 12 months:* Ophthalmologic monitoring (central visual fields (one eye only) and color vision)

CONTRAINDICATIONS & PRECAUTIONS
(a) Known hypersensitivity to chloroquine; (b) Chloroquine associated retinopathy

TOXICITY
Reversible: (a) Mucocut: Rash – variable; *(b) GI:* Anorexia, nausea & vomiting, dyspepsia, cramps, bloating, diarrhea; *(c) CNS:* Headaches, giddiness, insomnia, nervousness; *(d)Ocular:* Defects in accommodation & corneal deposits - reversible
Potentially Serious: (a) Ocular: Retinopathy – pigmentary changes, clumping, bull's eye lesion; *(b) CNS:* 8th cranial nerve toxicity; *(c) MSK:* Skeletal muscle palsies or skeletal muscle myopathy or neuromyopathy; *(d) CVS:* Conduction disturbances (long QT), congestive heart failure

PREGNANCY & LACTATION
Pregnancy: **RISK CANNOT BE RULED OUT. (CATEGORY C)** – Consensus document felt that chloroquine in pregnancy is safe because of the long half-life and the large number of successful pregnancies with the fetus exposed to an anti-malarial.
Lactation: Small amounts of chloroquine are excreted in breast milk. Nursing is not generally recommended; however, it is likely safe.

DRUG INTERACTIONS
Chloroquine may ⬆ *levels and toxicity of:* Digoxin, hydroxychloroquine

MECHANISM OF ACTION
Chloroquine phosphate is the active form. Chloroquine is found in high concentrations within cells. It is a basic compound which causes an elevation of intracellular pH, particularly within vacuoles, lysosomes, and endosomes. It is through this elevation of intracellular pH that chloroquine probably exerts its most important effects such as: (a) Lysosomotropic action: interference with cellular function in compartments in which there is an acid microenvironment. This reduces the ability of intracellular organelles to degrade and process proteins; (b) Reduced formation of MHC-peptide complexes in the presence of the basic intracellular pH. Chloroquine has numerous other actions such as: Inhibition of phospholipase A2 and other enzymes; Inhibition of several pro-inflammatory cytokines; Immune activity & Anti–infectious activity

PHARMACOKINETICS
Avail: Rapidly absorbed ; *1/2 Life:* 50 days; *Steady State:* 3-4 months; *Metab:* Hepatic with main metabolite desethylchloroquine; *Prot Bind:* 55% bound to plasma proteins; *Concn:* Mononuclear cells > neutrophils, Intracellular lysosomes and pigmented eye tissue; *Excret:* Predominantly renal - 90% (50% unchanged); Faeces - 10%

CYCLOPHOSPHAMIDE - INTRAVENOUS (CYTOXAN)

INDICATIONS
Approved: No approved rheumatologic indications. *Off-Label Uses:* Active vasculitis & SLE with mononeuritis multiplex, CNS disease, RPGN, mesenteric vasculitis, cardiac involvement, and alveolar hemorrhage.

DOSE & DRUG ADMINISTRATION

Given once monthly by intravenous route; **Initial Dose:** 0.5 - 0.75 mg/m2 IV infusion in saline over 30 - 60 minutes (500 mg); **Adjustments:** If WBC nadir at 10-14 days is >4000/mm3 increase dose 25%; If WBC nadir at 10-14 days is <1500/mm3 decrease dose 25%; Although the above is the standard dosing protocol, the induction of neutropenia is NOT essential to achieve remission - Granulocyte kinetics have found that marked suppression of granulocytopoiesis is not necessary for a favorable response. **Maximum Dose:** 1 mg/m2.

Example of orders for cyclophosphamide are as follows:

Initial Bloodwork: Bloodwork to be done prior to infusion: CBC with differential, creatinine, sodium, and potassium - ensure it is normal.

Cyclophosphamide Infusion: (a) Insert large bore IV into forearm and administer 200 mL normal saline over 30 minutes; (b) Ondansetron 8 mg PO one hour prior to cyclophosphamide, then, 8 mg PO BID for 24-48 hours; (c) If IV methylprednisolone is not going to be given with the cyclophosphamide give dexamethasone 10 mg one hour prior to infusion and 4 hours after infusion; (d) MESNA (bladder protection) 180 mg IV just prior to administration of cyclophosphamide and repeated 180 mg IV 4 and 8 hours post cyclophosphamide; (e) IV Cyclophosphamide 0.75-1.0 g/m2 (if normal renal function otherwise decrease by 50%) in 250 mL of D5W given over 1 hour; (f) IV normal saline 250 mL/hr for two hours after cyclophosphamide infusion;

Methylprednisolone Infusion (optional): After two hours of normal saline, administer IV methylprednisolone 1000 mg in 250 mL D5W over one hour; Record pulse and blood pressure every 15 minutes during the infusion and every 30 minutes following the infusion for two hours;

Cyclophosphamide Infusion (continued): Follow the IV methylprednisolone with normal saline 125 mL per hour until completion; For the following 24 hours ask the patient to drink 250 mL of fluid q1h; If the patient is to return for subsequent infusions of methylprednisolone the patient may be discharged with the saline lock in place;

Subsequent infusions of methylprednisolone (optional next 2 days): Draw blood for Na and K prior to infusion and ensure it is normal; Give IV methylprednisolone 1000 mg in 250 mL D5W over one (1) hour. Record pulse and blood pressure every 15 minutes during the infusion and then every 30 minutes for two hours.

Post-transfusion Bloodwork: CBC with differential and platelet count must be measured on day 7, 10, and 14 post infusion counting day 0 as the day of administration; If possible, IV cyclophosphamide is changed to oral cyclophosphamide after the first week at a dose of 2 mg/kg/day.

DOSE ADJUSTMENT

Hepatic Failure: Hepatic failure increases half-life; however, dose modifications are generally not required.

Renal Failure: **CrCl > 50 ml/min:** No initial dose adjustment; **CrCl 10-50 ml/min:** Reduce initial dose by 50-70%; **CrCl < 10 ml/min:** Reduce initial dose by 75%; **Dialysis:** 50% after dialysis

ONSET OF ACTION

Initial Response: 4 - 8 weeks; **Maximal Response:** Months

MONITORING

Baseline: CBC, creatinine, AST, ALT, ALP, urinalysis; **10 – 14 days after IV infusion:** CBC, urinalysis; **Prior to each subsequent infusion:** CBC, creatinine, AST, ALT, ALP, urinalysis; **Monthly:** CBC, creatinine, urinalysis; **Every 6 months to a year:** Urine cytology (should be done chronically even after discontinuation of the medication)

CONTRAINDICATIONS & PRECAUTIONS

(a) Hypersensitivity to cyclophosphamide; (b) Active infection – chronic and localized; (c) History of recurring infections or conditions which may predispose to infections (i.e. diabetes); (d) Previous malignancy; (e) Severe leukopenia or thrombocytopenia; (f) Hepatic or renal dysfunction

TOXICITY

Reversible: (a) GI: Nausea, vomiting, abdominal pain, diarrhea; *(b) Mucocut:* Alopecia, skin rash, oral ulcers;

Potentially Serious: (a) Hem: Reversible myelosuppression is common (leukopenia, thrombocytopenia, anemia); *(b) GU:* Hemorrhagic cystitis and bladder fibrosis; *(c) Reproductive:* Male and female infertility and amenorrhea; *(d) Infection:* Serious infections and sepsis, including fatality, have been reported with the use of cyclophosphamide; *(e) Malignancy:* ↑ Risk of myeloproliferative, lymphoproliferative, skin, and urinary bladder malignancies; *(f) Resp:* Interstitial pulmonary fibrosis (rare); *(g) CVS:* Rare reports of hemorrhagic myocarditis

Managing Toxicity: (a) Hydration with intravenous saline and administration of IV MESNA (dose of 20% of the total cyclophosphamide dose at 0, 4, and 8 hours) may help to reduce bladder toxicity; *(b) Anti-emetics:* Dexamethasone 10 mg PO and ondansetron 4-8 mg PO q4h x 3-4 doses; *(c) Septra:* Can be given concomitantly for Pneumocystis Carinii prophylaxis

PREGNANCY & LACTATION

Pregnancy: POSITIVE EVIDENCE OF RISK. (CATEGORY D)

Lactation: Contraindicated

DRUG INTERACTIONS

Cyclophosphamide may ↑ toxicity of: Succinylcholine (cyclophosphamide causes a marked and persistent inhibition of cholinesterase activity which potentiates the effects of succinylcholine), warfarin; *Drugs which may ↑ toxicity of cyclophosphamide:* Cimetidine (inhibits activity of hepatic enzymes and increases bone marrow toxicity in mouse-model); allopurinol (increases the half-life and frequency of leukopenia)

MECHANISM OF ACTION

Cyclophosphamide is an analogue of nitrogen mustard. Cyclophosphamide is biologically inactive and is rapidly metabolized by the liver to active metabolites 4-hydroxycyclophosphamide, aldophosphamide, phosphoramide mustard, and acrolein.

Cyclophosphamide works by alkylation of DNA by the active metabolites, such as phosphoramide mustard. Alkylation results in cross-linking of DNA, breaks in DNA, ↓ DNA synthesis, and apoptosis. The resulting effects include a reduction in numbers of T and B lymphocytes, ↓ lymphocyte proliferation, ↓ antibody production, and suppression of delayed hypersensitivity. Effects are not limited to any particular cell type, however, effects are more marked with rapidly dividing cells.

PHARMACOKINETICS

Bioavail: 100%; *Max Plasma Concn:* 1 hour; *Elim 1/2 Life:* 3 - 12 hours; *Metab:* Cytochrome P450 enzyme system in the liver; *Prot Bind:* 20%; *Excret:* Urine

CYCLOPHOSPHAMIDE - ORAL (CYTOXAN)

INDICATIONS

Approved: No approved rheumatologic indications. *Off-Label Uses:* Active vasculitis & SLE with mononeuritis multiplex, CNS disease, RPGN, mesenteric vasculitis, cardiac involvement, and alveolar hemorrhage.

DOSE & DRUG ADMINISTRATION

Initial Dose: 2 mg/kg OD; *Increase:* 25 mg at 1 - 2 week intervals; *Maximum Dose:* 5 mg/kg per day; *Supplied:* 25 & 50 mg tablets.

DOSE ADJUSTMENT

Hepatic Failure: Increase half-life; dose modifications are generally not required.
Renal Failure: CrCl ≥ 100: 2.0 mg/kg/day; *CrCl 50-99:* 1.5 mg/kg/day; *CrCl 25-49:* 1.2 mg/kg/d; *CrCl 15-24:* 1.0 mg/kg/d; *CrCl <15 or dialysis:* 0.8 mg/kg/d

ONSET OF ACTION

Initial Response: 4 - 8 weeks; *Maximal Response:* Months

MONITORING

Baseline: CBC, creatinine, AST, ALT, ALP, urinalysis; *Every 1 to 2 weeks for initial 2 months or with dose change:* CBC, Cr, urinalysis; *Monthly:* CBC, creatinine, urinalysis; *Every 6 months to a year:* Urine cytology (should be done chronically even after discontinuation of the medication)

CONTRAINDICATIONS & PRECAUTIONS

(a) Hypersensitivity to cyclophosphamide; (b) Active infection – chronic and localized; (c) History of recurring infections or conditions which may predispose to infections; (d) Previous malignancy; (e) Severe leukopenia or thrombocytopenia; (f) Hepatic or renal dysfunction

TOXICITY

Reversible: (a) GI: Nausea, vomiting, abdominal pain, diarrhea; *(b) Mucocut:* Alopecia, skin rash, oral ulcers
Potentially Serious: (a) Hem: Reversible myelosuppression is common (leukopenia, thrombocytopenia, anemia); *(b) GU:* Hemorrhagic cystitis and fibrosis; *(c) Reproductive:* Male and female infertility and amenorrhea; *(d) Infection:* Serious infections and sepsis, including fatality, have been reported with the use of cyclophosphamide; *(e) Malignancy:* ↑ Risk of myeloproliferative, lymphoproliferative, skin and urinary bladder malignancies; *(f) Resp:* Interstitial pulmonary fibrosis (rare)
Reducing Toxicity: (a) Administer as a single morning dose with plenty of water; (b) Dose for renal function and reduce dose by 1/2 for elderly patients; (c) Check the CBC every 2 weeks; (d) Pneumocystis carinii prophylaxis with septra

PREGNANCY & LACTATION

Pregnancy: POSITIVE EVIDENCE OF RISK. (CATEGORY D)
Conception & Fertility: Cyclophosphamide causes amenorrhea and may cause permanent ovarian failure (up to 70% with daily oral use & up to 45% with monthly pulse doses). Concomitant use of oral contraceptives or gonadotropin-releasing hormone agonists may protect ovarian follicle viability. *Fetal Effects:* Cyclophosphamide is a significant teratogen when administered during conception or within the first trimester. Use of cyclophosphamide in the second and third trimesters does not seem to place the fetus at risk for congenital defects and may be considered for a woman with life-threatening rheumatic disease.
Lactation: Cyclophosphamide is found in substantial amounts in breast milk and is therefore contraindicated during breast feeding.
Recommendations: Cyclophosphamide is generally contraindicated during pregnancy and lactation; It should be discontinued at least 3 months before the patient tries to conceive; Consideration should be given to protecting ovarian function with hormone therapy; For life-threatening rheumatic disease, cyclophosphamide may be considered in the 2 & 3rd trimesters.

DRUG INTERACTIONS

Cyclophosphamide may ↑ toxicity of: Succinylcholine (cyclophosphamide causes a marked and persistent inhibition of cholinesterase activity which potentiates the effects of succinylcholine), warfarin; **Drugs which may↑ toxicity of cyclophosphamide:** Cimetidine (inhibits activity of hepatic enzymes and increases bone marrow toxicity in mouse-model); allopurinol (increases the half-life and frequency of leukopenia)

MECHANISM OF ACTION

Cyclophosphamide is an analogue of nitrogen mustard. Cyclophosphamide is biologically inactive and is rapidly metabolized by the liver to active metabolites 4-hydroxycyclophosphamide, aldophosphamide, phosphoramide mustard, & acrolein. Cyclophosphamide works by alkylation of DNA by the active metabolites, such as phosphoramide mustard. Alkylation results in cross-linking of DNA, breaks in DNA, ↓ DNA synthesis, and apoptosis. The resulting effects include a reduction in numbers of T and B lymphocytes, ↓ lymphocyte proliferation, ↓ antibody production, and suppression of delayed hypersensitivity. Effects are not limited to any particular cell type, however, effects are more marked with rapidly dividing cells.

PHARMACOKINETICS

Bioavail: >75%; *Max Plasma Concn:* 1 hour; *Elim 1/2 Life:* 3 -12 hours; *Metab:* Cytochrome P450 enzyme system in the liver; *Prot Bind:* 20%; *Excret:* Urine

CYCLOSPORINE (NEORAL, SANDIMMUNE, GENGRAF)

INDICATIONS

Approved: Rheumatoid arthritis; psoriasis. *Off-Label Uses:* Autoimmune eye disease (uveitis, scleritis); vasculitis; autoimmune pulmonary disease; inflammatory myopathies; Behcet's disease; psoriatic arthritis

DOSE & DRUG ADMINISTRATION

Initial Dose: 2.5 mg/kg per day in 2 divided doses (i.e. 100 mg BID); *Increase:* 1 mg/kg per week. *Maximum Dose:* 4 mg/kg per day;
Supplied: 25, 50, & 100 mg capsules & 100 mg/mL oral suspension.

DOSE ADJUSTMENT

Hepatic Failure: Impairs excretion of cyclosporine metabolites; use with caution. *Renal Failure:* Contraindicated. Cyclosporine can be used with dialysis patients with no dose adjustment necessary.

ONSET OF ACTION

Initial Response: 2 - 4 months; *Maximal Response:* 6 - 8 months

MONITORING

Baseline: CBC, creatinine (average of 2 readings), liver function tests, uric acid, serum magnesium, blood pressure (average of 2 readings); *Every two weeks for initial 3 months:* Blood pressure and creatinine; *Monthly:* CBC, creatinine, liver function tests, serum magnesium, blood pressure; *Change in Dose:* Monitor blood pressure and creatinine every 2 weeks

CONTRAINDICATIONS & PRECAUTIONS

(a) Known hypersensitivity to cyclosporine; (b) Uncontrolled hypertension; (c) Malignancy within the last 5 years (except basal cell carcinoma); (d) Abnormal renal or liver function; (e) Uncontrolled infection; (f) Primary or secondary immunodeficiency excluding autoimmune disease

TOXICITY

Reversible: (a) Gen: Fatigue, weakness, cramps, bloating, flushing; *(b) GI:* Dyspepsia, nausea, abdominal pain; *(c) Mucocut:* Hirsutism/hypertrichosis, gingival hyperplasia; *(d) CNS:* Headache, paresthesias; *(e) MSK:* Arthropathy, muscle cramps, tremor; *(f) Lab:* Hypomagnesemia, hyperuricemia, hyperkalemia, hyperlipidemia

Potentially Serious: *(a) Renal:* Nephrotoxicity (reversibility if renal function <30% above baseline); *(b) GI:* Hepatotoxicity; *(c) CVS:* Hypertension (reversible); *(d) Infection:* Serious infections and sepsis have been reported with the use of cyclosporine; *(e) Malignancy:* May ↑ risk of lymphoproliferative disease (reversible & dose dependant)

Managing Toxicity: Patients must drink 1.5 liters of fluid per day; dehydration can have an adverse effect on renal function; If change in serum creatinine is >25% above patients baseline then ↓ cyclosporine by 25-50% (100 mg/day); if serum creatinine is > 30% above baseline stop cyclosporine; Cyclosporine dose should be ↓ by 25-50% (100 mg) with sustained hypertension (160/95 on two consecutive occasions). If hypertension persists dose can be further ↓ or anti-hypertensive therapy (B-blocker, ACE-inhibitor, adalat XL, amlodipine) can be started.

PREGNANCY & LACTATION

Pregnancy: RISK CANNOT BE RULED OUT – (CATEGORY C).

Conception & Fertility: Insufficient evidence. **Pregnancy Effects:** Pregnancy outcome data is largely derived from transplant patients. Most of these pregnancies were high-risk with an increased risk of abortion and low birth weight. It is very difficult to separate the effect of the disease on the pregnancy & fetus from the effect of the cyclosporine.

Lactation: Cyclosporine is excreted in human breast milk and is considered to be contraindicated during lactation.

Recommendations: In general, cyclosporine is contraindicated in the treatment of rheumatic disease during pregnancy; Breast feeding is not recommended.

DRUG INTERACTIONS

Contraindicated: STATINS, FLUCONAZOLE, ITRACONAZOLE, KETOCONAZOLE; **Cyclosporine may ↑ toxicity of:** Statins (myopathy), colchicine (neuromyopathy), digoxin, potassium-sparing diuretics; **Drugs which may ↑ levels and toxicity of cyclosporine:** Diltiazem, nicardipine, verapamil, clarithromycin, erythromycin, fluconazole, itraconazole, ketoconazole, methylprednisolone, allopurinol, bromocriptine, danazol, metoclopramide; **Drugs which may ↓ renal toxicity of cyclosporine:** NSAIDs, ACE-inhibitors, aminoglycosides, amphotericin B, quinolone antibiotics; **Drugs which may ↓ levels and efficacy of cyclosporine:** Nafcillin, rifampin, carbamazepine, phenobarbital, phenytoin, octreotide, ticlopidine

MECHANISM OF ACTION

Cyclosporine is a lipophilic endecapeptide derived from a fungus. Cyclosporine complexes with cyclophilin, a cytosolic binding protein. The cyclosporine-cyclophilin complex binds to, and inhibits calcineurin, a serine-threonine phosphatase. Inhibition of calcineurin phosphatase prevents the translocation of cytosolic nuclear factor into the nucleus of activated T-cells. This cytosolic nuclear factor is required for the transcription of genes for cytokines such as interleukin-2 and for T-cell activation. Thus, cyclosporine impairs the production of interleukin-2 and other cytokines which decreases lymphocyte proliferation.

PHARMACOKINETICS

Bioavail: 30%; **Max Plasma Concn:** 1 - 8 hrs; **Elim 1/2 Life:** 20 hrs in adults; **Metab:** Cytochrome P450 3A4 enzyme system in the intestinal mucosa and the liver. It is extensively metabolized to more than 20 metabolites; **Prot Bind:** 30%; **Excret:** Primarily biliary with 6% excreted in the urine

D-PENICILLAMINE (CUPRIMINE, DEPEN)

INDICATIONS
Approved: Rheumatoid arthritis. *Off-label Uses:* SSc; JIA

DOSE & DRUG ADMINISTRATION
Oral Medication – "go low & go slow"; *Initial Dose:* 125 - 250 mg PO OD; *Increments:* 125 - 250 mg every 1 to 3 months; *Maximum Dose:* 1000 mg/day; *Supplied:* 125 & 250 mg tablets.

DOSE ADJUSTMENT
Hepatic Failure: Use with caution.
Renal Failure: CrCl > 50 ml/min: No initial dose adjustment; *CrCl < 50 ml/min:* Avoid; *Dialysis:* 250 mg after dialysis

ONSET OF ACTION
Initial Response: 8 - 12 weeks; *Maximal Response:* Several months

MONITORING
Baseline: CBC, platelet count, Cr, urine dipstick for protein; *Until Dosage Stable (q2-4 weeks):* CBC, platelet count, Cr, urine dipstick for protein; *Then every 1 - 3 months:* CBC, platelet count, Cr, urine dipstick for protein

CONTRAINDICATIONS & PRECAUTIONS
(a) Known hypersensitivity to penicillamine; (b) Penicillamine related aplastic anemia or agranulocytosis; (c) Renal failure

TOXICITY
Reversible: (a) Gen: Drug fever; *(b) GI:* Anorexia, nausea & vomiting, hypogeusia, dysgeusia, metallic taste; *(c) Mucocut:* Rash, stomatitis, painful oral ulcers
Potentially Serious: (a) Hem: Leukopenia, thrombocytopenia, aplastic anemia; *(b) Renal:* Proteinuria, membranous nephropathy; *(c) CNS:* Myasthenia gravis; *(d) Autoimmune:* Drug-induced SLE (+ ANA); *(e) Resp:* Bronchiolitis

PREGNANCY & LACTATION
Pregnancy: POSITIVE EVIDENCE OF RISK. (CATEGORY D)
Fetal Effects: Exposure of the human fetus to penicillamine has resulted in serious disorders of connective tissue (cutis laxa, hernia, dislocated hips, & delayed growth)
Lactation: D-penicillamine is contraindicated during lactation.
Recommendations: Treatment with penicillamine should be discontinued at least 3 months before conception or as soon as pregnancy is confirmed.

DRUG INTERACTIONS
Drugs which may ↑ toxicity of d-penicillamine: Gold salts (increase hematologic toxicity); *Drugs which may chelate d-penicillamine and ↓ efficacy:* Iron supplements, aluminum salts; *D-penicillamine may ↓ levels of:* Digoxin

MECHANISM OF ACTION
The active form is thought to be unchanged d-penicillamine. Largely unknown but may work via: Reduction of rheumatoid factor, immune complexes, & T-cell activity

PHARMACOKINETICS
Bioavail: Relatively high (40-70%); *Mean abspn time:* 2 hours; *1/2 Life:* 1.7 - 3.2 hours; *Metab:* Small amounts of hepatic metabolism; *Prot Bind:* 80% bound to plasma proteins; *Excret:* Renal (30 - 60% as unchanged drug)

DAPSONE

INDICATIONS
Approved: Leprosy & dermatitis herpetiformis. *Off-label Uses:* Cutaneous vasculitis (Sweet's syndrome, leukocytoclastic vasculitis, urticarial vasculitis, erythema elevatum diuntinum, and cutaneous PAN), Cutaneous lesions of Behcet's disease,

Cutaneous lesions of SLE (bullous disease and panniculitis), relapsing polychondritis, and pyoderma gangrenosum.

DOSE & DRUG ADMINISTRATION
Initial Dose: 50-100 mg OD; *Increments:* 25-50 mg as tolerated; *Max Dose:* 300 mg/day
Supplied: 25 & 100 mg tablets.

DOSE ADJUSTMENT
Hepatic Failure: Use with caution as dapsone is metabolized in the liver.
Renal Failure: Metabolic products are excreted in the urine, however, no dosage adjustment is likely required

ONSET OF ACTION
Initial Response: Fairly prompt response to treatment within 1 to 3 week; *Maximal Response:* Several months

MONITORING
Baseline: CBC, platelet count, Cr, AST, ALT, ALP, & albumin; *Every month for the first six months:* CBC, reticulocyte count, AST, ALT, ALP, albumin; *Then every 3 - 6 months:* CBC, reticulocyte count, AST, ALT, ALP, albumin

CONTRAINDICATIONS & PRECAUTIONS
(a) Known hypersensitivity to Dapsone; (b) Prior allergy to sulfonamides; (c) Known G6PD deficiency; (d) Use with caution in patients with moderate to severe underlying anemia or known bone marrow dysfunction; (e) Use with caution in patients with severe hepatic impairment

TOXICITY
Reversible: (a) Gen: Drug fever; *(b) GI:* Anorexia, nausea & vomiting, abdominal pain; *(c) Mucocut:* Skin Rash; *(d) CNS:* Headache, insomnia
Potentially Serious: (a) Hem: Dose related hemolysis is seen in all patients with a typical fall in hemoglobin of 1-2 g/dL (10-20 g/L). Hemolysis can be severe in patients with G6PD deficiency. Agranulocytosis and leukopenia can rarely be seen (<1%); *(b) Neuro:* Peripheral neuropathy is a rare but well documented side effect of dapsone (motor weakness is more common). Reactional states (psychosis) can also be seen with the use of dapsone; *(c) Mucocut:* Exfoliative dermatitis (Stevens-Johnson Syndrome); *(d) GI:* Hepatotoxicity; *(e) Dapsone Syndrome:* Fever and eosinophilia - Dangerous as it may progress to exfoliative dermatitis, fall in albumin levels, psychosis, hepatitis, and death.
Managing Toxicity: Folic acid 1 mg PO OD to reduce the hem. toxicity of dapsone.

PREGNANCY & LACTATION
Pregnancy: RISK CANNOT BE RULED OUT. (CATEGORY C)
Conception & Fertility: Dapsone is not known to affect fertility. *Fetal Effects:* There have been no controlled animal or human studies regarding the safety of dapsone during pregnancy. Uncontrolled experience and two published surveys have not shown that dapsone increases the risk of fetal abnormalities if administered during all trimesters of pregnancy.
Lactation: Dapsone is excreted in breast milk in substantial amounts and is therefore not recommended during breast feeding. There are rare reports of hemolytic anemia developing in breastfeeding infants.
Recommendations: In general, dapsone is contraindicated in the treatment of rheumatic disease during pregnancy; Breast feeding is not recommended.

DRUG INTERACTIONS
Drugs which may ↑ levels/toxicity of dapsone: Probenecid (slows renal excretion), CYP3A4 inhibitors (azole antifungals, ciprofloxacin, clarithromycin,

diclofenac, doxycycline, erythromycin, imatinib, isoniazid, nefazodone, nicardipine, propofol, protease inhibitors, quinidine, and verapamil). Folic acid antagonists may increase the hematologic toxicity of dapsone, Trimethoprim. ***Drugs which may↓ levels/efficacy of dapsone:*** CYP3A4 inducers (aminoglutethimide, carbamazepine, nafcillin, nevirapine, phenobarbital, phenytoin, and rifamycins), didanosine, rifampin.

MECHANISM OF ACTION
The mechanism of action of dapsone in cutaneous vasculitis is unknown.

PHARMACOKINETICS
Bioavail: Relatively high (70-80%); ***Mean abs time:*** 4-8 hours to reach peak levels; ***1/2 Life:*** 10-50 hours; ***Metab:*** Hepatic metabolism via CYP; ***Prot Bind:*** 50-80% bound to plasma proteins; ***Excretn:*** Renal (water soluble metabolites)

GOLD SODIUM THIOMALATE (AUROLATE, ✚MYOCHRISINE)

INDICATIONS
Approved: Adult & juvenile rheumatoid arthritis; psoriatic arthritis; Felty's syndrome.

DOSE & DRUG ADMINISTRATION
Initial Dosing: 10 mg IM test dose, 25 mg IM one week later, then 50 mg IM weekly; ***Maintenance Dose:*** 50% of patients develop side effects requiring dose adjustment. Continue weekly injections (50 mg if tolerated) until the patient is in complete remission or no expectation of further improvement. Intervals between injections may be increased to 3 to 4 weeks in the event of remission. When RA flares, resume weekly regimen. The most effective regimen is every 1 - 2 weeks; ***Supplied:*** Boxes of 3 ampules of 1mL vials containing 10, 25, or 50 mg/mL.

DOSE ADJUSTMENT
Hepatic Failure: No formal studies; use with caution.
Renal Failure: Contraindicated.

ONSET OF ACTION
Initial Response: 3 months; ***Maximal Response:*** 6 - 18 months

MONITORING
Baseline: CBC, platelet count, and urinalysis; ***Every week for the first 4 weeks:*** CBC, platelet count, and urinalysis; ***Every 2 weeks until 20 weeks:*** CBC, platelet count, and urinalysis; ***Every 3 weeks until 52 weeks:*** CBC, platelet count, and urinalysis; ***Every 4-8 injections thereafter:*** CBC, platelet count, and urinalysis

CONTRAINDICATIONS & PRECAUTIONS
(a) Renal failure; (b) Gold induced thrombocytopenia, leukopenia, aplastic anemia; (c) Gold induced pneumonitis, nephrotic syndrome; (d) Systemic lupus erythematosus ➔ increased risk of toxicity; (e) Anticoagulants ➔ risk of hematoma (not a contraindication)

TOXICITY
Reversible: (a) Post-Injection Reactions: Myalgias or arthralgias; ***(b) Mucocut:*** Stomatitis, dermatitis with or without a rash; ***(c) Ophtho:*** Corneal or lens chrysiasis; ***(d) Misc:*** Metallic taste; ***(e) Nitritoid Reaction:*** Dizziness, nausea, fatigue or weakness within seconds to 30 minutes after injection; ***(f) Hem:*** Thrombocytopenia (1%), eosinophilia; ***(g) Renal:*** Proteinuria, hematuria, membranous nephropathy
Potentially Serious: (a) Hem: Aplastic anemia, leukopenia; ***(b) GI:*** Colitis, cholestatic hepatitis, pancreatitis; ***(c) Resp:*** Gold induced pneumonitis; ***(d) CNS:*** Encephalopathy, peripheral neuropathy
Managing Toxicity: The interval between injections can be modified once the maximal clinical efficacy has been achieved; Prior to each injection ask about: rash, pruritus, post-injection reactions, and any other unusual complaints; ***(a) Rash,***

prurItIs, stomatitis, and proteInuria ➔ hold gold until side effects subside and reintroduce at 50% lower dosage; *(b) Post-injection reactions* ➔ Reduce dose by 50% until reactions no longer occur or switch to gold sodium thioglucose (Solganal®); *(c) Thrombocytopenia* ➔ Discontinue gold; treat with prednisone 30-60 mg PO OD

PREGNANCY & LACTATION
Pregnancy: **RISK CANNOT BE RULED OUT. (CATEGORY C)**
Conception & Fertility: Gold does not seem to impair fertility. *Fetal Effects:* Gold compounds cross the placenta. There is no evidence of an increase in malformations.
Lactation: Gold is excreted in breast milk. The American Academy of Pediatrics considers gold salts to be compatible with breast feeding.
Recommendations: Since there are no known adverse effects in pregnancy, patients may choose to continue gold if it has been effective for controlling disease.

DRUG INTERACTIONS
Drugs which may ⬆ *toxicity of gold sodium thiomalate:* ACE inhibitors (increased risk of nitritoid reactions)

MECHANISM OF ACTION
The metabolism of sodium aurothiomalate is unknown but it is believed not to be broken down into elemental gold. The mechanism of action is largely unknown but may: Cause reductions in immunoglobulin synthesis, rheumatoid factor, & circulating immune complexes; Inactivates classical and alternative complement pathways; Inhibits phagocytic action of macrophages and fibroblast proliferation; Inhibits cytokine production (IL1, IL6, IFN) and cellular response to cytokines (IL1, IL2, IFN); Inhibits acid phosphatase, collagenases, protein kinase, and phospholipase C

PHARMACOKINETICS
IM mean abs time: 4 - 6 hrs; *1/2 life:* 6 - 25 days; *Metab:* Unknown; *Prot Bind:* Highly protein bound; *Excret:* 40% initial dose is excreted - renal 70% & faeces 30%

HYDROXYCHLOROQUINE (PLAQUENIL)

INDICATIONS
Approved: Discoid & systemic lupus erythematosus; rheumatoid arthritis. *Off-Label Uses:* Other inflammatory arthritides; juvenile polyarthritis

DOSE & DRUG ADMINISTRATION
Dose: 200 - 600 mg PO OD **not to exceed 6.5 mg/kg/day lean body weight** (can be divided into two daily doses)
Supplied: 200 mg tabs

DOSE ADJUSTMENT
Hepatic Failure: Use with caution. *Renal Failure: CrCl > 10 ml/min:* No initial dose adjustment; *CrCl <10 ml/min:* 50% initial dose reduction; *Dialysis:* No adjustment

ONSET OF ACTION
Initial Response: 8 - 12 weeks; *Maximal Response:* Several months

MONITORING
Baseline: Ophthalmologic monitoring (central visual fields (one eye only) and color vision) within the first 6 months; *Every 12 months:* Ophthalmologic monitoring (central visual fields (one eye only) and color vision)

CONTRAINDICATIONS & PRECAUTIONS
(a) Known hypersensitivity to hydroxychloroquine; (b) Hydroxychloroquine associated retinopathy

TOXICITY

Reversible: **(a) Mucocut:** Rash - variable; **(b) GI:** Anorexia, nausea & vomiting, dyspepsia, cramps, bloating, diarrhea; **(c) CNS:** Headaches, giddiness, insomnia, nervousness, tinnitus; **(d) Ocular:** Defects in accommodation & corneal deposits - reversible

Potentially Serious: **(a) Ocular:** Retinopathy – pigmentary changes, clumping, bull's eye lesion; **(b) MSK:** Skeletal muscle palsies or skeletal muscle myopathy or neuromyopathy; **(c) CVS:** Conduction disturbances, congestive heart failure

PREGNANCY & LACTATION

Pregnancy: RISK CANNOT BE RULED OUT. (CATEGORY C)

Conception & Fertility: No reports of adverse effects of hydroxychloroquine on fertility.

Maternal Effects: Available data suggests hydroxychloroquine can be continued safely throughout pregnancy.

Fetal Effects: Hydroxychloroquine does cross the placenta. There have been no reports of congenital malformations in children exposed to this drug.

Lactation: Low concentrations of hydroxychloroquine are found in breast milk. The American Academy of Pediatrics classifies the drug as compatible with breast feeding.

Recommendations: Hydroxychloroquine appears to be safe during pregnancy and compatible with breast feeding. Hydroxychloroquine withdrawal in patients with SLE may precipitate a disease flare; therefore, continued use during pregnancy and lactation may be justifiable.

DRUG INTERACTIONS

Hydroxychloroquine may ↑ levels and toxicity of: Digoxin

MECHANISM OF ACTION

Hydroxychloroquine is thought to be the active compound. Hydroxychloroquine is found in high concentrations within cells. It is a basic compound which causes an elevation of intracellular pH, particularly within vacuoles, lysosomes, and endosomes. It is through this elevation of intracellular pH that hydroxychloroquine probably exerts its most important effects such as: Lysosomotropic action – Interference with cellular function in compartments in which there is an acid microenvironment. This reduces the ability of intracellular organelles to degrade and process proteins; Reduced formation of MHC-peptide complexes in the presence of the basic intracellular pH; Hydroxychloroquine has numerous other actions such as: Inhibition of phospholipase A2 and other enzymes; Inhibition of several pro-inflammatory cytokines; Immune activity; Infectious activity

PHARMACOKINETICS

Abs: Rapidly absorbed; *1/2 Life:* 50 days; *Steady State:* 3 - 4 months; *Metab:* Hepatic; *Prot Bind:* 55% bound to plasma proteins; *Concn:* Mononuclear cells > neutrophils, intracellular lysosomes, and pigmented eye tissue; *Excret:* Predominantly renal - 90% (50% unchanged), Faeces - 10%

INTRAVENOUS IMMUNOGLOBULIN (IVIG)

INDICATIONS

Approved: No approved rheumatologic indications. *Off-Label Uses:* Beneficial effects have been established in controlled trials with corticosteroid resistant dermatomyositis; ANCA associated vasculitis; Kawasaki's disease; autoimmune uveitis. IVIG is used for other inflammatory autoimmune diseases (SLE, vasculitis) often when immunosuppressive medications are contraindicated (e.g. renal SLE in the presence of sepsis).

DOSE & DRUG ADMINISTRATION

Dose: 2.0 g/kg administered intravenously over 2 - 4 days (1g/kg/day x 2 days or 0.5 g/kg/day x 4 days). This regimen can be repeated at monthly intervals for 3 months. *Maximum Dose:* 5 g/kg

Supplied: 5% solution (5g per 100 mL) or 10% solution (10g per 100 mL).

DOSE ADJUSTMENT

Hepatic Failure: No dosage adjustment recommended; however, can worsen volume overload use with caution.

Renal Failure: No dosage adjustment recommended; however, use with caution pre-existing renal dysfunction – use with caution.

ONSET OF ACTION

Initial Response: Unknown & variable (1 - 3 months); *Maximal Response:* Unknown & variable (1 - 3 months)

MONITORING

Baseline: Serum immunoglobulin level to rule out IgA deficiency, AST, ALT, ALP, albumin, bilirubin, CBC, serum creatinine

CONTRAINDICATIONS

(a) Known anaphylactic or severe systemic response to IVIG; (b) IgA deficiency who have known antibodies against IgA; (c) Current congestive heart failure – may worsen with fluid load; (d) Renal dysfunction

TOXICITY

Reversible: (a) CNS: Headache; *(b) CVS:* Hypertension, chest tightness, chest pain, dyspnea; *(c) GI:* Nausea & vomiting; *(d) Mucocut:* Mild infusion site erythema; *(e) MSK:* Back or hip pain; *(f) Gen:* Fever, chills, feeling of faintness

Potentially Serious: (a) Hypersensitivity: Precipitous fall in BP and anaphylaxis; *(b) Renal:* Renal dysfunction, acute renal failure, osmotic nephrosis, and death (seen in elderly patients and patients with pre-existing renal disease or diabetes) – tubular damage by sucrose in the IVIG solution; *(c) Infection:* IVIG is a blood product, and although donors are carefully screened, there is a risk of transmission of infectious agents (such as viruses); *(d) CVS:* Worsening congestive heart failure due to fluid overload

Managing Toxicity: (a) Reduce infusion rate or temporarily stop infusion; (b) Premedicate 30 min prior to infusion with 650 mg acetaminophen (Tylenol®) and 25-50 mg of diphenhydramine (Benadryl®)

PREGNANCY & LACTATION

Pregnancy: **RISK CANNOT BE RULED OUT. (CATEGORY C)**

Lactation: Animal or human reproductive studies have not been performed. Should be given only if the benefit outweighs the risks to the fetus.

DRUG INTERACTIONS

May interfere with response to live viral vaccines (measles, mumps, rubella)

MECHANISM OF ACTION

Intravenous immunoglobulin is a solution containing neutralizing immunoglobulin G antibodies (IgG) collected from a large pool of donors. IVIG may work by the following mechanisms: Interferes with the selection of B-Cell repertoires; Modulates antibody production; Control of cellular proliferation (T-cells & B-cells); Modulation of activation and cytokine production (↓ IL-1); Neutralization of pathogenic autoantibodies (i.e. ANCA); Neutralization of T-cell superantigens; Binds to activated components of complement (C3b & C4b) preventing the generation of the membrane attack complex (C5b-C9)

PHARMACOKINETICS

Bioavail: 100%; *1/2 Life:* 3 weeks; *Metab:* Proteolysis; *Prot Bind:* None; *Excret:* Protein is lysed

LEFLUNOMIDE (ARAVA)

INDICATIONS

Approved: Active rheumatoid arthritis.   *Off-Label Uses:* Psoriatic arthritis and other inflammatory arthritides

DOSE & DRUG ADMINISTRATION

Loading Dose: 100 mg PO OD X 3 days (this can be omitted, if prepared to wait longer for onset of action); *Daily Dose:* 10 - 20 mg OD; *Maximum Dose:* 20 mg/day
Supplied: 10, 20, & 100 mg tablets

DOSE ADJUSTMENT

Hepatic Failure: Not recommended with significant hepatic impairment or with hepatitis B or C infection.
Renal Failure: Use with caution – limited clinical experience, contraindicated in moderate to severe renal impairment.

ONSET OF ACTION

Initial Response: 4 weeks; *Maximal Response:* 3 - 6 months

MONITORING

Baseline: AST, ALT, ALP, albumin, hepatitis B & C serology, CBC, serum creatinine;
Every 4 weeks for the first 6 months: CBC, AST, ALT, ALP, albumin, creatinine;
Every 1-2 months thereafter: CBC, AST, ALT, ALP, albumin, creatinine
Liver Biopsy: Pretreatment: Alcoholics, abnormal AST, chronic hepatitis B or C; Treatment: 5 of 9 abnormal AST within a given 12 month period if leflunomide is to be continued or if LFTs do not return to normal

CONTRAINDICATIONS

(a) Known hypersensitivity reaction to leflunomide; (b) Cirrhosis, hepatitis, active viral hepatitis B or C, or hepatic impairment; (c) Severe immunodeficiency, bone marrow dysplasia, severe infection; (d) Renal impairment; (e) PREGNANCY MUST BE EXCLUDED BEFORE THE START OF TREATMENT WITH LEFLUNOMIDE.

TOXICITY

Reversible: (a) GI: Nausea, diarrhea, elevated liver enzymes; *(b) Mucocut:* Rash, reversible alopecia; *(c) Gen:* Hypertension
Potentially Serious: (a) Infection; (b) Hem: Pancytopenia; *(c) Malignancy:* May increase risk of lymphoproliferative disorders; *(d) Hepatic:* Hepatotoxicity, hepatic failure, & death; (e) Mucocut: Stevens Johnson syndrome; cut. necrotizing vasculitis
Managing Toxicity: In most cases, diarrhea is usually mild to moderate and resolves spontaneously under continued leflunomide treatment. Treatment of diarrhea includes reducing the dose of leflunomide or giving an anti-diarrheal agent. In most cases, alopecia and rashes are usually mild to moderate and transient. Management involves dose reduction or cessation of treatment. Elevated liver enzymes (2-3 times normal) should result in careful monitoring and dose reduction. Enzymes >3 times normal should result in cessation of therapy. Hypertension should be managed by dose reduction, discontinuation, or anti-hypertensive treatment depending upon the clinical situation and severity.
Drug Elimination Procedure: Cholestyramine 8 g TID X 11 days or Activated Charcoal 50 grams QID X 11 days (For women wishing to become pregnant,

plasma levels < 0.02 mg/L should be verified by two separate tests performed 14 days apart. If plasma levels are > 0.02 mg/L additional cholestyramine should be considered). Plasma levels of leflunomide can be obtained by contacting a LabCorp service representative at 1-919-361-7147 or Aventis Pharma at 1-800-265-7927.

Drug elimination procedure is used for: (a) Severe reaction (Inflammation of the buccal or genital mucosa, fever, extensive body rash, including bullous reactions or other signs suggestive of Stevens-Johnson or similar syndromes), Anaphylaxis (e.g. angioedema); (b) Severe undesirable effect of leflunomide (hematologic, hepatotoxicity, allergic reaction, skin and/or mucosal reactions); (c) Switching to another hepatotoxic DMARD; (d) Desired pregnancy by either partner

PREGNANCY & LACTATION

Pregnancy: **CONTRAINDICATED IN PREGNANCY. (CATEGORY X)**
There is very little pregnancy experience with leflunomide. Animal data suggests that leflunomide may increase the risk of fetal death or have teratogenic effects.

Lactation: Unknown if leflunomide is excreted in breast milk. Breast feeding should be avoided if possible.

Recommendations: Patients of child bearing potential should consider the use of a different DMARD because of the long half life of leflunomide. If a patient taking leflunomide wishes to become pregnant or becomes pregnant, leflunomide should be discontinued and the drug elimination procedure followed.

DRUG INTERACTIONS

Leflunomide may ↑ toxicity of: Methotrexate (hepatic), alcohol; ***Drugs which may↑ toxicity of leflunomide:*** Methotrexate (hepatic), rifampin, tolbutamide, NSAIDs; ***Drugs which may↓ absorption of leflunomide:*** Cholestyramine

MECHANISM OF ACTION

Leflunomide is inactive. Initial metabolism occurs in both liver and GI tract to the active compound A77-1726. When lymphocytes are stimulated the de novo synthesis of pyrimidines is crucial for DNA replication and cellular proliferation. Dihydro-orotate dehydrogenase is an important enzyme involved in de novo pyrimidine synthesis. A77-1726 inhibits the activity of dihydro-orotate dehydrogenase arresting the activated lymphocyte in the G1 phase of the cell cycle. Through this mechanism, leflunomide may suppress autoimmune T-cell proliferation and the production of autoantibodies by B-cells.

PHARMACOKINETICS

Bioavail: Relatively high (80%); ***Mean abs time:*** 6 - 12 hours; ***1/2 Life (A77 1726):*** 2 weeks; ***Metab:*** Unknown – thought to occur in intestinal mucosa and hepatocyte; ***Prot Bind:*** 99% bound to plasma proteins; ***Excret:*** Faeces (48%) and urine (43%)

METHOTREXATE (RHEUMATREX, TREXALL)

INDICATIONS

Approved: Rheumatoid arthritis; psoriasis; seronegative arthritides. ***Off-Label Uses:*** Systemic lupus erythematosus; systemic sclerosis; Sjogren's syndrome; inflammatory myopathies; vasculitis as a steroid sparing agent (e.g. maintenance of remission in Wegener's granulomatosis)

DOSE & DRUG ADMINISTRATION

Given once weekly by oral or subcutaneous routes; ***Initial Dose:*** 10 - 15 mg / week PO or SC (PO dose can be divided q12h x 3 doses); ***Increments:*** 2.5 - 5 mg every 4 - 8 weeks; ***Maximum recommended Dose:*** 25 mg/wk PO or SC;

Supplied: 2.5 mg, Trexall 5, 7.5, 10, & 15 mg tabs, 10 & 25 mg/mL solution

DOSE ADJUSTMENT
Hepatic Failure: Contraindicated.
Renal Failure: CrCl 50 - 80: Reduce initial dose by 25%; *CrCl 10-50:* Reduce initial dose by 50%; *CrCl < 10:* Avoid

ONSET OF ACTION
Initial Response: 4 - 8 weeks; *Maximal Response:* Several months

MONITORING
Baseline: AST, ALT, ALP, albumin, hepatitis B & C serology, CBC, creatinine, and a chest X-ray if one has not been done in the past year; *Every 4- 8 weeks:* CBC, AST, ALT, ALP, albumin, creatinine; *Liver Biopsy:* Pretreatment: Alcoholics, abnormal AST, chronic hepatitis B or C;
Treatment: 5 of 9 abnormal AST within a given 12 month period if methotrexate is to be continued or if LFTs do not return to normal

CONTRAINDICATIONS & PRECAUTIONS
(a) Known hypersensitivity to methotrexate; (b) Cirrhosis, hepatitis, active viral hepatitis B or C, or hepatic impairment; (c) Methotrexate induced pneumonitis, hepatitis, & malignancy; (d) Blood dyscrasias (leukopenia, thrombocytopenia, significant anemia, bone marrow hypoplasia); (e) Active infectious disease; (f) Pregnant or nursing mothers

TOXICITY
Reversible: (a) Gen: General malaise, fatigue; *(b) GI:* Anorexia, nausea & vomiting, diarrhea, weight loss; *(c) Mucocut:* Stomatitis, painful oral ulcers
Potentially Serious: (a) Infection; (b) Hem: Pancytopenia, leukopenia, thrombocytopenia, megaloblastic anemia; *(c) Malignancy:* Non-Hodgkin's lymphoma – reversible with discontinuation; *(d) Resp:* Methotrexate pneumonitis (fever, cough, SOB); *(e) Hepatic:* Fibrosis & cirrhosis
Managing Toxicity: Giving methotrexate at bed time may reduce nausea as patient sleeps through it; Dividing the dose of methotrexate over a 24 hour period; Changing to subcutaneous methotrexate can reduce the GI side-effects; Folic acid given 1 mg/ day helps reduce toxicity; Folinic acid 5mg / week, 8 - 12 hours after methotrexate dose

PREGNANCY & LACTATION
Pregnancy: POSITIVE EVIDENCE OF RISK. (CATEGORY D)
Conception & Fertility: Does not appear to adversely affect female fertility. It can result in reversible sterility in men (case reports).
Fetal Effects: Methotrexate is contraindicated in pregnancy because of severe adverse effects on both the fetus and the course of the pregnancy.
Lactation: Methotrexate is found in low concentrations in breast milk. The American Academy of Pediatrics considers methotrexate to be contraindicated during breast feeding.
Recommendations: Patients of child bearing potential should receive concomitant folic acid. Both men and women taking methotrexate should discontinue the drug at least 3 months before conception. Methotrexate is contraindicated in a patient trying to conceive, during pregnancy, and during breastfeeding.

DRUG INTERACTIONS
Drugs which may ↑ toxicity of methotrexate: Alcohol (Increases hepatic toxicity), trimethoprim/sulfamethoxazole (hematologic toxicity), probenecid (inhibits tubular secretion of methotrexate), leflunomide (hepatotoxicity).   Use with caution with medications that may alter renal function. *Drugs which may ↓ efficacy of methotrexate:* Folic acid, neomycin, polymyxin B, nystatin, vancomycin

MECHANISM OF ACTION

Methotrexate is metabolized from a monoglutamate to a polyglutamate which have stronger cellular retention, remain within the cell, and are more potent than the monoglutamates. Synthesis of polyglutamates increases with duration of treatment. Methotrexate binds and inactivates the enzyme Dihydrofolate Reductase (DHFR) which depletes the active folate pool of the cell resulting in a reduction of de novo purine synthesis (thymidylate & inosinic acid). Reducing purine synthesis inhibits cellular proliferation. Methotrexate also inhibits AICAR transformylase which leads to the release of adenosine. Adenosine inhibits neutrophil function, inhibits production of TNF, IL-6, and IL-8, and has anti-inflammatory properties. Finally, methotrexate inhibits the synthesis of polyamines which are necessary for the proliferation and synthesis of macromolecules.

PHARMACOKINETICS

Oral Bioavail: Relatively high but variable (40 - 100%); *Mean abs time:* 1.2 hours *1/2 life:* 3 - 10 hours; *Maxi parental serum concn:* 2 hours; *Metab:* Some hepatic metabolism; *Prot Bind:* 50-60% bound to plasma proteins; *Excret:* Renal

MINOCYCLINE (MINOCIN)

INDICATIONS

Approved: No approved rheumatologic indications. *Off-Label Uses:* Inflammatory arthritis such as rheumatoid arthritis

DOSE & DRUG ADMINISTRATION

Initial Dose: 50 - 100 mg PO BID; *Maximum Dose:* 200 mg/day
Supplied: 50, 75, & 100 mg caps

DOSE ADJUSTMENT

Hepatic Failure: Use with caution, may worsen pre-existing liver disease.
Renal Failure: In patients with renal insufficiency, significant renal impairment may lead to accumulation and possible liver toxicity. The total dosage should be decreased by either reducing individual doses and/or extending dosing intervals.

ONSET OF ACTION

Initial Response: 4 - 8 weeks; *Maximal Response:* Several months

MONITORING

Baseline: AST, ALT, ALP, serum creatinine; *Periodically:* Patients receiving long term therapy should have renal and liver function monitored periodically

CONTRAINDICATIONS

(a) Known hypersensitivity to minocycline; (b) Pregnancy

TOXICITY

Reversible: (a) GI: Anorexia, nausea & vomiting, diarrhea, weight loss; *(c) CNS:* Dizziness & headaches; *(c) Mucocut:* Photosensitivity
Potentially Serious: (a) CNS: Increased intracranial pressure; *(b) Mucocut:* Pigmentation of the skin and mucous membranes; *(c) GI:* Pancreatitis, hepatitis, esophagitis; *(d) Rheum:* Drug induced SLE or exacerbation of SLE

PREGNANCY & LACTATION

Pregnancy: POSITIVE EVIDENCE OF RISK. (CATEGORY D)
Lactation: Tetracyclines are excreted in human breast milk; Generally not recommended.

DRUG INTERACTIONS

Minocycline may ↑ levels or toxicity of the following dugs: Warfarin (monitor closely, may require downward adjustment in their anticoagulant dosage); *Drugs which may ↓ levels or efficacy of minocycline:* Aluminum, calcium, & magnesium antacids and oral iron (impair absorption of minocycline)

MECHANISM OF ACTION

Minocycline is a synthetic derivative of tetracycline. There is no clear understanding of the mechanism of action of tetracycline antibiotics in rheumatoid arthritis, however, they have long been advocated as a treatment for RA, based originally on the belief that RA was caused by an infectious agent. This theory has been supported by the isolation of mycoplasma from the synovial fluid of patients with rheumatoid arthritis. Despite this belief, most researchers believe the immunologic effects of minocycline are the most important mechanism in the treatment of RA. Minocycline is known to induce lupus; this probably occurs because of a shift in the immune system in a Th2 direction. In rheumatoid arthritis, shifting the immune system from Th1 towards Th2 may be the mechanism by which minocycline exerts its effect as RA is dominated by Th1 cytokines. A third premise for their use comes from data which reveals the activity of collagenase, a matrix metalloproteinase, is reduced with minocycline.

PHARMACOKINETICS

Bioavail: 60%; *Mean abs time:* 1-4 hours; *1/2 life:* 11.1 - 22.1 hours; *Excret:* Hepatic & renal

MYCOPHENOLATE MOFETIL (CELLCEPT)

INDICATIONS

Approved: No approved rheumatologic indications. *Off-Label Uses:* Lupus nephritis, vasculitis

DOSE & DRUG ADMINISTRATION

Initial Dose: 500 - 1000 mg PO BID; *Maximum Dose:* 3000 mg/day
Supplied: 250 mg capsules, 500 mg tablets, 200 mg/mL oral suspension

DOSE ADJUSTMENT

Hepatic Failure: No dosage adjustment necessary.
Renal Failure: No dosage adjustment necessary in mild-moderate renal failure. Use smaller doses (< 2 g per day) with caution in severe renal failure (<25 mL/min). Use starting doses of 250 mg PO BID in dialysis patients.

ONSET OF ACTION

Initial Response: unknown; *Maximal Response:* unknown

MONITORING

Baseline: CBC, creatinine, AST, ALT, ALP, albumin, bilirubin; *Weekly for initial month:* CBC; *Twice monthly for the 2nd and 3rd months:* CBC; *Monthly thereafter:* CBC

CONTRAINDICATIONS & PRECAUTIONS

(a) Hypersensitivity to mycophenolate mofetil; (b) Renal failure; (c) Active PUD

TOXICITY

Reversible: (a) GI: Nausea, vomiting, diarrhea; *(b) Gen:* Drug-induced fever; *(c) CNS:* Headache, insomnia, dizziness, and tremor; *(d) MSK:* Back pain; *(e) Mucocut:* Acne
Potentially Serious: (a) Hem: Leukopenia, anemia, thrombocytopenia; *(b) GI:* Small increased risk of GI bleeding; *(c) Infection:* Serious infections and sepsis have been reported with the use of mycophenolate; *(d) Malignancy:* May ↑ risk of lymphoproliferative disease
Managing Toxicity: Reduction in dose

PREGNANCY & LACTATION

Pregnancy: **RISK CANNOT BE RULED OUT. (CATEGORY C)**

Lactation: Unknown if mycophenolate mofetil is excreted in breast milk. Due to the potential for serious adverse reactions in nursing infants, a decision should be made to discontinue nursing or discontinue the medication.

DRUG INTERACTIONS

Drugs which may ↑ levels and toxicity of mycophenolate: Probenecid, acyclovir, ganciclovir, high-dose salicylates (may increase free fraction of MMF); ***Drugs which may ↓ absorption of mycophenolate:*** Magnesium & aluminium hydroxide antacids, cholestyramine, iron supplements; ***Mycophenolate may ↑ toxicity of:*** Tacrolimus, azathioprine; ***Mycophenolate may ↓ efficacy of:*** Oral contraceptive pills

MECHANISM OF ACTION

Mycophenolate mofetil is the 2-morpholinoethyl ester of mycophenolic acid (MPA), and inhibitor of inosine monophosphate dehydrogenase (IMPDH). After absorption, mycophenolate mofetil is hydrolyzed in the plasma, liver, and kidney to mycophenolic acid (MPA), which is the active metabolite. Mycophenolic acid is a selective, non-competitive, and reversible inhibitor of inosine monophosphate dehydrogenase (IMPDH). By inhibiting IMPDH, mycophenolic acid inhibits the de-novo synthesis of guanosine nucleotides which results in: ↓ Proliferation of T & B lymphocytes; ↓ Antibody formation by B-cells; ↓ Glycosylation of adhesion molecules that are involved in the attachment of lymphocytes to endothelium

PHARMACOKINETICS

Bioavail: 94%; ***Max Plasma Concn:*** 1 - 2 hours; ***Elim 1/2 Life:*** 18 hours; ***Metab:*** Mycophenolate is hydrolyzed initially to mycophenolic acid. Mycophenolic acid (MPA) is inactivated through conjugation to glucuronide to MPAG; ***Prot Bind:*** 97%; ***Excret:*** Primarily urinary excretion with MPAG found in the urine;

SULFASALAZINE (AZULFIDINE, AZULFIDINE-EN ♣SALAZOPYRIN, SALAZOPYRIN-EN)

INDICATIONS

Approved: Active rheumatoid arthritis. ***Off-Label Uses:*** Seronegative spondyloarthropathies (ankylosing spondylitis; psoriatic arthritis; enteropathic arthritis; reactive arthritis)

DOSE & DRUG ADMINISTRATION

Initial Dose: 500 mg daily; ***Increments:*** 500 mg per week to maximum dose; ***Maintenance Dose:*** Most common dose for rheumatic disease is 2 grams daily (1000 mg PO BID); ***Maximum Dose:*** 3 grams per day (1500 mg PO BID)
Supplied: 500 mg tablets, 500 mg EN tabs (Enteric coated – EN).

DOSE ADJUSTMENT

Hepatic Failure: Contraindicated.
Renal Failure: CrCl > 50: No initial dose adjustment; ***CrCl 10-50:*** 50% initial dose reduction(500 mg BID); ***CrCl < 10:*** 75% initial dose reduction (500 mg OD)

ONSET OF ACTION

Initial Response: 4 - 6 weeks; ***Maximal Response:*** 12 weeks

MONITORING

Baseline: CBC, AST, ALT, ALP, serum creatinine; ***Every 2 weeks for 3 months:*** CBC, AST, ALT, INR/PTT; ***Every 1 - 3 months thereafter:*** CBC, AST, ALT, INR/PTT

CONTRAINDICATIONS & PRECAUTIONS

(a) Hypersensitivity to sulfonamides ; (b) ASA precipitated asthma, urticaria, rhinitis or other allergic manifestations; (c) Porphyria

TOXICITY

Reversible: (a) GI: Anorexia, nausea & vomiting, malaise, abdominal pain, dyspepsia; *(b) CNS:* Headache, fever, light-headedness, dizziness; *(d) Mucocut:* Rash; *(e) Hepatic:* Mild transaminase elevation; *(f) Hem:* Leukopenia, hemolysis, methemoglobinemia

Potentially Serious: (a) Gen: Hypersensitivity reactions; *(b) Hem:* Aplastic anemia, agranulocytosis; *(c) Resp:* Fibrosing alveolitis; *(d) CNS:* Neuromuscular and CNS effects (mood); *(e) Renal:* Worsening renal impairment; *(f) Hepatic:* Hepatitis; *(g) Fertility:* Reversible oligospermia in men

PREGNANCY & LACTATION

Pregnancy: **NO EVIDENCE OF RISK IN HUMANS. (CATEGORY B)**

Conception & Fertility: No reports of fertility problems in women taking sulfasalazine. In men, sulfasalazine may result in infertility which has been shown to be reversible.

Fetal Effects: Sulfasalazine does not appear to cause an increase in either the incidence of fetal abnormalities or spontaneous abortions.

Lactation: Anecdotal reports suggest sulfasalazine is compatible with breast feeding; however, the American Academy of Pediatrics suggests sulfasalazine be given with caution because substantial adverse events (one infant developed bloody diarrhea) may occur in some infants.

Recommendations: Sulfasalazine can probably be used safely during pregnancy. It may be the first choice of DMARDs in treating rheumatic diseases in women of child bearing age who are trying to conceive or are already pregnant.

DRUG INTERACTIONS

Drugs which may ↓ absorption of sulfasalazine: Broad spectrum antibiotics (may affect gut flora and result in decreased bioavailability); cholestyramine; *Drugs which may ↑ levels or toxicity of sulfasalazine:* Probenecid, sulfinpyrazone; *Sulfasalazine may ↑ toxicity of the following drugs:* Methotrexate, methenamine, phenylbutazone, photosensitizing medications, azathioprine; *Sulfasalazine may ↓ levels of the following drugs:* Digoxin, folic acid

MECHANISM OF ACTION

Sulfasalazine consists of salicylic acid and sulfapyridine joined by an azo bond. The azo bond is reduced by colonic bacteria releasing sulfapyridine – the active component in rheumatic diseases. Sulfasalazine may work by the following mechanisms: Scavenge reactive oxygen species and their products released from active polymorphs; Reduces circulating active lymphocytes, inhibits B cell activation, reduction in IgM and rheumatoid factor; Reduces interleukin 1, and TNF in patients with rheumatoid arthritis < 1 yr duration; Reduces basal interleukin-6 production

PHARMACOKINETICS

Abs: 10 - 20% of the drug. Most of drug reaches the colon where the azo bond is broken by colonic bacteria; *Max serum concn:* 4 - 6 hours; *Metab:* Sulfapyridine is extensively metabolized in the liver by N4-acetylation and ring hydroxylation with subsequent glucuronidation; *Excret:* Metabolites in the urine

TACROLIMUS (PROGRAF, FK506)

INDICATIONS

Approved: No approved rheumatologic indications, ♥Rheumatoid arthritis. *Off-Label Uses:* Rheumatoid arthritis; active vasculitis; SLE (nephritis & vasculitis)

DOSE & DRUG ADMINISTRATION

Initial Dose: 0.05 - 0.1 mg/kg per day in 2 divided doses (~ 3 - 7 mg PO BID);
Increase: 0.5 - 1 mg q2-4 months; *Maximum Dose:* Titrate to clinical effect and
toxicity; in RA 3mg PO BID
Supplied: 1 & 5 mg capsules

DOSE ADJUSTMENT

Hepatic Failure: Impairs excretion of tacrolimus metabolites; use with caution.
Renal Failure: No dosage adjustment, however, use with caution

ONSET OF ACTION

Initial Response: 2 - 4 months; *Maximal Response:* 6 months

MONITORING

Baseline: CBC, creatinine (average of 2 readings), AST, ALT, ALP, albumin,
bilirubin, serum magnesium, blood pressure (average of 2 readings), and electrolytes,
glucose; *Every two weeks for initial 3 months:* Blood pressure, creatinine, glucose,
and electrolytes; *Monthly:* Blood pressure, creatinine, serum magnesium, glucose,
and electrolytes; *Change in Dose:* Monitor blood pressure, creatinine, glucose, and
electrolytes every 2 weeks

CONTRAINDICATIONS & PRECAUTIONS

(a) Hypersensitivity to tacrolimus; (b) Abnormal renal function, hypertension, or
malignancies; (c) Renal impairment and mild hypertension; (d) Active infection or
frequent recurrent infections; (e) Hyperkalemia

TOXICITY

Reversible: (a) GI: Nausea, vomiting, diarrhea, constipation; (b) CNS: Tremor,
paresthesias, insomnia, headache, and other changes in mental function; (c) Lytes:
Hypokalemia, hypomagnesemia; (d) Hyperglycemia
Potentially Serious: (a) Renal: Nephrotoxicity; (b) GI: Hepatotoxicity; (c) CVS:
Hypertension, myocardial hypertrophy; (d) Lytes: Hyperglycemia, hyperkalemia; (f)
Infection: Serious infections and sepsis have been reported with the use of
tacrolimus; (g) Hem: Anemia, thrombocytopenia, leukopenia; (i) Malignancy: May
↑ risk of lymphoproliferative disease
Managing Toxicity: If change in serum creatinine is >25% above patients baseline,
tacrolimus should be ↓by 25-50%; Tacrolimus dose should be ↓by 25-50% with
sustained hypertension. If hypertension persists dose can be further ↓ or anti-
hypertensive therapy can be started

PREGNANCY & LACTATION

Pregnancy: RISK CANNOT BE RULED OUT. (CATEGORY C)
Lactation: Since tacrolimus is excreted in breast milk, nursing should be avoided.

DRUG INTERACTIONS

Contraindicated: STATINS, FLUCONAZOLE, ITRACONAZOLE,
KETOCONAZOLE, COLCHICINE; *Tacrolimus may ↑ toxicity of:* Statins
(myopathy), colchicine (neuromyopathy), digoxin, K-sparing diuretics (hyperkalemia),
cyclosporine; *Drugs which may ↑ toxicity of tacrolimus:* Diltiazem, nicardipine,
verapamil, clarithromycin, erythromycin, fluconazole, itraconazole, ketoconazole,
methylprednisolone, allopurinol, bromocriptine, danazol, metoclopramide,
cyclosporine; *Drugs which may ↑ renal toxicity of tacrolimus:* NSAIDs, ACE-
inhibitors, aminoglycosides, amphotericin B, quinolone antibiotics, cyclosporine;
Drugs which may ↓ levels and efficacy of tacrolimus: Nafcillin, rifampin,
carbamazepine, phenobarbital, phenytoin; Grapefruit juice ↑ concentration of
tacrolimus and should be avoided; Tacrolimus may cause prolongation of QT interval

MECHANISM OF ACTION

Tacrolimus is a macrolide immunosuppressant produced by streptomyces tsukubaenis. Tacrolimus complexes with the intra-cellular protein FKBP-12. This complex then binds to calcium, calmodulin, and calcineurin resulting in the inhibition of the serine-threonine phosphatase, calcineurin. Inhibition of calcineurin phosphatase prevents the translocation of cytosolic nuclear factor into the nucleus of activated T-cells. This cytosolic nuclear factor is required for the transcription of genes for cytokines such as interleukin-2 and for T-cell activation. Thus, tacrolimus impairs the production of interleukin-2 and other cytokines which decreases lymphocyte proliferation.

PHARMACOKINETICS

Bioavail: Incomplete and variable (17 - 34%); Max Plasma Concn: 1 - 3 hours; Elim 1/2 Life: 11.7 - 34.4 hours; Metab: Cytochrome P450 3A4 enzyme system in the intestinal mucosa and the liver. It is extensively metabolized to 8 metabolites; Prot Bind: 99%; Excret: Primarily biliary with 6% excreted in the urine

GASTROPROTECTION

Risk Factors for the Development of NSAID-Associated Gastroduodenal Ulcers: (a) Advanced Age (>65); (b) Current active peptic ulcer disease; (c) Previous history of peptic ulcer disease; (d) Concomitant use of corticosteroids; (e) Higher doses of NSAIDs, including multiple NSAIDs; (f) Concomitant administration of anticoagulants; (g) Serious systemic disorder

Possible risk factors: (a) Concomitant infection with helicobacter pylori; (b) Cigarette smoking; (c) Consumption of alcohol

FAMOTIDINE (PEPCID)

INDICATIONS
Approved: Gastroesophageal reflux (treatment & maintenance); gastric & duodenal ulcer treatment; duodenal ulcer prophylaxis; Zollinger-Ellison syndrome

★ Famotidine is the only H2-receptor antagonist with supporting evidence for protection of NSAID induced ulceration (N Engl J Med. 1996 May 30;334(22):1435-9.)

DOSE & DRUG ADMINISTRATION
Initial Dose: 40 mg PO BID for prevention of NSAID induced ulceration otherwise 20 – 40 mg PO OD. *Maximum Dose:* 640 mg/day;

Supplied: 10, 20, & 40 mg tablets.

DOSE ADJUSTMENT
Hepatic Failure: No dosage reduction is required.

Renal Failure: CrCl > 50 ml/min: Reduce initial dose by 50%t; *CrCl 10-50 ml/min:* Reduce initial dose by 75%; *CrCl < 10 ml/min:* Reduce initial dose by 90%

ONSET OF ACTION
Initial Response: 60 minutes

MONITORING
No specific laboratory monitoring is necessary

CONTRAINDICATIONS & PRECAUTIONS
(a) Known hypersensitivity to famotidine; (b) Caution in advanced renal disease

TOXICITY
Reversible: (a) GI: Constipation, diarrhea; *(b) CNS:* Headache, dizziness

PREGNANCY & LACTATION
Pregnancy: NO EVIDENCE OF RISK IN HUMANS. (CATEGORY B)

Lactation: Famotidine is secreted in breast milk; however, is thought to be compatible with breast feeding

DRUG INTERACTIONS
Famotidine may ↓ absorption of: Cefuroxime, cefditoren, cefpodoxime, fluoroquinolone antibiotics, delavirdine, ketoconazole, itraconazole; *Famotidine may ↑ concentration of:* Cyclosporine

MECHANISM OF ACTION
Famotidine is the active compound. Histamine is an Important stimulant of gastric acid secretion and histamine receptors are found on the base of parietal cells in the gastric mucosa. Famotidine is a competitive inhibitor of histamine H2 type receptors. This inhibition results in a reduction in acid and pepsin concentration and a reduction of the volume of basal, nocturnal, and stimulated gastric secretion.

PHARMACOKINETICS
Bioavail: 40-50%; *Max Plasma Concn:* 1-4 hours; *1/2 Life:* 2.5-4 hours; *Metab:* Hepatic; *Prot Bind:* Low (15-20%); *Excret:* Renal (60-70%), other metabolic routes (30-40%)

MISOPROSTOL (CYTOTEC)

INDICATIONS
Approved: Indicated for the prevention of NSAID-induced gastric ulcers in patients at high risk of complications from gastric ulcer, as well as patients at high risk of developing gastric ulceration. Cytotec has not been shown to prevent duodenal ulcers in patients taking NSAIDs;

DOSE & DRUG ADMINISTRATION
Initial Dose: 200 mcg PO QID (200 mcg TID may have the best balance of efficacy to toxicity); *Maximum Dose:* 800 mcg/day; *Supplied:* 100 & 200 mcg tablets

DOSE ADJUSTMENT
Hepatic Failure: No dosage reduction is required.
Renal Failure: Use smallest dose possible; starting dose of 100 mcg QID recomm.

ONSET OF ACTION
Initial Response: 30-60 minutes

MONITORING
Baseline: In women of child-bearing potential a negative pregnancy test should be performed within 2 weeks prior to the initiation of therapy

CONTRAINDICATIONS & PRECAUTIONS
(a) Known hypersensitivity to misoprostol; (b) Known sensitivity to prostaglandins or prostaglandin analogues; (c) Pregnancy; (d) Epilepsy

TOXICITY
Reversible: (a) GI: Abdominal pain, diarrhea, dyspepsia, nausea, flatulence, vomiting, constipation; *(b) Gyne:* Spotting, uterine cramps, menorrhagia, menstrual disorder, dysmenorrhea, vaginal hemorrhage and post-menopausal vaginal bleeding; *(c) CNS:* Confusion, headaches, dizziness

PREGNANCY & LACTATION
Pregnancy: CONTRAINDICATED IN PREGNANCY. (CATEGORY X)
Lactation: Unknown if misoprostol is excreted in breast milk; gen. not recommended.

DRUG INTERACTIONS
No clinically significant drug interactions attributable to misoprostol have been shown

MECHANISM OF ACTION
Misoprostol is a prodrug which is rapidly converted to its active form misoprostol acid which occurs rapidly in the stomach. NSAIDs inhibit prostaglandin synthesis, and a deficiency of prostaglandins within the gastric mucosa may lead to diminishing bicarbonate and mucous secretion which may contribute to the mucosal damage caused by these medications. Misoprostol is a synthetic prostaglandin E1 analog with gastric antisecretory and (in animals) mucosal protective properties.

PHARMACOKINETICS
Bioavail: 7%; *Max Plasma Concn:* 30 minutes; *1/2 Life:* 30 min; *Metab:* Hepatic; *Prot Bind:* High (<90%); *Excret:* Urine 90%

PROTON PUMP INHIBITORS: ESOMEPRAZOLE (NEXIUM), LANSOPRAZOLE (PREVACID), OMEPRAZOLE (LOSEC, PRILOSEC), PANTOPRAZOLE (PANTOLOC, PROTONIX), RABEPRAZOLE (ACIPHEX, PARIET)

INDICATIONS
Approved: Duodenal ulcer, gastric ulcer, gastroesophageal reflux disease (GERD), pathologic hypersecretory conditions (Zollinger-Ellison)

DOSE & DRUG ADMINISTRATION
Dose: Esomeprazole: 10-40 mg OD; Lansoprazole: 15-30 mg OD; Omeprazole: 20-40 mg OD; Pantoprazole: 40 mg OD; Rabeprazole: 20 mg OD

Supplied: Esomeprazole: 20 & 40 mg tablets; Lansoprazole: 15 & 30 mg tablets, 15 & 30 mg granules for oral suspension; Omeprazole: 20 mg tablets; Pantoprazole: 40 mg tablets; Rabeprazole: 20 mg tablets

DOSE ADJUSTMENT
Hepatic Failure: No dose reduction required
Renal Failure: No dose reduction required

ONSET OF ACTION
Initial Response: 0.5 - 3 hours

MONITORING
No routine monitoring is recommended with the use of this medication

CONTRAINDICATIONS
(a) Known hypersensitivity to proton pump inhibitors

TOXICITY
Reversible: (a) GI: Diarrhea, nausea, abdominal pain, constipation, flatulence; **(b) CNS:** Headache; **(c) Mucocut:** Rash

PREGNANCY & LACTATION
Pregnancy: Omeprazole - **RISK CANNOT BE RULED OUT. (CATEGORY C);** Esomeprazole, Lansoprazole, Pantoprazole, Rabeprazole - **NO EVIDENCE OF RISK IN HUMANS. (CATEGORY B)**
Lactation: It is not known if proton pump inhibitors are excreted in human breast milk and therefore should be avoided. Used only if the potential benefit justifies the potential risk to the baby.

DRUG INTERACTIONS
Proton pump inhibitors can have prolonged and profound effects on gastric acid secretion, therefore, they can affect medications whose absorption is dependant upon gastric pH;
Esomeprazole may ↑ efficacy/toxicity of: Benzodiazepines & carbamazepine;
  May ↓ absorption of: Cefuroxime, indinavir, itraconazole, ketoconazole, iron
Lansoprazole may ↓ absorption of: Cefuroxime, indinavir, itraconazole, ketoconazole;
Omeprazole may ↑ efficacy/toxicity of: Carbamazepine, benzodiazepines, warfarin; **May ↓ absorption of:** Indinavir, ketoconazole, itraconazole;
Pantoprazole may ↓ absorption of: Indinavir, ketoconazole, itraconazole;
Rabeprazole may ↓ absorption of: Cefuroxime, indinavir, itraconazole, ketoconazole

MECHANISM OF ACTION
Proton pump inhibitors inhibit the gastric enzyme H+,K+ - ATPase which catalyzes the exchange of H+ and K+.

PHARMACOKINETICS
Esomeprazole: Bioavail: 64-90%; Max Plasma Conc'n: 1.5 h; 1/2 Life: 1-1.5 h; Hepatic Metab: CYP2C19 CYP3A4; Excret: Urine (80%), Feces (20%)
Lansoprazole: Bioavail: 50-80%; Max Plasma Conc'n: 1.7 h; 1/2 Life: 2-3 h; Hepatic Metab: CYP2C19 CYP3A4; Excret: Feces (67%) Urine (33%)
Omeprazole: Bioavail: 30-40%; Max Plasma Conc'n: 0.5-3.5 h; 1/2 Life: 0.5-1 h; Hepatic Metab: CYP2C19 CYP450; Excret: Urine (77%)
Pantoprazole: Bioavail: 77%; Max Plasma Conc'n: 2.5 h; 1/2 Life: 1.0 h; Hepatic Metab: CYP2C19 CYP3A4; Excret: Urine (71%); Feces (18%)
Rabeprazole: Bioavail: 52%; Max Plasma Conc'n: 2-5 h; 1/2 Life: 0.85-2 h; Hepatic Metab: CYP2C19 CYP3A4; Excret: Urine (90%); Feces (10%)

MEDICATIONS USED FOR THE TREATMENT OF GOUT & HYPERURICEMIA

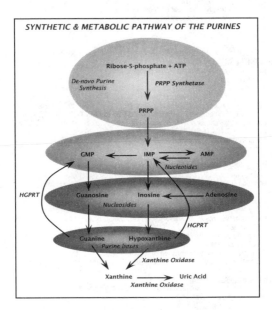

SYNTHETIC & METABOLIC PATHWAY OF THE PURINES

ALLOPURINOL (ZYLOPRIM)

INDICATIONS

Approved: The management of patients with signs and symptoms of primary or secondary gout (acute attacks, tophi, joint destruction, uric acid lithiasis and/or nephropathy). The management of patients with leukemia, lymphoma and malignancies who are receiving cancer therapy which causes elevations of serum and urinary uric acid levels. The management of patients with recurrent calcium oxalate calculi whose daily uric acid excretion exceeds 800 mg/day in male patients and 750 mg/day in female patients.

DOSE & DRUG ADMINISTRATION
Initial Dose: Start low 50 - 300 mg PO OD; *Increments:* Increase by 50 - 100 mg q1-3 weeks until serum uric acid is reduced to lower limit of normal lab range. For doses greater than 300 mg/day use divided doses; *Average Maintenance Dose:* Doses of 200 - 300 mg/day are typically used for prevention of gout attacks. However, the maintenance dose should be adjusted for the individual patient and doses of 400 - 600 mg/day are sometimes required; *Maximum Dose:* 800 mg/day
Supplied: 100 & 300 mg tabs

DOSE ADJUSTMENT
Hepatic Failure: Generally tolerated but liver enzymes should be followed closely as allopurinol can cause hepatotoxicity; adjust dose for the individual patient.
Renal Failure: CrCl >60: 200 mg/d; *CrCl >30:* 100 mg/d; *CrCl 10-30:* 50-100 mg/d; *CrCl <10:* 100 mg/ q2-3d; *Dialysis:* <100 mg/d after dialysis

ONSET OF ACTION
Initial Response: 2 - 3 days; *Maximal Response:* 1 - 3 weeks

MONITORING
Baseline: Serum uric acid, AST, ALT, ALP, albumin, bilirubin, CBC, serum creatinine.
Every 3 weeks: Serum uric acid should be measured every 3 weeks and dose of allopurinol adjusted accordingly until the serum uric acid level is reduced to the lower limit of the normal laboratory range

CONTRAINDICATIONS & PRECAUTIONS
(a) Previous hypersensitivity reaction to allopurinol, (b) Current acute gouty attack

TOXICITY
Reversible: (a) MSK: Increase in acute gout attacks when starting or stopping. Myopathy, arthralgias; *(b) Mucocut:* Pruritic maculopapular skin eruption, sometimes scaly or exfoliative; *(c) GI:* Diarrhea, nausea; *(d) CNS:* Drowsiness
Potentially Serious: (a) GI: Hepatotoxicity; *(b) Mucocut:* Stevens-Johnson syndrome (erythema multiforme exudativum); *(c) Hem:* Bone marrow suppression; *(d) Neuro:* Peripheral neuropathy; *(e) Renal:* Worsening renal failure
Managing Toxicity: Use the lowest dose possible; Imp. tolerated if taken with meals

PREGNANCY & LACTATION
Pregnancy: RISK CANNOT BE RULED OUT. (CATEGORY C)
Lactation: Allopurinol has been detected in the breast milk of nursing mothers. Although generally considered safe, allopurinol should be used only if the potential benefit justifies the potential risk to the baby.

DRUG INTERACTIONS
Drugs which may ↑ toxicity of allopurinol: ACE-inhibitors (hypersensitivity), amoxicillin & ampicillin (rash), thiazide diuretics; *Drugs which may ↓ efficacy of allopurinol:* Uricosuric agents; *Allopurinol may ↑ toxicity of the following drugs:* Azathioprine, cyclosporine, chlorpropamide (hypoglycemia), vidarabine (CNS tox)

MECHANISM OF ACTION
Allopurinol is rapidly oxidized in the liver to oxypurinol the active metabolite. Xanthine oxidase is the enzyme responsible for converting hypoxanthine to xanthine and xanthine to uric acid. By inhibiting the enzyme xanthine oxidase, oxypurinol reduces the production of uric acid.

PHARMACOKINETICS
Bioavail: 80 - 90%; *Allopurinol 1/2 Life:* 1 - 3 hours; *Oxypurinol 1/2 Life:* 12 - 30 hours; *Max Serum Concn:* 0.5 - 2 hours; *Metab:* Some hepatic metabolism; *Prot Bind:* None; *Excret:* Allopurinol (7%) and oxypurinol (70%) are excreted in the urine; The remaining is excreted in the faeces.

COLCHICINE

INDICATIONS

Approved: Colchicine is specifically indicated for treatment and relief of pain in attacks of acute gouty arthritis. It is also recommended for regular use between attacks as a prophylactic measure, and is often effective in aborting an attack when taken at the first sign of articular discomfort; *Off-Label Uses:* Behcet's disease; Familial Mediterranean Fever; Sweets syndrome; palindromic rheumatism

DOSE & DRUG ADMINISTRATION

Acute Gout Attack Initial Dose: 0.6 - 1.2 mg; *Acute Gout Attack Increments:* Continue 0.6 mg q2-3 hours after initial dose until pain is relieved or diarrhea ensues, whichever comes first.; *Maintenance Dose:* 0.6 mg OD/BID; *Maximum Dose:* 6 mg/day (if, during an acute gout attack, the maximum dose is administered, it should not be given for 7 days to avoid cumulative toxicity)
Supplied: 0.5 & 0.6 mg tablets

DOSE ADJUSTMENT

Hepatic Failure: Generally tolerated but should be monitored closely; use the lowest dose possible.
Renal Failure: CrCl > 50: No dose adjustment; *CrCl 10-50:* Reduce maintenance dose by 50%; *CrCl < 10:* Reduce maintenance dose by 75% (<0.6 mg/d)

ONSET OF ACTION

Initial Response: 12 hours; *Maximal Response:* 1 - 2 days

MONITORING

Baseline: CBC, serum creatinine; *Periodic:* CBC, serum creatinine

CONTRAINDICATIONS & PRECAUTIONS

(a) Previous hypersensitivity reaction to colchicine; (b) Serious gastrointestinal, cardiac, hepatic, or renal disorders; (c) Blood dyscrasias

TOXICITY

Reversible: (a) GI: Dose related – nausea, vomiting, abdominal pain, diarrhea; *(b) Mucocut:* Urticaria, dermatitis, purpura, alopecia
Potentially Serious: (a) MSK: Muscular weakness (reversible with discontinuation); *(b) Hem:* Agranulocytosis, aplastic anemia; *(c) Neuro:* Peripheral neuropathy; *(d) Renal:* May cause renal damage at toxic doses; *(e) CVS:* Myopathy;
Managing Toxicity: Use the lowest dose possible

PREGNANCY & LACTATION

Pregnancy: POSITIVE EVIDENCE OF RISK. (CATEGORY D)
Lactation: It is not known if colchicine is excreted in breast milk; however, it is generally felt to be compatible with breast feeding.

DRUG INTERACTIONS

Drugs which may ↑ levels of colchicine: Sodium bicarbonate, cyclosporine; *Drugs which may ↑ toxicity of colchicine:* Alcohol (GI toxicity), phenylbutazone (bone m.); *Drugs which may ↓ levels of colchicine:* Antacids, ascorbic acid (Vitamin C); *Colchicine may ↑ sensitivity to the following drugs:* CNS depressants (opiates, sedative hypnotics, benzodiazepines, alcohol), sympathomimetics (epinephrine, dopamine, dobutamine, isoprenaline, ephedrine); *Colchicine may ↑ toxicity of the following drugs:* Cyclosporine; *Colchicine may ↓ levels of the following drugs:* Vitamin B12

MECHANISM OF ACTION

Colchicine is the active compound. The mechanism of action of colchicine is unknown. It is thought to decrease lactic acid production by leukocytes and thereby decrease urate crystal precipitation in the joint and the subsequent inflammatory response. Colchicine binds to the leukocyte intracellular protein tubulin → inhibits tubulin polymerization to form microtubules → inhibition of leukocyte migration/ phagocytosis and leukotriene B4 formation.

PHARMACOKINETICS

Bioavail: Absorbed well; **Max Serum Concn:** 2 hours; **1/2 Life:** plasma (20 minutes), tissue (10 - 31 hours); **Metab:** Partly deacetylated in the liver, the nature of various other metabolites is unknown; **Prot Bind:** Low; **Excret:** Primarily by biliary and renal routes; Urine - 28% as unchanged colchicine, 8% as metabolites

PROBENECID

INDICATIONS

Approved: Prevention of gouty arthritis; hyperuricemia; prolongation of beta-lactam effect (ie, serum levels); Usually used after failure of or intolerance to allopurinol

DOSE & DRUG ADMINISTRATION

Patients must drink 1 - 2 L of water per day while taking probenecid. **Initial Dose:** 250 mg BID x 1 week; **Maintenance Dose:** 500 mg BID thereafter and may be increased to 1000 mg BID; **Maximum Recommended Dose:** 3000 mg per day **Supplied:** Comb. tablet Colchicine/Probenecid (0.5 mg / 500 mg), ♥500 mg tablets

DOSE ADJUSTMENT

Hepatic Failure: No dosage reduction required.

Renal Failure: Efficacy of probenecid is reduced in renal failure due to the reduction in glomerular filtration rate. **CrCl < 50:** No dose adjustment; **CrCl < 50:** Avoid

ONSET OF ACTION

Initial Response: 0.5 - 2 hours

MONITORING

Baseline: CBC, creatinine, AST, ALT, ALP, albumin, 24hr urine for uric acid; **Yearly:** CBC, creatinine, AST, ALT, ALP, albumin, 24 hr urine for uric acid

CONTRAINDICATIONS & PRECAUTIONS

(a) Known hypersensitivity to probenecid; (b) Known blood dyscrasia; (c) Renal calculi; (d) Current acute gouty attack

TOXICITY

Reversible: (a) Mucocut: Alopecia, rash; (b) GI: Anorexia, nausea, vomiting; (c) Gen: Flushing; (d) CNS: Dizziness, headache; (e) MSK: Precipitate acute gout **Potentially Serious:** (a) Hepatic: Associated with hepatic necrosis; (b) Renal: Hematuria, renal colic, CV pain; (c) Hem: Anemia, leukopenia, hemolytic anemia

PREGNANCY & LACTATION

Pregnancy: RISK CANNOT BE RULED OUT. (CATEGORY C) **Lactation:** Safety during breast feeding has not been established – Used only if potential benefit justifies the potential risk to the baby.

DRUG INTERACTIONS

Probenecid may ↑ levels of the following drugs: Sulfonamides, sulfonylureas, indomethacin, rifampin, cephalosporins, penicillins; **Probenecid may ↑ toxicity of the following drugs:** Ganciclovir, zidovudine, diflunisal, methotrexate; **Drugs which may ↓ efficacy of probenecid:** ASA & pyrazinamide (interfere with uricosuric actn.)

MECHANISM OF ACTION

Probenecid is a uricosuric and renal tubular blocking agent. It inhibits the tubular reabsorption of urate, thus increasing the urinary excretion of uric acid and decreasing serum urate levels. Effective uricosuria reduces the miscible urate pool, retards urate deposition, and promotes resorption of urate deposits.

PHARMACOKINETICS
Bioavail: 60%; *Max Plasma Concn:* 0.5-6 hours; *1/2 Life:* 3-12 hours; *Metab:* Extensively metabolized via hydroxylation; *Prot Bind:* High (98 - 99%); *Excret:* Renal

SULFINPYRAZONE

INDICATIONS
Approved: Treatment of chronic gouty arthritis and intermittent gouty arthritis. Sulfinpyrazone is usually used after failure of or intolerance to allopurinol

DOSE & DRUG ADMINISTRATION
Initial Dose: 100 - 200 mg PO BID x 1 week; *Maintenance Dose:* 200 mg PO BID thereafter and may be increased to 400 mg PO BID; *Maximum Recommended Dose:* 800 mg per day.
Supplied: 100 & 200 mg tablets.

DOSE ADJUSTMENT
Hepatic Failure: No dosage reduction required; monitor closely (see toxicity).
Renal Failure: Efficacy of sulfinpyrazone is reduced in renal failure due to the reduction in GFR. *CrCl > 10:* No dose adjustment; *CrCl < 10:* Avoid

ONSET OF ACTION
Initial Response: Not available

MONITORING
Initial: Serum uric acid levels, 24hr urine for uric acid levels

CONTRAINDICATIONS & PRECAUTIONS
(a) Known hypersensitivity to sulfinpyrazone; (b) Acute attack of gout; (c) ASA sensitive asthma, urticaria or acute rhinitis; (d) Active peptic ulcer disease; (e) Known blood dyscrasias, porphyria, coagulopathies; (f) Severe renal or liver disease; (g) Uric acid renal calculi

TOXICITY
Reversible: (a) Mucocut: Skin rashes; *(b) GI:* Nausea, vomiting, diarrhea, elevated transaminases, jaundice, hepatitis
Potentially Serious: (a) Resp: May worsen ASA sensitive asthma; *(b) Renal:* Worsening of renal function and overt renal failure (rare); *(c) Hem:* Blood dyscrasias (anemia, leukopenia, agranulocytosis, thrombocytopenia, aplastic anemia – rare); *(d) GI:* Aggravate GI ulceration

PREGNANCY & LACTATION
Pregnancy: RISK CANNOT BE RULED OUT. (CATEGORY C)
Lactation: Safety during breast feeding has not been established; used only if potential benefit justifies the potential risk to the baby.

DRUG INTERACTIONS
Drugs which may ↑ toxicity of sulfinpyrazone: ASA or NSAIDs (platelets and GI toxicity); *Drugs which may ↓ efficacy of sulfinpyrazone:* ASA (antagonizes uricosuric effect); *Sulfinpyrazone may ↑ toxicity of the following drugs:* Warfarin (INR); *Sulfinpyrazone may ↓ efficacy of the following drugs:* Cyclosporine

MECHANISM OF ACTION
Sulfinpyrazone is a uricosuric and renal tubular blocking agent. It inhibits the tubular reabsorption of urate, thus increasing the urinary excretion of uric acid and decreasing serum urate levels. Effective uricosuria reduces the miscible urate pool, retards urate deposition, and promotes resorption of urate deposits.

PHARMACOKINETICS
Bioavail: 60%; *Max Plasma Concn:* Unknown; *1/2 Life:* 4 - 6 hours; *Metab:* Unknown; *Prot Bind:* Unknown, *Excret:* Renal

NON-STEROIDAL ANTI-INFLAMMATORY DRUGS (NSAIDs)
GENERAL INFORMATION

INDICATIONS
In general, the NSAIDs have a wide variety of uses in the field of rheumatology and are used for their anti-inflammatory, anti-pyretic, and analgesic effects.

DOSE ADJUSTMENT
Hepatic Failure: Most NSAIDs are metabolized in the liver. In general, small dosage decreases may be required in the setting of hepatic impairment. Some NSAIDs are contraindicated in severe hepatic impairment.

Renal Failure: All NSAIDs should be used with caution in the setting of renal impairment.

MONITORING
In general, short term use of NSAIDs in healthy patients is typically safe. Otherwise, the following monitoring strategy may be advisable. *Baseline:* CBC, creatinine, electrolytes, AST, ALT, ALP, albumin; *One week:* CBC, creatinine, electrolytes, AST, ALT, ALP, albumin; *Yearly:* CBC, creatinine, electrolytes, AST, ALT, ALP, albumin

CONTRAINDICATIONS & PRECAUTIONS
(a) Known hypersensitivity to any NSAID; (b) Asthma, urticaria, or allergic-type reactions after ASA or other NSAIDs; (c) Active peptic ulcer, a history of recurrent ulceration, or active inflammatory disease of the gastrointestinal tract; (d) History of peptic ulcer disease (especially if age >65, concomitant steroid use); (e) Significant hepatic impairment or active liver disease; (f) Advanced renal disease; (g) Congestive heart failure or hypertension; (h) Concomitant anticoagulants, chronic alcohol abuse.

TOXICITY
Reversible: (a) CVS: Hypertension, fluid retention, and edema; *(b) GI:* Dyspepsia, nausea, abdominal pain, diarrhea; *(c) Ophtho:* Blurred vision; *(d) CNS:* Drowsiness, dizziness, vertigo, insomnia, or depression; *(e) Mucocut:* Rash

Potentially Serious: (a) Resp: Worsening of asthma; *(b) Mucocut:* Almost all of the NSAIDs have been associated with adverse cutaneous reactions including erythema multiforme, Stevens-Johnson syndrome, or toxic epidermal necrolysis; *(c) Hepatic:* Up to 15% of patients experience borderline ↑ in liver enzymes with rare cases of associated fulminant hepatitis, liver necrosis, and fatal hepatic failure; *(d) Renal:* Worsening of renal function through a reduction in glomerular blood flow by prostaglandin inhibition or by an idiosyncratic acute interstitial nephritis with hematuria, proteinuria, and nephritic syndrome; hyperkalemia (rare); *(e) Hem:* Aplastic anemia, agranulocytosis, and thrombocytopenia are rare associations; *(f) GI:* Complicated GI ulceration with perforation, obstruction, and bleeding; *(g) CNS:* Aseptic meningitis

MECHANISM OF ACTION
The exact mechanism of action of NSAIDs is unknown; many mechanisms have been proposed. The primary mechanism of action of the NSAIDs is thought to be via inhibition of prostaglandin synthesis by blocking the enzymes cyclooxygenase 1 and 2 (COX-1, COX-2). COX-1 is expressed constitutively and is responsible for producing protective prostaglandins (i.e. in the gastric mucosa). COX-2 is induced by tissue insult and sets off the inflammatory cascade. Most NSAIDs preferentially inhibit COX-1. The anti-pyretic effect of NSAIDs is thought to be through the inhibition of prostaglandin E1 synthesis in the CNS. Some NSAIDs also have anti-platelet activity through inhibition of thromboxane A2 synthesis (i.e. ASA).

NSAID COMPARISON CHART

Generic Name (Trade Name)	Class	Usual Starting Dose	Max Dose
ACETYLSALICYLIC ACID (ASA) (Aspirin)	Salicylates	325-650 mg q4-6h	5400 mg
DICLOFENAC (Voltaren, DVoltaren-SR, Voltaren-XR, Cataflam)	Acetic Acid	50 mg TID	200 mg
DICLOFENAC / MISOPROSTOL (Arthrotec)	Acetic Acid	Arthrotec 50-75 mg TID	200 mg
DIFLUNISAL (Dolobid)	Salicylates	250 - 500 mg BID-TID	1500 mg
ETODOLAC (Ultradol, Lodine, Lodine-XL)	Acetic Acid	200 - 300 mg BID-TID	1200 mg
FENOPROFEN (Nalfon)	Propionic Acid	600 mg TID-QID	3000 mg
FLURBIPROFEN (Ansaid, DFroben, DFroben-SR)	Propionic Acid	100 mg BID	300 mg
IBUPROFEN (Motrin, Advil)	Propionic Acid	400 - 800 mg TID-QID	3200 mg
INDOMETHACIN (Indocid, Indocid-SR)	Acetic Acid	25 - 75 mg BID-TID	200 mg
KETOPROFEN (Orudis, Oruvail, DRhodis, Rhovail)	Propionic Acid	50 mg TID-QID	300 mg
KETOROLAC (Toradol)	Acetic Acid	10 mg q4-6h or 10-30 mg IM q4-6h	PO - 40 mg IM - 120 mg
MECLOFENAMATE (Meclomen)	Fenamate	50 - 100 mg TID-QID	400 mg
MEFENAMIC ACID (Ponstel, Ponstan)	Fenamate	250 mg QID	1000 mg
MELOXICAM (Mobic, DMobicox)	Oxicam	7.5 - 15 mg OD	15 mg
NABUMETONE (Relafen)	Naphthylalkanones	1000 - 2000 mg OD	2000 mg
NAPROXEN (Aleve, Anaprox, Naprosyn, EC-Naprosyn, Naprelan)	Propionic Acid	250 - 500 BID	1500 mg
OXAPROZIN (Daypro)	Propionic Acid	1200 mg OD	1800 mg
PIROXICAM (Feldene)	Oxicam	10 - 20 mg OD	20 mg
SALSALATE (Disalcid, Salflex, Amigesic)	Salicylates	1000 mg BID	3000 mg
SULINDAC (Clinoril)	Acetic Acid	150 - 200 mg BID	400 mg
TENOXICAM (DMobiflex)	Oxicam	10 - 20 mg OD	20 mg
TIAPROFENIC ACID (DSurgam, DAlbertTiafen)	Propionic Acid	200 mg TID	600 mg
TOLMETIN (Tolectin)	Acetic Acid	400 mg TID	2000 mg

ACETYLSALICYLIC ACID (ASA) (ASPIRIN)

INDICATIONS
Approved: Treatment of mild to moderate pain, inflammation, and fever; may be used as prophylaxis of myocardial infarction; prophylaxis of stroke and/or TIA.

DOSE & DRUG ADMINISTRATION
Dose: 325 - 650 mg PO q4-6h; *Max Dose:* 5400 mg/day;
Supplied: Tablets: 81, 325, 500, 650, & 975 mg; Suppositories: 60, 120, 125, 200, 300, 325, 600, 650

DOSE ADJUSTMENT
Hepatic Failure: No dosage reduction required but give with caution
Renal Failure: Use with caution as ASA may exacerbate renal dysfunction

ONSET OF ACTION
Initial Response: 30 minutes

PREGNANCY & LACTATION
Pregnancy: 1st & 2nd trimesters: **NO EVIDENCE OF RISK IN HUMANS. (CATEGORY B).** Contraindicated in the 3rd trimester - risk of premature closure of ductus arteriosus.
Lactation: Salicylates are excreted in breast milk. No adverse effects have been reported in infants of mothers taking usual analgesic doses; however, close supervision of the baby is required with chronic dosing.

DRUG INTERACTIONS
ASA may ↑ toxicity of: Warfarin (monitor INR), cyclosporine, NSAIDS (GI), methotrexate; anti-platelet agents; *ASA may ↑ levels of:* Lithium, digoxin; *ASA may ↓ efficacy of:* ACE-Inhibitors, angiotensin receptor blockers, furosemide, hydralazine, thiazide diuretics; *Drugs which ↑ levels of ASA:* Probenecid

PHARMACOKINETICS
Active Form & Initial Metab: ASA is hydrolyzed to salicylic acid which is the active metabolite; *Bioavail:* 90%; *Max Plasma Concn:* 2 hours; *ASA plasma 1/2 Life:* 15 minutes; *Salicylic Acid 1/2 Life:* 3 - 6 hours; *Metab:* Hydrolyzed in the liver to salicylic acid which is conjugated to glycine and glucuronic acid; *Prot Bind:* High (99%); *Excret:* Metabs. in the urine

DICLOFENAC (VOLTAREN, ♣VOLTAREN-SR, VOLTAREN-XR, CATAFLAM)

INDICATIONS
Approved: Ankylosing spondylitis; rheumatoid arthritis; dysmenorrhea; osteoarthritis; mild to moderate pain.

DOSE & DRUG ADMINISTRATION
Oral Dose: 75 - 150 mg/day PO in three divided doses (i.e. 50 mg PO TID) or Slow-Release (SR/XR) preparation of 75 - 150 mg PO OD; *Rectal Dose:* 75 - 150 mg/day PR in three divided doses (i.e. 50 mg PO TID); *Max Dose:* 200 mg/day
Supplied: 25, 50, & 75 mg tablets; 100 mg XR tablets; ♣75 & 100 mg SR tablets; ♣50 & 100 mg suppositories

DOSE ADJUSTMENT
Hepatic Failure: No dosage reduction required but give with caution
Renal Failure: Use with caution as diclofenac may worsen renal impairment

ONSET OF ACTION
Initial Response: 1 - 2 hours

PREGNANCY & LACTATION
Pregnancy: 1st & 2nd trimester: **NO EVIDENCE OF RISK IN HUMANS (CAT B)**
Contraindicated in 3rd trimester: Risk of premature closure of ductus arteriosus.

Lactation: Unknown safety. Some experts think that diclofenac may be safely used during breast feeding.

DRUG INTERACTIONS

Diclofenac may ↑ toxicity of: Warfarin (monitor INR), cyclosporine, NSAIDS (GI), methotrexate; anti-platelet agents; *Diclofenac may ↑ levels of:* Lithium, digoxin; *Diclofenac may ↓ efficacy of:* ACE-Inhibitors, angiotensin receptor blockers, furosemide, hydralazine, thiazide diuretics

PHARMACOKINETICS

Active Form & Initial Metab: Diclofenac is a member of the phenylacetic acid class of NSAIDs (Acetic Acid Derivative). Diclofenac is a non-steroidal anti-inflammatory drug that exhibits anti-inflammatory, analgesic, and anti-pyretic activities. Diclofenac is the active compound; *Bioavail:* 50%; *Max Plasma Concn:* 1 hours; *1/2 Life:* 1-2 hours; *Metab:* Hepatic via cytochrome P4502C9; *Prot Bind:* High (99%); *Excret:* Urine 65% & bile 35%

DICLOFENAC / MISOPROSTOL (ARTHROTEC)

INDICATIONS

Approved: Rheumatoid arthritis; osteoarthritis

DOSE & DRUG ADMINISTRATION

Oral Dose: Arthrotec 50 PO TID or Arthrotec 75 PO TID; *Max Dose:* 200 mg/day
Supplied: Arthrotec 50: 50 mg diclofenac & 200 µg misoprostol; *Arthrotec 75:* 75 mg Diclofenac & 200 µg Misoprostol.

DOSE ADJUSTMENT

Hepatic Failure: No dosage reduction required but give with caution
Renal Failure: Use with caution as diclofenac may worsen renal function

ONSET OF ACTION

Initial Response: 1 - 2 hours

PREGNANCY & LACTATION

Pregnancy: CONTRAINDICATED IN PREGNANCY. (CATEGORY X)
Lactation: Use during breast feeding is not advisable.

DRUG INTERACTIONS

Arthrotec may ↑ toxicity of: Warfarin (monitor INR), cyclosporine, NSAIDS (GI), methotrexate; anti-platelet agents; *Arthrotec may ↑ levels of:* Lithium; *Arthrotec may ↓ efficacy of:* ACE-Inhibitors, angiotensin receptor blockers, furosemide, hydralazine, thiazide diuretics

PHARMACOKINETICS

Active Form & Initial Metab: Arthrotec is a combination product containing diclofenac sodium, a non-steroidal anti-inflammatory drug (NSAID) and misoprostol, a gastrointestinal (GI) mucosal protective prostaglandin E1 analog. Diclofenac is a member of the phenylacetic acid class of NSAIDs and is a non-steroidal anti-inflammatory drug that exhibits anti-inflammatory, analgesic, and anti-pyretic activities. Diclofenac is the active anti-inflammatory compound with no initial metabolism. Misoprostol is a prodrug which is rapidly converted to its active form misoprostol acid which has gastric antisecretory and mucosal protective properties. *Bioavail of Diclofenac:* 50%; *Bioavail of Misoprostol:* rapid and extensive; *Max Plasma Concn of Diclofenac:* 2 hours; *Max Plasma Concn of Misoprostol:* 20 min; *1/2 Life of Diclofenac:* 1 - 2 hours; *1/2 Life of Misoprostol:* 30 minutes; *Metab of Diclofenac:* Hepatic via cytochrome P450 2C9; *Metab of Misoprostol:* Hepatic; *Prot Bind of Diclofenac:* High (99%); *Prot Bind of Misoprostol:* High (90%); *Excret of Diclofenac:* Urine 65% & bile 35%; *Excret of Misoprostol:* Urine 90%

DIFLUNISAL (DOLOBID)

INDICATIONS
Approved: Mild to moderate pain; osteoarthritis; rheumatoid arthritis

DOSE & DRUG ADMINISTRATION
Initial Loading Dose: 500 - 1000 mg PO; *Maintenance Dose:* 250 - 500 mg PO q 8-12 hours; *Max Dose:* 1500 mg per day
Supplied: 250 & 500 mg tablets

DOSE ADJUSTMENT
Hepatic Failure: No dosage reduction required but give with caution.
Renal Failure: Use with caution as diflunisal may worsen renal impairment

ONSET OF ACTION
Initial Response: Up to 3 days

PREGNANCY & LACTATION
Pregnancy: 1st & 2nd trimesters - **RISK CANNOT BE RULED OUT. (CAT C)** Contraindicated in the 3rd trimester - Risk of premature closure of ductus arteriosus.
Lactation: Unknown safety, diflunisal is secreted in breast milk - Used only if potential benefit justifies the potential risk to the fetus.

DRUG INTERACTIONS
Diflunisal may ↑ *levels of:* Acetaminophen, hydrochlorothiazide, lithium; *Diflunisal may* ↑ *toxicity of:* Warfarin (monitor INR), cyclosporine, NSAIDS (GI), methotrexate; anti-platelet agents; *Diflunisal may* ↓ *efficacy of:* ACE-Inhibitors, angiotensin receptor blockers, furosemide, hydralazine, thiazide diuretics

PHARMACOKINETICS
Active Form & Initial Metab: Diflunisal is a difluorophenyl derivative of salicylic acid (Salicylate), a non-steroidal anti-inflammatory drug that exhibits anti-inflammatory, analgesic, and anti-pyretic activities. *Bioavail:* High, *Max Plasma Concn:* 2 - 3 hours *1/2 Life:* 8 - 12 hours; *Metab:* Hepatic glucuronide conjugation; *Prot Bind:* High (99%); *Excret:* Glucuronide metabolites in the urine

ETODOLAC (ULTRADOL, LODINE, LODINE-XL)

INDICATIONS
Approved: Mild to moderate pain; osteoarthritis

DOSE & DRUG ADMINISTRATION
Dose: 200 - 300 mg PO BID to QID; *Max Dose:* 1200 mg per day.
Supplied: 200 & 300 mg tablets or capsules; 400, 500, & 600 mg XL tablets

DOSE ADJUSTMENT
Hepatic Failure: No dosage reduction required but give with caution.
Renal Failure: Use with caution as etodolac may worsen renal impairment.

ONSET OF ACTION
Initial Response: 30 minutes

PREGNANCY & LACTATION
Pregnancy: 1st & 2nd trimesters - **RISK CANNOT BE RULED OUT. (CAT C)** Contraindicated in the 3rd trimester - Risk of premature closure of ductus arteriosus.
Lactation: Unknown safety. Long elimination 1/2-life other NSAIDs usually used.

DRUG INTERACTIONS
Etodolac may ↑ *toxicity of:* Warfarin (monitor INR), cyclosporine, NSAIDS (GI), methotrexate; anti-platelet agents; *Etodolac may* ↑ *levels of:* Lithium; *Etodolac may* ↓ *efficacy of:* ACE-Inhibitors, angiotensin receptor blockers, furosemide, hydralazine, thiazide diuretics

PHARMACOKINETICS
Active Form & Initial Metab: Etodolac is a mixture of R- and S- racemic etodolac. The biologically active form is the S-form. Etodolac is a member of the pyranocarboxylic acid class of NSAIDs (Acetic Acid Derivative), a non-steroidal anti-inflammatory drug that exhibits anti-inflammatory, analgesic, and anti-pyretic activities. ***Bioavail:*** 80%; ***Max Plasma Concn:*** 1.7 hours; ***1/2 Life:*** 7 hours; ***Metab:*** Extensively metabolized in the liver via glucuronidation and hydroxylation conjugation; ***Prot Bind:*** High (99%); ***Excret:*** Glucuronide metabolites in the urine

FENOPROFEN (NALFON)

INDICATIONS
Approved: Osteoarthritis; rheumatoid arthritis; mild to moderate pain
DOSE & DRUG ADMINISTRATION
Initial Dose: 600 mg PO TID to QID; ***Maintenance Dose:*** Reduce in increments of 300 mg until minimal effective dose is established; ***Max Dose:*** 3000 mg per day.
Supplied: 200, 300, & 600 mg tablets
DOSE ADJUSTMENT
Hepatic Failure: No dosage reduction required but give with caution
Renal Failure: Use with caution as fenoprofen may worsen renal impairment.
ONSET OF ACTION
Initial Response: 2 days; ***Max Response:*** 2 - 3 weeks
PREGNANCY & LACTATION
Pregnancy: 1st & 2nd trimester: **NO EVIDENCE OF RISK IN HUMANS (CAT B)** Contraindicated in 3rd trimester: Risk of premature closure of ductus arteriosus and fenoprofen may prolong parturition.
Lactation: Unknown safety, fenoprofen is secreted in breast milk. Used only if potential benefit justifies the potential risk to the baby.
DRUG INTERACTIONS
Fenoprofen may ↑ toxicity of: Warfarin (monitor INR), cyclosporine, NSAIDS (GI), methotrexate; anti-platelet agents; ***Fenoprofen may ↑ levels of:*** Lithium; ***Fenoprofen may ↓ efficacy of:*** ACE-Inhibitors, angiotensin receptor blockers, furosemide, hydralazine, thiazide diuretics; ***Drugs which may ↓ levels and efficacy of fenoprofen:*** ASA (decreases half-life), phenobarbital (decreases half-life)
PHARMACOKINETICS
Active Form & Initial Metab: Fenoprofen is a member of the propionic acid class of NSAIDs, a non-steroidal anti-inflammatory drug that exhibits anti-inflammatory, analgesic, and anti-pyretic activities. ***Bioavail:*** High; ***Max Plasma Concn:*** 2 hours; ***1/2 Life:*** 3 hours; ***Metab:*** Metabolized in the liver via glucuronidation & hydroxylation conjugation; ***Prot Bind:*** High (99%); ***Excret:*** Glucuronide metabolites in the urine

FLURBIPROFEN (ANSAID, ✦FROBEN, ✦FROBEN-SR)

INDICATIONS
FDA Approved: Rheumatoid arthritis; osteoarthritis
DOSE & DRUG ADMINISTRATION
Oral Dose: 200 - 300 mg/day PO in 2 to 4 divided doses (100 mg PO BID); ***Rectal Dose:*** 50 - 100 mg PR qhs (as part of maximum daily dose); ***Max Dose:*** 300 mg/day
Supplied: 50 & 100 mg tablets; ✦Froben 200 mg SR formulation.
DOSE ADJUSTMENT
Hepatic Failure: Dosage reduction of 50% in moderate hepatic impairment. Not recommended in severe hepatic impairment.

Renal Failure: Use with caution as flurbiprofen may worsen renal impairment.
ONSET OF ACTION
Initial Response: 1 - 2 hours
PREGNANCY & LACTATION
Pregnancy: 1st & 2nd trimester: **NO EVIDENCE OF RISK IN HUMANS (CAT B)**
  Contraindicated in 3rd trimester: Risk of premature closure of ductus arteriosus.
Lactation: Compatible with breast feeding.
DRUG INTERACTIONS
Flurbiprofen may ↑ *toxicity of:* Warfarin (monitor INR), cyclosporine, NSAIDS (GI), methotrexate; anti-platelet agents; *Flurbiprofen may* ↑ *levels of:* Lithium; *Flurbiprofen may* ↓ *efficacy of:* ACE-Inhibitors, angiotensin receptor blockers, furosemide, hydralazine, thiazide diuretics
PHARMACOKINETICS
Active Form & Initial Metab: Flurbiprofen is a member of the propionic acid class of NSAIDs, a non-steroidal anti-inflammatory drug that exhibits anti-inflammatory, analgesic, and anti-pyretic activities. Flurbiprofen is the active compound with no initial metabolism. *Bioavail:* Well absorbed; *Max Plasma Concn:* 3 - 4 hours; *1/2 Life:* 3 - 5 hours; *Metab:* Hepatic via oxidation and conjugation; *Prot Bind:* High (99%); *Excret:* Urine 95%

IBUPROFEN (Motrin, Advil)

INDICATIONS
Approved: Inflammatory diseases and rheumatoid disorders
DOSE & DRUG ADMINISTRATION
Dose: 400 - 800 mg/dose PO TID-QID; *Max Dose:* 3200 mg/day
Supplied: 100, 200, 400, 600, & 800 mg tablets; 200 mg capsules
DOSE ADJUSTMENT
Hepatic Failure: Dosage reduction of 50% in moderate hepatic impairment. Not recommended in severe hepatic impairment.
Renal Failure: Use with caution as ibuprofen may worsen renal impairment.
ONSET OF ACTION
Initial Response: 24 - 48 hours
PREGNANCY & LACTATION
Pregnancy: 1st & 2nd trimester: **NO EVIDENCE OF RISK IN HUMANS (CAT B)**
  Contraindicated in 3rd trimester: Risk of premature closure of ductus arteriosus.
Lactation: Compatible with breast feeding.
DRUG INTERACTIONS
Ibuprofen may ↑ *toxicity of:* Warfarin (monitor INR), cyclosporine, NSAIDS (GI), methotrexate; anti-platelet agents; *Ibuprofen may* ↑ *levels of:* Digoxin, Lithium; *Ibuprofen may* ↓ *efficacy of:* ACE-Inhibitors, angiotensin receptor blockers, furosemide, hydralazine, thiazide diuretics
PHARMACOKINETICS
Active Form & Initial Metab: Ibuprofen is a member of the propionic acid class of NSAIDs, a non-steroidal anti-inflammatory drug that exhibits anti-inflammatory, analgesic, and anti-pyretic activities. Ibuprofen is the active compound with no initial metabolism. *Bioavail:* 85%; *Max Plasma Concn:* 1 - 2 hours; *1/2 Life:* 2 - 4 hours; *Metab:* Hepatic; *Prot Bind:* High (90 - 99%); *Excret:* Urine (only 1% as free drug)

INDOMETHACIN (INDOCID, INDOCID-SR)

INDICATIONS
Approved: Moderate pain; acute gouty arthritis, acute bursitis/tendonitis, moderate to severe osteoarthritis, rheumatoid arthritis, ankylosing spondylitis

DOSE & DRUG ADMINISTRATION
Oral Dose: 25 - 75 mg/dose PO BID-TID or sustained release (SR) 75 mg PO OD-BID; *Rectal Dose:* 50 - 100 mg PR qhs (as part of maximum daily dose); *Max Dose:* 200 mg/day;
Supplied: 25 & 50 mg capsules; 75 mg SR capsules; 50 & ♣100 mg suppositories

DOSE ADJUSTMENT
Hepatic Failure: Dosage reduction of 50% in moderate hepatic impairment. Not recommended in severe hepatic impairment.
Renal Failure: Use with caution as indomethacin may worsen existing renal impairment.

ONSET OF ACTION
Initial Response: 30 minutes

PREGNANCY & LACTATION
Pregnancy: 1st & 2nd trimester: NO EVIDENCE OF RISK IN HUMANS (CAT B)
Contraindicated in 3rd trimester: Risk of premature closure of ductus arteriosus.
Lactation: Compatible with breast feeding.

DRUG INTERACTIONS
Indomethacin may ↑ *toxicity of:* Warfarin (monitor INR), cyclosporine, NSAIDS (GI), methotrexate; anti-platelet agents; *Indomethacin may* ↑ *levels of:* Lithium; *Indomethacin may* ↓ *efficacy of:* ACE-Inhibitors, angiotensin receptor blockers, furosemide, hydralazine, thiazide diuretics

PHARMACOKINETICS
Initial Response: Indomethacin is a member of the indole acetic acid class of NSAIDs, a non-steroidal anti-inflammatory drug that exhibits anti-inflammatory, analgesic, and anti-pyretic activities. Indomethacin is the active compound with no initial metabolism. *Bioavail:* 100%; *Max Plasma Concn:* 3 - 4 hours; *1/2 Life:* 4.5 hours; *Metab:* Hepatic with significant enterohepatic circulation; *Prot Bind:* High (99%); *Excret:* Urine 60% & Faeces 33%

KETOPROFEN (ORUDIS, ORUVAIL, ♣RHODIS, RHOVAIL)

INDICATIONS
Approved: Rheumatoid arthritis; dysmenorrhea; osteoarthritis; pain; ♣Ank Spond

DOSE & DRUG ADMINISTRATION
Dose: 50 mg PO TID - QID (150 - 200 mg/day) or 150 – 200 mg (SR) PO OD; *Max Dose:* 300 mg per day.
Supplied: 25, 50, & 75 mg capsules & tablets; 100, 150, & 200 mg extended release capsules; ♣100 mg suppositories

DOSE ADJUSTMENT
Hepatic Failure: No dosage reduction required but give with caution.
Renal Failure: Ketoprofen may worsen existing renal impairment. *CrCl < 50:* 150 mg/day initial dose; *CrCl < 25:* 100 mg/day initial dose

ONSET OF ACTION
Initial Response: 2 days; *Max Response:* 2 - 3 weeks

PREGNANCY & LACTATION
Pregnancy: 1st & 2nd trimester: NO EVIDENCE OF RISK IN HUMANS (CAT B)
Contraindicated in 3rd trimester: Risk of premature closure of ductus arteriosus.

Lactation: Unknown safety, used only if potential benefit justifies the potential risk.
DRUG INTERACTIONS
Ketoprofen may ↑ toxicity of: Warfarin (monitor INR), cyclosporine, NSAIDS (GI), methotrexate; anti-platelet agents; *Ketoprofen may ↑ levels of:* Lithium; *Ketoprofen may ↓ efficacy of:* ACE-Inhibitors, angiotensin receptor blockers, furosemide, hydralazine, thiazide diuretics; *Drugs which may ↑ toxicity of ketoprofen:* ASA or NSAIDs (GI), diuretic use (renal), probenecid
PHARMACOKINETICS
Active Form & Initial Metab: Ketoprofen is a member of the propionic acid class of NSAIDs, a non-steroidal anti-inflammatory drug that exhibits anti-inflammatory, analgesic, and anti-pyretic activities. *Bioavail:* 90%; *Max Plasma Concn:* 0.5 - 2 hours; *1/2 Life:* 2 hours; *Metab:* Extensively metabolized in the liver via hydroxylation & conjugation; *Prot Bind:* High (99%); *Excret:* Urine 25% - 90%

KETOROLAC (TORADOL)

INDICATIONS
Approved: Short-term management of moderately-severe acute pain requiring opioid level analgesia
DOSE & DRUG ADMINISTRATION
Dose: 10 mg PO q4-6h; 10-30 mg IM q4-6h; *Max Dose:* 40 mg PO daily; 120 mg IM daily;
Supplied: 10 mg tablets; 15 & 30 mg/mL solution for injection
DOSE ADJUSTMENT
Hepatic Failure: No dosage reduction required but give with caution.
Renal Failure: Ketorolac may worsen existing renal impairment. *CrCl 50-100:* Reduce initial dose by 50%; *CrCl < 50:* Avoid
ONSET OF ACTION
Initial Response: 10 minutes with IM dose; *Max Response:* 2 - 3 hours
PREGNANCY & LACTATION
Pregnancy: 1st & 2nd trimesters - **RISK CANNOT BE RULED OUT. (CAT C)**
   Contraindicated in the 3rd trimester - Risk of premature closure of ductus arteriosus.
Lactation: Unknown safety, used only if potential benefit justifies the potential risk.
DRUG INTERACTIONS
Ketorolac may ↑ toxicity of: Warfarin (monitor INR), cyclosporine, NSAIDS (GI), methotrexate; *Ketorolac may ↑ levels of:* Lithium; *Ketorolac may ↓ efficacy of:* ACE-Inhibitors, angiotensin receptor blockers, furosemide, anti-convulsants (phenytoin, carbamazepine); *Drugs which may ↑ toxicity of ketorolac:* Probenecid
PHARMACOKINETICS
Active Form & Initial Metab: Ketorolac is a member of the phenylacetic acid class of NSAIDs (Acetic Acid Derivative). Ketorolac is a non-steroidal anti-inflammatory drug that exhibits anti-inflammatory, analgesic, and anti-pyretic activities. *Oral Bioavail:* Well absorbed; *Max Plasma Concn:* 2 - 3 hours; *1/2 Life:* 2 - 8 hours; *Metab:* Extensively metabolized in the liver; *Prot Bind:* High (99%); *Excret:* Urine (60% as unchanged drug)

MECLOFENAMATE (MECLOMEN)

INDICATIONS
Approved: Rheumatoid arthritis; dysmenorrhea; osteoarthritis; pain

DOSE & DRUG ADMINISTRATION
Dose: 50 - 100 mg PO q4-6h; *Max Dose:* 400 mg per day.
Supplied: 50 & 100 mg capsules
DOSE ADJUSTMENT
Hepatic Failure: No dosage reduction required but give with caution.
Renal Failure: Meclofenamate may worsen existing renal impairment.
ONSET OF ACTION
Initial Response: 1 - 2 hours
PREGNANCY & LACTATION
Pregnancy: 1st & 2nd trimester: **NO EVIDENCE OF RISK IN HUMANS (CAT B)**
Contraindicated in 3rd trimester: Risk of premature closure of ductus arteriosus.
Lactation: Unknown safety, used only if potential benefit justifies the potential risk.
DRUG INTERACTIONS
Meclofenamate may ↑ toxicity of: Warfarin (monitor INR), cyclosporine, NSAIDS
(GI), methotrexate; anti-platelet agents; *Meclofenamate may ↑ levels of:* Lithium;
Meclofenamate may ↓ efficacy of: ACE-Inhibitors, angiotensin receptor blockers,
furosemide, hydralazine, thiazide diuretics
PHARMACOKINETICS
Active Form & Initial Metab: Meclofenamate is a member of the fenamate class of
NSAIDs, a non-steroidal anti-inflammatory drug that exhibits anti-inflammatory,
analgesic, and anti-pyretic activities. Meclofenamic acid is extensively metabolized
to an active metabolite (Metabolite I; 3-hydroxymethyl metabolite of meclofenamic
acid) and at least six other less well characterized minor metabolites. Only this
Metabolite I has been shown in vitro to inhibit cyclooxygenase activity with
approximately one fifth the activity of meclofenamate sodium. *Bioavail:* 90%; *Max
Plasma Concn:* 0.5 - 1.5 hours; *1/2 Life:* 2 - 3.3 hours; *Metab:* Extensively
metabolized in the liver via hydroxylation & conjugation; *Prot Bind:* High (99%);
Excret: Metabolites in urine and faeces

MEFENAMIC ACID (PONSTEL, PONSTAN)
INDICATIONS
Approved: Mild to moderate pain including primary dysmenorrhea
DOSE & DRUG ADMINISTRATION
Dose: 500 mg initial dose followed by 250 mg q6h; *Max Dose:* 1250 mg per day - Not
to exceed on week treatment.
Supplied: 250 mg capsules
DOSE ADJUSTMENT
Hepatic Failure: No dosage reduction required but give with caution.
Renal Failure: Mefenamic acid may worsen existing renal impairment.
ONSET OF ACTION
Initial Response: 2 - 4 hours
PREGNANCY & LACTATION
Pregnancy: 1st & 2nd trimesters - **RISK CANNOT BE RULED OUT. (CAT C)**
Contraindicated in the 3rd trimester - Risk of premature closure of ductus arteriosus.
Lactation: Not compatible with breast feeding.
DRUG INTERACTIONS
Mefenamic acid may ↑ toxicity of: Warfarin (monitor INR), cyclosporine, NSAIDS
(GI), methotrexate; anti-platelet agents; *Mefenamic acid may ↑ levels of:* Lithium;
Mefenamic acid may ↓ efficacy of: ACE-Inhibitors, angiotensin receptor blockers,
furosemide, hydralazine, thiazide diuretics

PHARMACOKINETICS
Active Form & Initial Metab: Mefenamic acid is a member of the fenamate class of NSAIDs, a non-steroidal anti-inflammatory drug that exhibits anti-inflammatory, analgesic, and anti-pyretic activities. *Bioavail:* Well absorbed; *Max Plasma Concn:* 2 - 4 hours; *1/2 Life:* 3.5 hours; *Metab:* Extensively metabolized in the liver ; *Prot Bind:* High; *Excret:* Urine 50%, Faeces 20%

MELOXICAM (MOBIC, ♣MOBICOX)

INDICATIONS
Approved: Rheumatoid arthritis; osteoarthritis
DOSE & DRUG ADMINISTRATION
Oral Dose: 7.5 - 15 mg PO OD; *Max Dose:* 15 mg/day
Supplied: 7.5 & 15 mg tablets
DOSE ADJUSTMENT
Hepatic Failure: No dosage reduction in mild-moderate hepatic impairment. It has not been studied in severe hepatic impairment but should likely be avoided.
Renal Failure: No dosage adjustment in mild-moderate renal impairment (CrCl>15); however, use with caution as meloxicam may worsen existing renal impairment.
ONSET OF ACTION
Initial Response: Within 24 hours
PREGNANCY & LACTATION
Pregnancy: 1st & 2nd trimesters - RISK CANNOT BE RULED OUT (CAT C)
Contraindicated in the 3rd trimester - Risk of premature closure of ductus arteriosus.
Lactation: Unknown whether meloxicam is excreted in breast milk. Caution should be used if meloxicam is given to a nursing mother.
DRUG INTERACTIONS
Meloxicam may ↑ toxicity of: Warfarin (monitor INR), cyclosporine, NSAIDS (GI), methotrexate; anti-platelet agents; *Meloxicam may ↑ levels of:* Lithium; *Meloxicam may ↓ efficacy of:* ACE-Inhibitors, angiotensin receptor blockers, furosemide, hydralazine, thiazide diuretics; *Drugs which may ↓ absorption of meloxicam:* Cholestyramine
PHARMACOKINETICS
Active Form & Initial Metab: Meloxicam is a member of the enolic acid class of NSAIDs (Oxicam Derivative), a non-steroidal, anti-inflammatory drug that exhibits anti-inflammatory, analgesic, and anti-pyretic activities. Meloxicam has been shown to have preferential selectivity for COX-2 in several in-vitro and ex-vivo test systems. Prospective, controlled, long-term (>3 months) studies to establish the clinical significance of these results have not been performed. *Bioavail:* 89%; *Max Plasma Concn:* 4 - 5 hours; *1/2 Life:* 15 - 20 hours; *Metab:* Hepatic via cytochrome P450 2C9; *Prot Bind:* High (99%); *Excret:* Metabolites in the urine & faeces

NABUMETONE (RELAFEN)

INDICATIONS
Approved: Rheumatoid arthritis & osteoarthritis
DOSE & DRUG ADMINISTRATION
Oral Dose: 1000 - 2000 mg PO OD; *Max Dose:* 2000 mg/day
Supplied: 500 & 750 mg tablets
DOSE ADJUSTMENT
Hepatic Failure: No dosage reduction required but give with caution.
Renal Failure: Use with caution, may worsen existing renal impairment.

ONSET OF ACTION
Initial Response: 30+ minutes
PREGNANCY & LACTATION
Pregnancy: 1st & 2nd trimesters - **RISK CANNOT BE RULED OUT (CAT C)**
Contraindicated in the 3rd trimester - Risk of premature closure of ductus arteriosus.
Lactation: Unknown safety.
DRUG INTERACTIONS
Nabumetone may ↑ toxicity of: Warfarin (monitor INR), cyclosporine, NSAIDS (GI), methotrexate; anti-platelet agents; *Nabumetone may ↑ levels of:* Lithium; *Nabumetone may ↓ efficacy of:* ACE-Inhibitors, angiotensin receptor blockers, furosemide, hydralazine, thiazide diuretics
PHARMACOKINETICS
Active Form & Initial Metab: Nabumetone is a member of the naphthylalkanone class of NSAIDs, a non-steroidal anti-inflammatory drug that exhibits anti-inflammatory, analgesic, and anti-pyretic activities. Nabumetone is an inactive prodrug which is hepatically converted to 6-methoxy-2-naphthylacetic acid (6MNA), that is a potent inhibitor of prostaglandin synthesis. *Bioavail:* 35%; *Max Plasma Concn:* 3 hours; *1/2 Life:* 24 hours;
Metab: Hepatic; *Prot Bind:* High (99%); *Excret:* Urine 90% & faeces 10%

NAPROXEN (ALEVE, ANAPROX, NAPROSYN, EC-NAPROSYN, NAPRELAN)
INDICATIONS
Approved: Ankylosing spondylitis; rheumatoid arthritis; dysmenorrhea; non-rheumatoid inflammation; osteoarthritis; pain
DOSE & DRUG ADMINISTRATION
Oral Dose: 250 - 500 mg PO BID OR 750 mg PO OD Sustained Release (SR);
Rectal Dose: 500 mg PR BID; *Max Dose:* 1500 mg/day.
Supplied: 250, 375, & 500 mg tablets; 375 & 500 mg EC tablets; 125mg/5mL suspension; ♣500 mg suppositories; ♣750 mg SR tablets
DOSE ADJUSTMENT
Hepatic Failure: No dosage reduction required but give with caution.
Renal Failure: Use with caution as naproxen may worsen existing renal impairment.
ONSET OF ACTION
Initial Response: 1 - 2 hours
PREGNANCY & LACTATION
Pregnancy: 1st & 2nd trimester: **NO EVIDENCE OF RISK IN HUMANS (CAT B)**
Contraindicated in 3rd trimester: Risk of premature closure of ductus arteriosus.
Lactation: Compatible with breast feeding, weakly excreted in breast milk.
DRUG INTERACTIONS
Naproxen may ↑ toxicity of: Warfarin (monitor INR), cyclosporine, NSAIDs (GI), methotrexate; anti-platelet agents; *Naproxen may ↑ levels of:* Lithium; *Naproxen may ↓ efficacy of:* ACE-Inhibitors, angiotensin receptor blockers, furosemide, hydralazine, thiazide diuretics
PHARMACOKINETICS
Active Form & Initial Metab: Naproxen is a member of the propionic acid class of NSAIDs, a non-steroidal anti-inflammatory drug that exhibits anti-inflammatory, analgesic, and anti-pyretic activities. Naproxen is the active compound with no initial metabolism. *Bioavail:* 95%; *Max Plasma Concn:* 2 - 4 hours; *1/2 Life:* 13 hours;
Metab: Hepatic; *Prot Bind:* High (99%); *Excret:* Urine 95%

OXAPROZIN (DAYPRO)

INDICATIONS
Approved: Rheumatoid arthritis; osteoarthritis; juvenile rheumatoid arthritis
DOSE & DRUG ADMINISTRATION
Dose: 1200 mg PO OD; *Max Dose:* 1800 mg/day.
Supplied: 600 mg tablets
DOSE ADJUSTMENT
Hepatic Failure: No dosage reduction required but give with caution.
Renal Failure: Use with caution as oxaprozin may worsen existing renal impairment.
ONSET OF ACTION
Initial Response: 1 - 2 hours
PREGNANCY & LACTATION
*Pregnancy:*1st & 2nd trimesters - **RISK CANNOT BE RULED OUT. (CAT C)**
Contraindicated in the 3rd trimester - Risk of premature closure of ductus arteriosus.
Lactation: Unknown safety. Because of its long elimination half-life other NSAIDs
are preferred.
DRUG INTERACTIONS
Oxaprozin may ⬆ *toxicity of:* Warfarin (monitor INR), cyclosporine, NSAIDS (GI),
methotrexate; anti-platelet agents; *Oxaprozin may* ⬆ *levels of:* Lithium; *Oxaprozin
may* ⬇ *efficacy of:* ACE-Inhibitors, angiotensin receptor blockers, furosemide,
hydralazine, thiazide diuretics, beta blockers; *Drugs which may*⬆ *oxaprozin levels:*
H2-receptor antagonists
PHARMACOKINETICS
Active Form & Initial Metab: Oxaprozin is a member of the propionic acid class of
NSAIDs, a non-steroidal anti-inflammatory drug that exhibits anti-inflammatory,
analgesic, and anti pyrotic activities. Oxaprozin is the active compound with no initial
metabolism. *Bioavail:* 95%; *Max Plasma Concn:* 3 - 5 hours; *1/2 Life:* 50 hours;
Metab: Hepatic microsomal oxidation and glucuronide conjugation; *Prot Bind:* High
(99%); *Excret:* Urine 65% & faeces 35%

PIROXICAM (FELDENE)

INDICATIONS
Approved: Rheumatoid arthritis; osteoarthritis; ✽Ank Spond
DOSE & DRUG ADMINISTRATION
Oral Dose: 10 - 20 mg OD; *Rectal Dose:* 10 - 20 mg PR OD; *Max Dose:* 20 mg/d
Supplied: 10 & 20 mg capsules; ✽20 mg suppositories.
DOSE ADJUSTMENT
Hepatic Failure: No dosage reduction but give with caution.
Renal Failure: Use with caution, piroxicam may worsen existing renal impairment.
ONSET OF ACTION
Initial Response: 1 - 2 hours
PREGNANCY & LACTATION
*Pregnancy:*1st & 2nd trimesters - **RISK CANNOT BE RULED OUT. (CAT C)**
Contraindicated in the 3rd trimester - Risk of premature closure of ductus arteriosus.
Lactation: Compatible with breast feeding.
DRUG INTERACTIONS
Piroxicam may ⬆ *toxicity of:* Warfarin (monitor INR), cyclosporine, NSAIDS (GI),
methotrexate; anti-platelet agents; *Piroxicam may* ⬆ *levels of:* Lithium; *Piroxicam
may* ⬇ *efficacy of:* ACE-Inhibitors, angiotensin receptor blockers, furosemide,
hydralazine, thiazide diuretics

PHARMACOKINETICS
Active Form & Initial Metab: Piroxicam is a member of the enolic acid class of NSAIDs (Oxicam Derivative), a non-steroidal anti-inflammatory drug that exhibits anti-inflammatory, analgesic, and anti-pyretic activities. Piroxicam is the active compound with no initial metabolism. ***Bioavail:*** 95%; ***Max Plasma Concn:*** 3 - 5 hours; ***1/2 Life:*** 50 hours; ***Metab:*** Hepatic; ***Prot Bind:*** High (99%); ***Excret:*** Urine & faeces

SALSALATE (DISALCID, SALFLEX, AMIGESIC)
INDICATIONS
FDA Approved: Rheumatoid arthritis; osteoarthritis
DOSE & DRUG ADMINISTRATION
Dose: 1000 mg PO TID; ***Max Dose:*** 3000 mg/day.
Supplied: 500 & 750 mg tablets
DOSE ADJUSTMENT
Hepatic Failure: No dosage reduction required but give with caution.
Renal Failure: Use with caution as salsalate may exacerbate renal dysfunction.
ONSET OF ACTION
Initial Response: 3 - 4 days of continuous dosing
PREGNANCY & LACTATION
Pregnancy: 1st & 2nd trimesters - **RISK CANNOT BE RULED OUT. (CAT C)**
  Contraindicated in the 3rd trimester - Risk of premature closure of ductus arteriosus.
Lactation: Not compatible with breast feeding.
DRUG INTERACTIONS
Salsalate may ↑ toxicity of: Warfarin (monitor INR), methotrexate; oral hypoglycemics; ***Salsalate may ↓ efficacy of:*** ACE-Inhibitors, angiotensin receptor blockers, furosemide, thiazide diuretics
PHARMACOKINETICS
Active Form & Initial Metab: Salsalate is hepatically hydrolyzed to two moles of salicylic acid, the active form. ***Bioavail:*** Very Good; ***1/2 Life:*** 7-8 hours; ***Metab:*** Hydrolyzed in the liver to 2 molecules of salicylic acid which is conjugated to glycine and glucuronic acid;
Prot Bind: Unknown; ***Excret:*** Metabolites in the urine

SULINDAC (CLINORIL)
INDICATIONS
Approved: Ankylosing spondylitis; rheumatoid arthritis; gout; osteoarthritis; acute painful shoulder (bursitis/tendonitis);
DOSE & DRUG ADMINISTRATION
Dose: 150 mg PO BID; ***Max Dose:*** 400 mg/day.
Supplied: 150 & 200 mg tablets
DOSE ADJUSTMENT
Hepatic Failure: No dosage reduction required but give with caution.
Renal Failure: Use with caution as sulindac may worsen renal impairment.
ONSET OF ACTION
Initial Response: 1 - 2 hours
PREGNANCY & LACTATION
Pregnancy: 1st & 2nd trimester: **NO EVIDENCE OF RISK IN HUMANS (CAT B)**
  Contraindicated in 3rd trimester: Risk of premature closure of ductus arteriosus.
Lactation: Unknown safety. Because of its long elimination half-life other NSAIDs are preferred.

DRUG INTERACTIONS
Sulindac may ⬆ *toxicity of:* Warfarin (monitor INR), cyclosporine, NSAIDS (GI); methotrexate; anti-platelet agents; *Sulindac may* ⬆ *levels of:* Lithium; *Sulindac may* ⬇ *efficacy of:* ACE-Inhibitors, angiotensin receptor blockers, furosemide, hydralazine, thiazide diuretics

PHARMACOKINETICS
Active Form & Initial Metab: Sulindac is a member of the indole acetic acid class of NSAIDs, a non-steroidal anti-inflammatory drug that exhibits anti-inflammatory, analgesic, and anti-pyretic activities. Sulindac is an inactive prodrug which is hepatically reduced to a sulfide metabolite which is felt to be the biologically active component. *Bioavail:* 80%; *Max Plasma Concn:* 2 hours; *1/2 Life:* 8 hours; *Metab:* Hepatic; *Prot Bind:* High (99%); *Excret:* Urine (75%) & faeces (25%)

TENOXICAM (✦MOBIFLEX)

INDICATIONS
Approved: ✦Canada Only: Ank Spond; RA; non-rheumatoid inflamm; osteoarthritis.

DOSE & DRUG ADMINISTRATION
Dose: 10 - 20 mg PO OD; *Max Dose:* 20 mg per day.
Supplied: 20 mg tablets.

DOSE ADJUSTMENT
Hepatic Failure: No dosage reduction required but give with caution.
Renal Failure: No dosage reduction required, however, use with caution as tenoxicam may worsen existing renal impairment.

ONSET OF ACTION
Initial Response: Unknown; *Max Response:* Unknown

PREGNANCY & LACTATION
Pregnancy: 1st & 2nd trimester: **NO EVIDENCE OF RISK IN HUMANS (CAT B)**
Contraindicated in 3rd trimester: Risk of premature closure of ductus arteriosus.
Lactation: Unknown safety, used only if potential benefit justifies the potential risk.

DRUG INTERACTIONS
Tenoxicam may ⬆ *toxicity of:* Methotrexate, lithium, warfarin (may prolong INR), cyclosporine, NSAIDs (GI); *Tenoxicam may* ⬇ *levels of:* ASA (reduces Concn); *Drugs which may* ⬆ *toxicity of tenoxicam:* ASA or NSAIDs (GI toxicity), diuretics

PHARMACOKINETICS
Active Form & Initial Metab: Tenoxicam is a member of the enolic acid class of NSAIDs (Oxicam Derivative), a non-steroidal anti-inflammatory drug that exhibits anti-inflammatory, analgesic, and anti-pyretic activities. *Bioavail:* 100%; *Max Plasma Concn:* 0.5 - 6 hours; *1/2 Life:* 72 hours; *Metab:* Extensively metabolized via hydroxylation; *Prot Bind:* High (98 - 99%); *Excret:* Urine

TIAPROFENIC ACID (✦SURGAM, ✦ALBERTTIAFEN)

INDICATIONS
Approved: ✦Canada Only: Rheumatoid arthritis; osteoarthritis.

DOSE & DRUG ADMINISTRATION
Dose: 200 mg PO TID / 300 mg PO BID OR 600 mg PO OD Sustained Release (SR);
 Max Dose: 600 mg/day.
Supplied: 200 & 300 mg tablets; 300 mg SR capsules.

DOSE ADJUSTMENT
Hepatic Failure: No dosage reduction required but give with caution.

Renal Failure: Use with caution as tiaprofenic acid may worsen existing renal impairment.

ONSET OF ACTION

Initial Response: 1 - 2 hours

PREGNANCY & LACTATION

Pregnancy: 1st & 2nd trimester: **NO EVIDENCE OF RISK IN HUMANS (CAT B)**
Contraindicated in 3rd trimester: Risk of premature closure of ductus arteriosus.

Lactation: Unknown safety.

DRUG INTERACTIONS

Tiaprofenic acid may ↑ toxicity of: Warfarin (monitor INR), cyclosporine, NSAIDS (GI), methotrexate; anti-platelet agents; *Tiaprofenic acid may ↑ levels of:* Lithium; *Tiaprofenic acid may ↓ efficacy of:* ACE-Inhibitors, angiotensin receptor blockers, furosemide, hydralazine, thiazide diuretics

PHARMACOKINETICS

Active Form & Initial Metab: Tiaprofenic acid is a member of the propionic acid class of NSAIDs, a non-steroidal anti-inflammatory drug that exhibits anti-inflammatory, analgesic, and anti-pyretic activities. Tiaprofenic acid is the active compound with no initial metabolism. *Bioavail:* Well absorbed; *Max Plasma Concn:* 0.5 - 1 hours; *1/2 Life:* 1.7 hours; *Metab:* Hepatic; *Prot Bind:* High (99%); *Excret:* Urine 95% - largely as unchanged tiaprofenic acid

TOLMETIN (TOLECTIN)

INDICATIONS

Approved: Rheumatoid arthritis; juvenile rheumatoid arthritis; osteoarthritis

DOSE & DRUG ADMINISTRATION

Dose: 400 mg PO TID; *Max Dose:* 2000 mg/day.

Supplied: 200, 400, & 600 mg tablets

DOSE ADJUSTMENT

Hepatic Failure: No dosage reduction required but give with caution.

Renal Failure: Use with caution, tolmetin may worsen existing renal impairment.

ONSET OF ACTION

Initial Response: 3 - 7 days

PREGNANCY & LACTATION

*Pregnancy:*1st & 2nd trimesters - **RISK CANNOT BE RULED OUT. (CAT C)**
Contraindicated in the 3rd trimester - Risk of premature closure of ductus arteriosus.

Lactation: Compatible with breast feeding

DRUG INTERACTIONS

Tolmetin may ↑ toxicity of: Warfarin (monitor INR), cyclosporine, NSAIDS (GI), methotrexate; anti-platelet agents; *Tolmetin may ↑ levels of:* Lithium; *Tolmetin may ↓ efficacy of:* ACE-Inhibitors, angiotensin receptor blockers, furosemide, hydralazine, thiazide diuretics

PHARMACOKINETICS

Active Form & Initial Metab: Tolmetin is a member of the indole acetic acid class of NSAIDs, a non-steroidal anti-inflammatory drug that exhibits anti-inflammatory, analgesic, and anti-pyretic activities. Tolmetin is the active compound with no initial metabolism. *Bioavail:* 95%; *Max Plasma Concn:* 30 - 60 minutes; *1/2 Life:* 5 hours; *Metab:* Hepatic oxidation and conjugation; *Prot Bind:* High (99%); *Excret:* Urine 100%

OSTEOPOROSIS & METABOLIC BONE DISEASE
ALENDRONATE (FOSAMAX)

INDICATIONS
Approved: Treatment & prevention of postmenopausal osteoporosis; treatment of male osteoporosis; treatment & prevention of steroid-induced osteoporosis in men and women; Paget's disease;

DOSE & DRUG ADMINISTRATION
Drug Administration: Alendronate should only be swallowed upon arising for the day with a full glass of water; Patients should not lie down for at least 30 minutes <u>and</u> until after their first food of the day to facilitate delivery to the stomach and to reduce the potential for esophageal irritation; To enhance absorption, patients should take alendronate at least 30 minutes (1-2 hours if possible) before the first food, beverage or medication of the day. *(Since the mean bioavailability of alendronate is only 0.64% when administered after an overnight fast and 2 hours before a standard breakfast, many rheumatologists suggest waiting up to 1-2 hours before the first food, beverage, or medication of the day);* ***Dose: Treatment of Osteoporosis:*** 10 mg PO OD OR 70 mg PO qweekly; ***Prevention of Osteoporosis:*** 5 mg PO OD OR 35 mg PO qweekly; ***Prevention of Glucocorticoid-Induced Osteoporosis:*** 5 mg PO OD or 35 mg PO qweekly, except for postmenopausal women not receiving estrogen – 10 mg PO OD or 70 mg PO qweekly; ***Treatment of Paget's Disease:*** 40 mg PO OD for up to 6 months
Supplied: 5, 10, 35, 40, & 70 mg tablets.

DOSE ADJUSTMENT
Hepatic Failure: No dosage adjustment necessary.
Renal Failure: CrCl > 60: No dose adjustment; CrCl 35-60: No dose adjustment; CrCl < 35: Not Recommended

ONSET OF ACTION
Not Applicable

MONITORING
Baseline Osteoporosis Screening: CBC, Cr, Ca, albumin, ALP, SPEP, BMD
Intermittent: BMD follow-up as indicated

CONTRAINDICATIONS & PRECAUTIONS
(a) Known hypersensitivity to alendronate; (b) Pregnancy; (c) Hypocalcemia; (d) Inability to stand or sit upright for 30 minutes; (e) Abnormalities of the esophagus which delay esophageal emptying such as achalasia; (f) Renal insufficiency

TOXICITY
Reversible: (a) GI: Abdominal pain, dyspepsia, nausea, esophagitis, esophageal erosions, esophageal ulcers; *(b) MSK:* Bone, muscle, and joint pain; *(c) Mucocut:* Rash (rare)
Potentially Serious: (a) GI: Associated with complicated GI ulceration with perforation, obstruction, and bleeding; *(b) MSK:* Osteonecrosis of the jaw

PREGNANCY & LACTATION
Pregnancy: RISK CANNOT BE RULED OUT. (CATEGORY C)
Lactation: It is unknown if alendronate is excreted in breast milk. Alendronate has not been studied in nursing mothers and therefore is not recommended during nursing.

DRUG INTERACTIONS
Drugs which may ↓ levels of alendronate: Calcium, iron, & aluminum containing products interfere with absorption (vitamins, minerals, antacids, laxatives);

Alendronate may ↑ toxicity of: ASA and NSAIDs (alendronate may be associated with an increase in upper gastrointestinal adverse events)

MECHANISM OF ACTION

Alendronate is chemically described as (4-amino-1-hydroxybutylidene) bisphosphonic acid monosodium salt trihydrate. Alendronate is the biologically active form. Alendronate is a bisphosphonate that binds to bone hydroxyapatite and specifically inhibits the activity of osteoclasts, the bone-resorbing cells. Alendronate reduces bone resorption with no direct effect on bone formation, although the latter process is ultimately reduced because bone resorption and formation are coupled during bone turnover.

PHARMACOKINETICS

Bioavail: 0.6 - 0.7% (very low secondary to poor absorption); *Plasma 1/2 Life:* 72 hours; *Bone 1/2-Life:* 10 years (time to dissociate from bone matrix); *Metab:* Not metabolized; *Prot Bind:* High (78%); *Excret:* Urine 100%

CALCITONIN (MIACALCIN, CALCIMAR)

INDICATIONS

Approved: Treatment of postmenopausal osteoporosis, Paget's disease, hypercalcemia. *Off-Label Uses:* Complex Regional Pain Syndrome

DOSE & DRUG ADMINISTRATION

Nasal Dose (Miacalcin®): 200 IU intra-nasally per day alternating nostrils daily; *SC Dose (Calcimar®):* Give a 1 IU test dose to rule out allergy. 100 IU SC 3 times/ week to 100 IU SC OD. Administer at bedtime to reduce the severity of nausea and flushing. Start with a low-dose and increase gradually over a two-week period to help alleviate side effects;

Supplied: Spray bottle which delivers at least 14 metered doses of 200 IU; Injectable solution of 200 IU/ml.

DOSE ADJUSTMENT

Hepatic Failure: Unknown.
Renal Failure: Unknown

MONITORING

Baseline Osteoporosis Screening: CBC, Cr, Ca, albumin, ALP, SPEP, BMD; *Intermittent:* BMD follow-up as indicated, calcium, albumin

CONTRAINDICATIONS & PRECAUTIONS

(a) Known hypersensitivity to calcitonin-salmon; (b) Hypocalcemia

TOXICITY

Reversible: (a) Gen: Flushing (with SC route); *(b) ENT:* Rhinitis, nasal dryness, epistaxis, and sinusitis (with nasal route); *(c) MSK:* Bone, muscle, and joint pain; *(d) Lab:* Mild, asymptomatic reduction in serum calcium and phosphorus levels (nasal); *(e) GI:* Metallic taste & nausea (SC route); *(f) Mucocut:* Injection site reactions (SC route)

Potentially Serious: (a) ENT: Nasal ulceration (nasal route)

PREGNANCY & LACTATION

Pregnancy: RISK CANNOT BE RULED OUT. (CATEGORY C)
Lactation: It is unknown if calcitonin is excreted in breast milk. Calcitonin has been shown to inhibit lactation in animals and should not be given to nursing mothers.

DRUG INTERACTIONS

Formal studies to evaluate drug interactions have not been performed

MECHANISM OF ACTION

Miaclacin® is a synthetic polypeptide of 32 amino acids in the same linear sequence that is found in calcitonin of salmon origin. Calcimar® is a polypeptide hormone of animal origin (salmon). Calcitonin is the biologically active form. The actions of calcitonin and its role in normal human bone physiology are still not completely elucidated, although calcitonin receptors have been discovered in osteoblasts and osteoclasts. In-vitro studies have shown that calcitonin causes inhibition of osteoclast function with loss of the ruffled osteoclast border responsible for resorption of bone. Bone formation may be augmented further through increased osteoblastic activity

PHARMACOKINETICS

Nasal Bioavail: 3 - 50%; *Nasal Elim 1/2 Life:* 45 minutes; *Nasal Bone 1/2 Life:* unknown; *Parental Peak Effect:* 2 hours; *Parental 1/2 Life:* 1.5 hours; *Metab:* unknown; *Prot Bind:* unknown; *Excret:* Mainly renal

CALCIUM SUPPLEMENTS

INDICATIONS

Off-Label Uses: Postmenopausal osteoporosis; male osteoporosis; steroid-induced osteoporosis

DOSE & DRUG ADMINISTRATION

Only 500 mg of elemental calcium can be absorbed at a time, therefore, it must be given in divided doses; *Dose:* **Prepubertal children (age 4 - 8):** 800 mg of elemental calcium per day; **Adolescents (age 9 - 18):** 1300 mg of elemental calcium per day; **Women (age 19 - 50):** 1000 of elemental calcium per day (500 mg PO BID); **Women (age >50):** 1500 mg of elemental calcium per day (500 mg PO TID); **Men (age 19 - 50):** 1000 mg of elemental calcium per day; **Men (age >50):** 1500 mg of elemental calcium per day; *Maximum Dose:* 2500 mg of elemental calcium per day;

Supplied: **Calcium Carbonate:** Inexpensive and contains the most elemental calcium. Generally, calcium carbonate is taken with a meal since the amount of acid in the stomach increases, which will help with absorption; **Calcium Citrate:** It does not require acid to be easily absorbed. This product is recommended for patients who have low stomach acidity (such as the elderly or those taking acid blocking drugs); **Calcium Lactate & Gluconate:** Are also soluble but provide less elemental calcium per tablet.

DOSE ADJUSTMENT

Hepatic Failure: No dosage adjustment necessary
Renal Failure: No dosage adjustment necessary

CONTRAINDICATIONS & PRECAUTIONS

(a) Hypercalcemia

TOXICITY

Reversible: **(a) GI:** Dyspepsia, constipation; **(b) Renal:** Possible increase in nephrolithiasis (controversial, measure 24hr urinary calcium excretion)

PREGNANCY & LACTATION

Considered safe in Pregnancy & Lactation

DRUG INTERACTIONS

Drugs which may ↓ calcium absorption: Drugs which lower stomach acidity (i.e. proton pump inhibitors & H2 antagonists), lack of vitamin D; *Calcium may ↓ absorption of:* Tetracycline antibiotics (chelation)

MECHANISM OF ACTION

Elemental calcium

VITAMIN D: CALCIFEROL & CALCITRIOL (ROCALTROL)

INDICATIONS

Approved (Calcitriol): Management of hypocalcemia in patients on chronic renal dialysis; management of secondary hyperparathyroidism in moderate to severe chronic renal failure; management of hypocalcemia in hypoparathyroidism and pseudohypoparathyroidism. *Off-Label Uses:* Postmenopausal osteoporosis; male osteoporosis; steroid-induced osteoporosis

DOSE & DRUG ADMINISTRATION

Vitamin D for Osteoporosis prevention and treatment: 800 – 1000 IU PO OD (especially in winter months). *Calcitriol (Rocaltrol) for Osteoporosis prevention and treatment:* Initial dose of 0.25 µg PO OD increasing to 0.25 µg PO BID.

Supplied: Vitamin D supplements of 1000 IU, Calcitriol 0.25 µg & 0.5 µg capsules and 1.0 µg/mL solution.

DOSE ADJUSTMENT

Hepatic Failure: No dosage adjustment necessary.
Renal Failure: No dosage adjustment necessary

CONTRAINDICATIONS & PRECAUTIONS

(a) Hypercalcemia

TOXICITY

Symptoms of Hyper-Vitaminosis D Include: (a) GI: Nausea, vomiting, anorexia, constipation; *(b) MSK:* Osteoporosis; *(c) Soft-Tissue:* Widespread calcification; *(d) Renal Impairment:* Polyuria, polydipsia, hypercalciuria; *(e) Lytes:* Hypercalcemia

PREGNANCY & LACTATION

Pregnancy: RISK CANNOT BE RULED OUT. (CATEGORY C)
Lactation: Vitamin D is considered safe, calcitriol is not recommended.

DRUG INTERACTIONS

Thiazide diuretics: Concomitant administration may result in hypercalcemia

MECHANISM OF ACTION

Vitamin D is formed in the skin after exposure to ultraviolet radiation and is also absorbed from the gastrointestinal tract. It is hydroxylated in the liver to 25-hydroxyvitamin D and then in the kidney to 1,25 dihydroxyvitamin D which is the active form. Calcitriol is 1,25 dihydroxyvitamin D.

The major role of vitamin D is to maintain normal blood levels of calcium and phosphorous. It increases the intestinal absorption of calcium and phosphorous and also has a role in stimulating osteoclasts. Vitamin D may also be important in muscle strength.

CONJUGATED ESTROGEN (PREMARIN, CENESTIN, CES, CONGEST) ESTROGEN/PROGESTERONE (PREMPRO, ✦PREMPLUS) TRANSDERMAL ESTROGEN (ALORA, CLIMARA, ESCLIM, ESTRADERM, ✦EST RADOT, FEMPATCH, OESCLIM, VIVELLE, VIVELLE-DOT) ESTRADIOL (ESTRACE, ESTRADIOL, GYNODIOL) ESTROPIPATE (OGEN)

INDICATIONS

Approved: Prevention and/or treatment of osteoporosis in naturally occurring or surgically induced estrogen-deficiency states

DOSE & DRUG ADMINISTRATION

Dose: Treatment and/or Prevention of Osteoporosis: Conjugated Estrogen: 0.625 - 3 mg PO OD with progesterone if intact uterus; **Estrogen/Progesterone:** 0.45 - 0.625 mg of estrogen with 1.5 - 5 mg progesterone; **Estropipate:** 0.625 - 2.5

mg PD OD with progesterone if intact uterus; *Prevention of Osteoporosis:*
Transdermal Estrogen: 25 - 100 mcg/day; Estradiol: **0.5 mg/day;**
Supplied: ***CONJUGATED ESTROGEN (Premarin, Cenestin, CES, Congest):*** 0.3,
0.45, 0.625, 0.9, 1.25, 2.5 mg; ***ESTROGEN/PROGESTERONE (Prempro,***
Premplus): E/P 0.45/1.5, 0.625/2.5, 0.625/5 mg); ***TRANSDERMAL ESTROGEN:***
Alora: 50, 75, & 100 mcg/day patches 2X/wk; ***Climara:*** 25, 50, 75, & 100 mcg/day
patches qweek; ***Esclim:*** 25, 37.5, 50, 75, 100 mcg/day patches 2X/wk; ***Estraderm:***
50 & 100 mcg/day patches 2X/wk; ***Estradot:*** 25, 50, 75, & 100 mcg/day patches 2X/
wk; ***FemPatch:*** 25 mcg/day patches qweek; ***Oesclim:*** 25, 37.5, 50, 75, 100 mcg/
day patches 2X/wk; ***Vivelle:*** 25, 37.5, 50, 75, 100 mcg/day patches 2X/wk; ***Vivelle-***
Dot: 25, 37.5, 50, 75, & 100 mcg/day patches 2X/wk; ***ESTRADIOL: Estrace:*** 0.5,1,
& 2 mg tablets; ***Gynodiol:*** 1.5 mg tablets; ***ESTROPIPATE: Ogen:*** 0.625, 1.25, 2.5
mg tablets;
Progesterone Supplements: In women with an intact uterus, progesterone MUST
be administered with estrogen to reduce the risk of hyperplastic endometrial
changes. **Provera** (2.5 – 5 mg PO OD continuously)

DOSE ADJUSTMENT
Hepatic Failure: Use with caution as estrogens may be poorly metabolized.
Renal Failure: No dosage adjustment is necessary.

MONITORING
Baseline Osteoporosis Screening: CBC, creatinine, calcium, albumin, ALP, SPEP,
BMD; *Yearly:* Creatinine, calcium, albumin, ± BMD

CONTRAINDICATIONS & PRECAUTIONS
(a) Known hypersensitivity to estrogen; (b) Pregnancy; (c) Abnormal undiagnosed
vaginal bleeding; (d) Myocardial infarction, cerebrovascular accident,
thrombophlebitis & thrombophlebitic disorders; (e) Previous history of breast or
uterine cancer; (f) Family history (first degree relative) of breast cancer; (g) Gall
bladder disease

TOXICITY
Reversible: (a) CVS: Fluid retention; *(b) Gyne:* Uterine bleeding, increase in size of
fibroids, breast tenderness & enlargement, vaginal candidiasis; *(c) Mucocut:*
Cholasma or melasma that may persist once drug is discontinued, alopecia; *(d)*
CNS: Headache, migraine, dizziness, mental depression, chorea; *(e) Gen:* Weight
loss or gain, reduced carbohydrate tolerance, changes in libido; *(f) Ophtho:*
Steepening of corneal curvature, intolerance to contact lenses
Potentially Serious: (a) Endo: Massive increases in plasma triglycerides leading to
pancreatitis; *(b) CVS:* Venous thromboembolism, pulmonary embolism

PREGNANCY & LACTATION
Pregnancy: CONTRAINDICATED IN PREGNANCY. (CATEGORY X)
Lactation: Use is not recommended because estrogens may inhibit lactation.

DRUG INTERACTIONS
Estrogens may ✔ *efficacy of:* Warfarin, oral hypoglycemics, anti-hypertensives;
Drugs which may ✔ *toxicity of estrogen:* Barbiturates, hydantoins,
carbamazepine, meprobamate, phenylbutazone, rifampin (can affect liver enzymes)

MECHANISM OF ACTION
Estrogen undergoes extensive first-pass metabolism and circulate primarily as
estrone sulphate, with smaller amounts of other conjugated and unconjugated
estrogenic species.   The transdermal route delivers estradiol, the principal
intracellular human estrogen which is substantially more potent than estrone or estriol
at the receptor.

Estrogens act by regulating the transcription of a limited number of genes. They diffuse through the cell membrane and bind to and activate the nuclear estrogen receptor which is a DNA-binding protein. The activated estrogen receptor binds to specific DNA sequences, or hormone response elements, which enhance the transcription of adjacent genes. Estrogen receptors have been identified in tissues of the reproductive tract, breast, pituitary, hypothalamus, liver, and bone of women.

PHARMACOKINETICS
Bioavail: Absorbed well, slowly released over several hours; *Plasma 1/2 Life:* unknown; *Bone 1/2 Life:* unknown; *Metab:* Predominantly hepatic; *Prot Bind:* Bound to sex hormone binding globulin; *Excret:* unknown

ETIDRONATE (DIDRONEL, ✤DIDROCAL)

INDICATIONS
Approved: Paget's disease; hypercalcemia; Heterotopic ossification following hip replacement or spinal cord injury. ✤Treatment & prevention of postmenopausal osteoporosis; Prevention of steroid-induced osteoporosis

DOSE & DRUG ADMINISTRATION
Etidronate should only be swallowed on an empty stomach with a full glass of water 2 hours prior to or after a meal. Food may decrease the absorption of etidronate.

Dose: Treatment & Prevention of Osteoporosis: Cyclical therapy consisting of 400 mg etidronate for 14 days followed by 76 days of 500 mg elemental calcium supplements; *Prevention of Glucocorticoid-Induced Osteoporosis:* Cyclical therapy consisting of 400 mg etidronate for 14 days followed by 76 days of 500 mg elemental calcium supplements; *Treatment of Paget's Disease:* 5 - 10 mg/kg/day for 6 months **OR** 11 – 20 mg/kg/day for 3 months; *Heterotopic Ossification following Hip Arthroplasty:* 20 mg/kg/day for 4 months; *Heterotopic Ossification following Spinal Cord Injury:* 20 mg/kg/day for 2 weeks followed by 10 mg/kg/day for 10 weeks;

Supplied: Didronel: 200 & 400 mg etidronate tablets; ✤*Didrocal:* 90 day cyclical therapy blister pack with a 14 day supply of 400 mg etidronate tablets and 76 day supply of 500 mg elemental calcium tablets

DOSE ADJUSTMENT
Hepatic Failure: No dosage adjustment necessary.

Renal Failure: CrCl > 60: No dose adjustment; CrCl 35-60: No dose adjustment; CrCl < 35: Not Recommended

MONITORING
Baseline Osteoporosis Screening: CBC, creatinine, calcium, albumin, ALP, SPEP, BMD; *Intermittent:* BMD follow-up as indicated

CONTRAINDICATIONS & PRECAUTIONS
(a) Known hypersensitivity to etidronate; (b) Pregnancy; (c) Clinically overt osteomalacia; (d) Hypocalcemia; (e) Abnormalities of the esophagus which delay esophageal emptying such as achalasia; (f) Renal insufficiency

TOXICITY
Reversible: (a) GI: Abdominal pain, dyspepsia, nausea, esophagitis, esophageal erosions, esophageal ulcers; *(b) MSK:* Bone, muscle, and joint pain; *(c) Mucocut:* Rash (rare); *(d) Lab:* Mild, asymptomatic reduction in serum calcium and phosphate levels

Potentially Serious: (a) GI: Associated with complicated GI ulceration with perforation, obstruction, and bleeding; *(b) Hem:* Rare reports of agranulocytosis, pancytopenia, and one report of leukemia; *(c) MSK:* Osteonecrosis of the jaw

PREGNANCY & LACTATION
Pregnancy: RISK CANNOT BE RULED OUT (CATEGORY C)
Lactation: It is unknown if etidronate is excreted in breast milk and therefore is generally not recommended.

DRUG INTERACTIONS
Drugs which may ↓ levels of etidronate: Calcium, iron, & aluminum containing products interfere with absorption (vitamins, minerals, antacids, laxatives);
Etidronate may ↑ toxicity of: Warfarin (may prolong INR)

MECHANISM OF ACTION
Etidronate is chemically described as the disodium salt of 1-hydroxyethylidene bisphosphonic acid. Etidronate is the biologically active form. Etidronate is a bisphosphonate that binds to bone hydroxyapatite and specifically inhibits the activity of osteoclasts, the bone-resorbing cells. Etidronate slows the accelerated bone-turnover in pagetic bone. Etidronate chemiabsorbs to calcium hydroxyapatite crystals and their amorphous precursors, blocking the aggregation, growth, and mineralization of these crystals. This is thought to be the mechanism by which etidronate prevents or retards heterotopic ossification.

PHARMACOKINETICS
Bioavail: 3.5%; *Plasma 1/2 Life:* 1 - 6 hours; *Bone 1/2 Life:* > 90 days; *Metab:* Not metabolized; *Prot Bind:* 24%; *Excret:* Urine (absorbed) & faeces (not absorbed)

IBANDRONATE (BONIVA)

INDICATIONS
Approved: Treatment & prevention of postmenopausal osteoporosis; ✚ Not approved in Canada

DOSE & DRUG ADMINISTRATION
Drug Administration: Ibandronate should only be swallowed upon arising for the day with a full glass of water; Patients should not lie down for at least 30 minutes and until after their first food of the day to facilitate delivery to the stomach and to reduce the potential for esophageal irritation; To enhance absorption, patients should take ibandronate at least 60 minutes before the first food, beverage or medication of the day. *Dose:* 2.5 mg OD OR 150 mg qmonthly; *Supplied:* 2.5 & 150 mg tablets.

DOSE ADJUSTMENT
Hepatic Failure: No dosage adjustment necessary.
Renal Failure: CrCl > 30: No dose adjustment; CrCl < 30: Not Recommended

ONSET OF ACTION
Not Applicable

MONITORING
Baseline Osteoporosis Screening: CBC, Cr, Ca, albumin, ALP, SPEP, BMD
Intermittent: BMD follow-up as indicated

CONTRAINDICATIONS & PRECAUTIONS
(a) Known hypersensitivity to ibandronate; (b) Pregnancy; (c) Hypocalcemia; (d) Inability to stand or sit upright for 30 minutes; (e) Abnormalities of the esophagus which delay esophageal emptying such as achalasia; (f) Renal insufficiency

TOXICITY
Reversible: (a) GI: Abdominal pain, dyspepsia, nausea, esophagitis, esophageal erosions, esophageal ulcers; *(b) MSK:* Bone, muscle, and joint pain
Potentially Serious: (a) GI: Associated with complicated GI ulceration with perforation, obstruction, and bleeding; *(b) MSK:* Osteonecrosis of the jaw

PREGNANCY & LACTATION
***Pregnancy:* RISK CANNOT BE RULED OUT. (CATEGORY C)**
Lactation: It is unknown if ibandronate is excreted in human breast milk. It has not been studied in nursing mothers and therefore is not recommended during nursing.

DRUG INTERACTIONS
Drugs which may ↓ levels of ibandronate: Calcium, iron, & aluminum containing products interfere with absorption (vitamins, minerals, antacids, laxatives); ***Ibandronate may ↑ toxicity of:*** ASA and NSAIDs (ibandronate may be associated with an increase in upper gastrointestinal adverse events)

MECHANISM OF ACTION
Ibandronate is chemically described as (3-(N-methyl-N-pentyl) amino-1-hydroxypropane-1,1-diphosphonic acid, monosodium salt. Ibandronate is the biologically active form. Ibandronate is a bisphosphonate that binds to bone hydroxyapatite and specifically inhibits the activity of osteoclasts, the bone-resorbing cells. Ibandronate reduces bone resorption with no direct effect on bone formation, although the latter process is ultimately reduced because bone resorption and formation are coupled during bone turnover.

PHARMACOKINETICS
Bioavail: 0.6 % (very low secondary to poor absorption); ***Terminal 1/2 Life:*** 37-157 hours (150 mg); ***Metab:*** None; ***Prot Bind:*** High (80-99%); ***Excret:*** Urine 100%

PAMIDRONATE (AREDIA)

INDICATIONS
Approved: Paget's disease; hypercalcemia of malignancy; bone metastases; multiple myeloma. ***Off-label Uses:*** Osteoporosis, glucocorticoid-induced osteoporosis, Ankylosing Spondylitis.

DOSE & DRUG ADMINISTRATION
Dose: 30 - 90 mg IV given at a maximum rate of 15 mg/hour; ***Treatment of Osteoporosis:*** Possible regimen - 30 mg IV infused over a 2 hour period every 3 months; ***Treatment of Paget's Disease:*** 30 mg IV once a week for 6 weeks, OR 30 mg on the first week and 60 mg every 2 weeks for another 3 cycles, OR 60 mg every 2 weeks for 3 cycles;
Supplied: 30 & 90 mg powder for reconstitution.

DOSE ADJUSTMENT
Hepatic Failure: No dosage adjustment necessary.
Renal Failure: CrCl > 60: No dose adjustment; CrCl 35-60: No dose adjustment; CrCl < 35: Not Recommended

MONITORING
Baseline Osteoporosis Screening: CBC, creatinine, calcium, albumin, ALP, SPEP, BMD; ***During Treatment:*** Calcium, albumin; ***Intermittent:*** BMD as indicated

CONTRAINDICATIONS & PRECAUTIONS
(a) Known hypersensitivity to pamidronate; (b) Pregnancy; (c) Monitor closely in hypocalcemia; (d) Renal insufficiency; (e) Use with other bisphosphonates

TOXICITY
Reversible: *(a) Gen:* Mild fever, flu-like symptoms; (b) ***Local reactions:*** Thrombophlebitis, pain, swelling redness, induration; (c) ***Lytes:*** Asymptomatic mild hypocalcemia, hypophosphatemia, hypomagnesemia; (d) ***GI:*** Nausea, anorexia; (e) ***MSK:*** Bone, muscle, and joint pain; osteonecrosis of the jaw *(f) Hem:* Mild transient lymphopenia, anemia; *(g) CNS:* Headache
Potentially Serious: *(a) Lyte:* Hypocalcemia, hypophosphatemia, hypomagnesemia

PREGNANCY & LACTATION
Pregnancy: RISK CANNOT BE RULED OUT. (CATEGORY C)
Lactation: No clinical experience and unknown if pamidronate is excreted in breast
   milk; therefore, it is generally not recommended.

DRUG INTERACTIONS
No known drug interactions

MECHANISM OF ACTION
Pamidronate is chemically described as (4-amino-1-hydroxybutylidene)
bisphosphonic acid monosodium salt trihydrate. Pamidronate is the biologically
active form. Pamidronate is a bisphosphonate that binds to bone hydroxyapatite and
specifically inhibits the activity of osteoclasts, the bone-resorbing cells. Pamidronate
reduces bone resorption with no direct effect on bone formation, although the latter
process is ultimately reduced because bone resorption and formation are coupled
during bone turnover.

PHARMACOKINETICS
Bone 1/2 Life: 300 days; *Metab:* Not metabolized; *Prot Bind:* 54%; *Excret:* Urine

RALOXIFENE (EVISTA)

INDICATIONS
Approved: Treatment and prevention of osteoporosis in post-menopausal women;

DOSE & DRUG ADMINISTRATION
Dose: 60 mg PO OD
Supplied: 60 mg tablets

DOSE ADJUSTMENT
Hepatic Failure: Concentrations increase in mild hepatic dysfunction but not studied
   in more severe hepatic dysfunction.
Renal Failure: No dosage adjustment necessary.

MONITORING
Baseline Osteoporosis Screening: CBC, creatinine, calcium, albumin, ALP, SPEP,
BMD, monitor triglyceride levels if known to be previously elevated*; Intermittent:*
BMD follow-up as indicated

CONTRAINDICATIONS & PRECAUTIONS
(a) Active or past history of venous thromboembolic events such as deep vein
thrombosis, pulmonary embolism, and retinal vein thrombosis; (b) Known
hypersensitivity to raloxifene

TOXICITY
Reversible: Hot flashes, leg cramps, weight gain
Potentially Serious: Venous thromboembolic events

PREGNANCY & LACTATION
Pregnancy: CONTRAINDICATED IN PREGNANCY. (CATEGORY X)
Lactation: Contraindicated

DRUG INTERACTIONS
Drugs which may ↓ efficacy of raloxifene: Ampicillin and amoxicillin,
cholestyramine, colestipol; *Raloxifene may ↓ efficacy of:* Warfarin (reduces
prothrombin time)

MECHANISM OF ACTION
Raloxifene is a selective estrogen receptor modulator that belongs to the
benzothiophene class of compounds. Raloxifene undergoes extensive first pass
metabolism to glucuronide conjugates which are likely the biologically active forms.
Raloxifene is a selective estrogen receptor modulator (SERM) with the biological

actions largely mediated through binding to estrogen receptors. Raloxifene decreases resorption of bone and reduces biochemical markers of bone turnover to the premenopausal range. Raloxifene also reduces total and LDL cholesterol levels but does not increase triglyceride levels. Clinical trial data suggest raloxifene lacks estrogen-like effects on the uterus and breast tissue.

PHARMACOKINETICS
Bioavail: 2%; *Max Plasma Concn:* Variable; *1/2 Life:* 27 hours; *Metab:* Undergoes extensive first pass hepatic metabolism to glucuronide conjugates; *Prot Bind:* 95%; *Excret:* Primarily in the faeces; Negligible amounts unchanged in the urine

RISEDRONATE (ACTONEL)

INDICATIONS
Approved: Treatment & prevention of post-menopausal osteoporosis; treatment & prevention of steroid-induced osteoporosis; Paget's disease;

DOSE & DRUG ADMINISTRATION
Drug Administration: Risedronate should only be swallowed upon arising for the day with a full glass of water; Patients should not lie down for at least 30 minutes and until after their first food of the day to facilitate delivery to the stomach and to reduce the potential for esophageal irritation; To enhance absorption, patients should take risedronate at least 30 minutes (1-2 hours if possible) before the first food, beverage or medication of the day. (Since the mean bioavailability of risedronate is only 0.63% when administered in the fasting state, many rheumatologists suggest waiting up to 1-2 hours before the first food, beverage, or medication of the day); *Dose:*
Treatment of Osteoporosis: 5 mg PO OD OR 35 mg PO qweekly; *Prevention of Osteoporosis:* 5 mg PO OD OR 35 mg PO q weekly; *Prevention of Glucocorticoid-Induced Osteoporosis:* 5 mg PO OD ; *Treatment of Paget's disease:* 30 mg PO OD for 2 months. Re-treatment with same dose and duration; *Supplied:* 5, 30, & 35 mg tablets.

DOSE ADJUSTMENT
Hepatic Failure: No dosage adjustment necessary.
Renal Failure: CrCl > 60: No dose adjustment; CrCl 35-60: No dose adjustment; CrCl < 35: Not Recommended

MONITORING
Baseline Osteoporosis Screening: CBC, creatinine, calcium, albumin, ALP, SPEP, BMD *Intermittent:* BMD follow-up as indicated

CONTRAINDICATIONS & PRECAUTIONS
(a) Known hypersensitivity to risedronate; (b) Pregnancy; (c) Hypocalcemia; (d) Inability to stand or sit upright for 30 minutes; (e) Abnormalities of the esophagus which delay esophageal emptying such as achalasia; (f) Renal insufficiency

TOXICITY
Reversible: (a) GI: Abdominal pain, dyspepsia, nausea, esophagitis, esophageal erosions, esophageal ulcers; (b) *MSK:* Bone, muscle, and joint pain; (c) *Mucocut:* Rash (rare); *(d) Lab:* Mild, asymptomatic reduction in serum calcium and phosphate levels
Potentially Serious: (a) GI: Associated with complicated GI ulceration with perforation, obstruction, and bleeding; *(b) MSK:* Osteonecrosis of the jaw

PREGNANCY & LACTATION
Pregnancy: RISK CANNOT BE RULED OUT. (CATEGORY C)

Lactation: It is unknown if risedronate is excreted in breast milk; therefore, it is generally not recommended for nursing mothers.

DRUG INTERACTIONS
Drugs which may ↓ levels of risedronate: Calcium, iron, & aluminum containing products interfere with absorption (vitamins, minerals, antacids, laxatives)

MECHANISM OF ACTION
Risedronate is chemically described as a pyridinyl bisphosphonate. Risedronate is the biologically active form. Risedronate is a bisphosphonate that binds to bone hydroxyapatite and specifically inhibits the activity of osteoclasts, the bone-resorbing cells. Risedronate reduces bone resorption with no direct effect on bone formation, although the latter process is ultimately reduced because bone resorption and formation are coupled during bone turnover.

PHARMACOKINETICS
Bioavail: 0.6%; *Plasma 1/2 Life:* 1.5 hours; *Bone 1/2 Life:* 480 hours (time to dissociate from osteoclasts); *Metab:* Not metabolized; *Prot Bind:* 24%; *Excret:* Urine

TERIPARATIDE (FORTEO)

INDICATIONS
Approved: Treatment of post-menopausal women with osteoporosis who are at a high risk for fracture, treatment of men with primary or hypogonadal osteoporosis who are at a high risk for fracture

DOSE & DRUG ADMINISTRATION
Dose: 20 mcg sc injection once weekly;
Supplied: Supplied in a pre-filled 3 mL (teriparatide 250 mcg/mL) glass cartridge which is pre-assembled into a disposable pen device. Each pen device delivers 20 mcg of teriparatide per dose for up to 28 days.

DOSE ADJUSTMENT
Hepatic Failure: No studies have been performed, however, non-specific proteolytic enzymes in the liver cleave PTH(1-34) into fragments that are cleared from the circulation by the kidney.
Renal Failure: No change in pharmacokinetics with mild to moderate renal insufficiency (CrCl 30 - 72 ml/min). With severe renal insufficiency (CrCl <30 ml/min) the half-life of teriparatide was increased by ~ 75%.

MONITORING
Baseline Osteoporosis Screening: CBC, creatinine, calcium, albumin, ALP, SPEP, BMD. *Intermittent:* BMD follow-up as indicated

CONTRAINDICATIONS & PRECAUTIONS
(a) Known hypersensitivity to teriparatide; Paget's disease of bone; (c) Unexplained elevations of serum alkaline phosphatase (may indicate Paget's); (d) Pediatric populations or young adults with open epiphyses; (e) Patients who have received prior skeletal radiation therapy; (f) Patients with bone metastases or a prior history of bone malignancy; (g) Patients with metabolic bone diseases other than osteoporosis; (h) Hypercalcemia; (i) Active urolithiasis or preexisting hypercalciuria; (j) Orthostatic hypotension; (k) Current digoxin use (hypercalcemia may predispose to digitalis toxicity); (l) Limited information available about patients with hepatic, renal, or cardiac disease

TOXICITY
Reversible: *(a) GI:* Nausea; *(b) MSK:* Leg Cramps, arthralgia, weakness; *(c) CNS:* Dizziness, transient headaches, depression, vertigo; *(d) Mucocut:* Local injection site reactions, rash; *(e) Lab:* Transient increase in serum calcium to hypercalcemia (likely

dose dependant). If hypercalcemia does not occur within the first six months of treatment it rarely develops later on. Increase in uric acid levels; *(f) CVS:* Transient episodes of mild symptomatic orthostatic hypotension (within 4 hours of a dose), chest pain

Potentially Serious: (a) Malignancy: Teriparatide has caused osteosarcoma in rats, however, the clinical relevance of these findings is unknown. Primate models have not shown this effect and, in humans, hyperparathyroidism is not a risk factor for osteosarcoma.

PREGNANCY & LACTATION
Pregnancy: **RISK CANNOT BE RULED OUT. (CATEGORY C)**
Lactation: It is unknown if teriparatide is excreted in breast milk; therefore, it is generally not recommended for nursing mothers.

DRUG INTERACTIONS
Teriparatide may ↑ increase toxicity of: Digoxin (transient hypercalcemia may increase the risk of digitalis toxicity)

MECHANISM OF ACTION
Teriparatide (rDNA origin) injection is a recombinant human parathyroid hormone, which has an identical sequence to the 34 N-terminal amino acids (the biologically active region) of the 84-amino acid human parathyroid hormone. Teriparatide is the biologically active form. Parathyroid hormone is an important regulator of bone metabolism, renal tubular reabsorption of calcium and phosphate, and intestinal calcium absorption. Continuous exposure to elevated levels of endogenous parathyroid hormone (hyperparathyroidism) can be detrimental to the skeleton because of an imbalance between bone resorption and formation. However, when teriparatide is given only once daily, new bone formation is stimulated on both trabecular and cortical surfaces.

PHARMACOKINETICS
Bioavail: 95%; *Plasma 1/2 Life:* 1 hour with sc injection; *Metab:* No studies have been performed; *Excret:* No studies have been performed

ZOLEDRONIC ACID (ZOMETA)
INDICATIONS
Approved: Treatment of hypercalcemia of malignancy following adequate fluid rehydration. *Off Label Uses:* Treatment of osteoporosis

DOSE & DRUG ADMINISTRATION
Dose: Treatment of Hypercalcemia: 4 mg IV dose given over 15 minutes; *Treatment of Osteoporosis:* 4 mg IV single dose given once yearly or 2 mg IV single dose given twice yearly;
Supplied: 4 mg powder for reconstitution; 4 mg/5 mL solution

DOSE ADJUSTMENT
Hepatic Failure: No dosage adjustment necessary.
Renal Failure: CrCl > 60: No dose adjustment; CrCl 35-60: Use cautiously; CrCl < 35: Not Recommended

MONITORING
Baseline Osteoporosis Screening: CBC, creatinine, calcium, albumin, ALP, SPEP, BMD; *Intermittent:* BMD follow-up as indicated

CONTRAINDICATIONS & PRECAUTIONS
(a) Known hypersensitivity to zoledronic acid; (b) Pregnancy; (c) Hypocalcemia; (d) Renal insufficiency

TOXICITY

Reversible. *(a) CV3.* Leg edema (19%), *(b) CNS.* Fatigue, fever, headaches, insomnia, anxiety, dizziness, agitation, depression; *(c) GI:* Abdominal pain, nausea, vomiting, diarrhea, constipation; *(d) MSK:* Bone, muscle, and joint pain, paresthesias; *(e) Mucocut:* Alopecia, rash; *(f) Lab:* Mild, asymptomatic reduction in serum calcium and phosphate levels, hypokalemia, hypomagnesemia

Potentially Serious: (a) Hem: Granulocytopenia, pancytopenia, thrombocytopenia; *(b) MSK:* Osteonecrosis of the jaw

PREGNANCY & LACTATION

Pregnancy: POSITIVE EVIDENCE OF RISK. (CATEGORY D)

Lactation: It is unknown if zoledronic acid is excreted in breast milk; therefore, it is generally not recommended for nursing mothers.

DRUG INTERACTIONS

Drugs which may ↑ toxicity of zoledronic acid: Aminoglycosides (hypocalcemia); Loop diuretics (hypocalcemia); Thalidomide (worsen renal function)

MECHANISM OF ACTION

Zoledronic acid is an imidazole derivative which contains a second nitrogen atom in the ring structure. It is currently the most potent bisphosphonate. Zoledronic acid is a potent bisphosphonate that binds to bone hydroxyapatite and specifically inhibits the activity of osteoclasts, the bone-resorbing cells. Zoledronic acid reduces bone resorption with no direct effect on bone formation, although the latter process is ultimately reduced because bone resorption and formation are coupled during bone turnover. In addition, zoledronic acid exerts direct anti-tumor effects on cultured human myeloma and breast cancer cells, inhibiting their proliferation and inducing apoptosis.

PHARMACOKINETICS

Bioavail: 100%; *Terminal Plasma 1/2 Life:* 167 hours; *Metab:* Not metabolized; *Prot Bind:* Low 22%; *Excret:* Eliminated intact primarily via the kidney 97%, <3% found in the feces

PULMONARY HYPERTENSION
BOSENTAN (TRACLEER)

INDICATIONS
Approved: Pulmonary hypertension in patients with class III and IV symptoms to improve exercise capacity and reduce the rate of clinical deterioration

DOSE & DRUG ADMINISTRATION
Initial Dose: 62.5 mg PO BID x 4 weeks then increase to maintenance dose (Patients < 40 kg should remain on 62.5 mg PO BID). **Maintenance Dose:** 125 mg PO BID;
Supplied: 62.5 & 125 mg tablets.

DOSE ADJUSTMENT
Hepatic Failure: Use with extreme caution in patients with mild hepatic impairment provided the benefits can justify the risks. Contraindicated in moderate to severe hepatic impairment.
Renal Failure: No adjustment is necessary as less than 3% of administered dose is excreted in the urine.

ONSET OF ACTION
Initial Response: Studies have shown improvement in functional outcomes (6 minute walk test) at 12 weeks.

MONITORING
Baseline: CBC, creatinine, AST, ALT, ALP, albumin, & a negative pregnancy test in women; **Every month for the first 6 months:** CBC, AST, ALT, ALP, albumin; **Every 2-3 months thereafter:** CBC, AST, ALT, ALP, albumin

CONTRAINDICATIONS & PRECAUTIONS
(a) Known hypersensitivity to bosentan; (b) Moderate to severe hepatic impairment; (c) Baseline liver enzymes (AST, ALT) greater than 3 times the upper limit of normal; (d) Pregnancy; (e) Concurrent cyclosporine or glyburide use due to potential drug interactions

TOXICITY
Reversible: (a) Gen: Flushing, fatigue, pruritis; **(b) CNS:** Headache; **(c) CVS:** Palpitations, edema; **(d) GI:** Dyspepsia; **(e) Resp:** Nasopharyngitis
Potentially Serious: (a) Hepatic: Dose related increased in serum transaminases (11%) usually within the first 6 weeks, 97% normalize upon drug withdrawal (within 8 weeks); **(b) Hem:** Anemia - typically in the first 6 weeks of therapy.

PREGNANCY & LACTATION
Pregnancy: CONTRAINDICATED IN PREGNANCY (CATEGORY X): Based on animal models, may result in significant teratogenicity and should be discontinued prior to conception. Caution - may reduce the efficacy of OCP
Lactation: Unknown whether bosentan is excreted in breast milk.

DRUG INTERACTIONS
Use bosentan with caution with medications which induce CYP3A4 & CYP2C9 Drugs which may ↑ toxicity of bosentan: Cyclosporine (possibly tacrolimus); glyburide (increased hepatotoxicity); amiodarone, cimetidine, clarithromycin, erythromycin, fluoxetine, delavirdine, diltiazem, dirithromycin, disulfiram, fluoxetine, fluvoxamine, grapefruit juice, indinavir, itraconazole, ketoconazole, nefazodone, nevirapine, propoxyphene, quinupristin, dalfopristin, ritonavir, saquinavir, sulfonamides, verapamil, zafirlukast, zileuton; **Bosentan may ↑ metabolism and ↓ levels/efficacy of:** Anti-convulsants; anti-psychotics; corticosteroids; doxycycline; estrogens; oral contraceptives; methadone; warfarin, atorvastatin, simvastatin, & lovastatin.

MECHANISM OF ACTION

Bosentan is an endothelin receptor antagonist. After absorption, bosentan is metabolized in the liver to 3 metabolites. One of these metabolites is biologically active and may contribute up to 10-20% of the total clinical effect of the medication. Endothelin 1 is a potent endogenous vasoconstrictor and smooth muscle mitogen that is over-expressed in the plasma and lung tissue of patients with primary pulmonary hypertension and scleroderma. It is secreted by endothelial cells and acts by binding to the receptors ETA (vascular smooth muscle) & ETB (vascular smooth muscle, endothelial cells, fibroblasts). Endothelin-1 is thus capable of inducing vasoconstriction, fibrosis, hypertrophy, & hyperplasia. Bosentan is a low molecular weight oral endothelin-1 receptor antagonist which works by blocking both receptors (ETA & ETB). Bosentan improves symptoms (NYHA functional class) and the 6-minute walk time due to: Decreased pulmonary vascular resistance, Decrease in pulmonary arterial pressure, Decrease in pulmonary vascular hypertrophy and right ventricular hypertrophy, Decrease in pulmonary fibrosis and inflammation

PHARMACOKINETICS

Bioavail: 50%; **Max Plasma Concn:** 3 - 5 hours; **1/2 Life:** 5 hours; **Metab:** Hepatic via CYP3A4 & CYP2C9; **Prot Bind:** High (98%) **Excret:** Biliary excretion following hepatic metabolism

EPOPROSTENOL (Flolan)

INDICATIONS

Approved: For the long-term treatment of primary pulmonary hypertension (PPH) and secondary pulmonary hypertension due \o scleroderma spectrum of diseases (SSD) in NYHA functional class III and IV patients who did not respond adequately to conventional therapy.

DOSE & DRUG ADMINISTRATION

Initial Dose: < 2 ng/kg/min as initial infusion rate; **Dose Increments:** Dose should be escalated slowly trying to ameliorate symptoms and have the fewest side effects possible. Patients are initially hospitalized for a few days and doses are increased to 4-6 ng/kg/min (if tolerable). Dose increases are very individual but generally range from 1-2 ng/kg/min a week. In most centers, once symptoms are under control, dose increments are reduced to every 2 weeks and then to every month. When a dose is reached which achieves a balance of symptomatic improvement and minimal side-effects dose increments are generally stopped. *Ann Int Med 2000;132(6):425-435* had average dose increments as follows (ng/kg/min): baseline (2.2), week 3 (5.4), week 6 (7.4), week 9 (9.5), week 12 (11.2). **Maintenance Dose:** Individualized maintenance doses vary from 20 - 60 ng/kg/min;
Supplied: Vials of 0.5 mg epoprostenol powder & 50 mL sterile diluent

DOSE ADJUSTMENT

Hepatic Failure: None.
Renal Failure: None

ONSET OF ACTION

Initial Response: Studies have shown improvement in survival in NYHA functional class III and IV PPH patients treated for 12 weeks.

MONITORING

Patients require very close follow-up titrating the dose of epoprostenol to maximize the benefits while monitoring for adverse events.

CONTRAINDICATIONS & PRECAUTIONS

(a) Known hypersensitivity to epoprostenol; (b) Congestive heart failure due to severe left ventricular systolic dysfunction

TOXICITY
Reversible: (a) Gen: Flushing, dizziness, administration site pain; *(b) CNS:* Headache, anxiety, hyperesthesia, paresthesia; *(c) CVS:* Hypotension, chest pain, bradycardia, tachycardia; *(d) GI:* Nausea, vomiting, abdominal pain; *(e) Resp:* Dyspnea; *(f) MSK:* Jaw pain, back pain, myalgias, non-specific pain;
Potentially Serious: (a) Infection: Epoprostenol requires an indwelling central venous catheter which may be a portal of entry for infection with symptoms of chills, fever, and sepsis; *(b) Withdrawal:* Abrupt withdrawal or sudden large reductions in dosage may result in symptoms associated with rebound pulmonary hypertension, including dyspnea, dizziness, asthenia, and rarely death; *(c) Hem:* Thrombocytopenia; *(d) Pulmonary edema*

PREGNANCY & LACTATION
Pregnancy: NO EVIDENCE OF RISK IN HUMANS. (CATEGORY B)
Lactation: Unknown whether epoprostenol is excreted in breast milk.

DRUG INTERACTIONS
Drugs which may ↑ toxicity of epoprostenol: Anti-hypertensives (may exacerbate hypotension), anti-platelet agents (bleeding); *Epoprostenol may ↑ toxicity of:* Anti-platelet agents (bleeding), warfarin (bleeding); *Epoprostenol may ↑ levels of:* Digoxin, furosemide.

MECHANISM OF ACTION
Epoprostenol is a naturally occurring metabolite of arachidonic acid also known as prostacyclin (PGI2). Epoprostenol has 2 primary mechanisms of action: Direct vasodilation of pulmonary and systemic arterial vascular beds & Inhibition of platelet aggregation via activation of intracellular adenylate cyclase with the resulting increase in cyclic adenosine monophosphate concentration within the platelets.

PHARMACOKINETICS
Bioavail: 100%; *Steady State Plasma Concn:* 15 minutes; *1/2 Life:* 2.7 minutes; *Metab:* Rapidly hydrolyzed at neutral blood pH and subject to enzymatic degradation; *Prot Bind:* None *Excret:* Metabolites in the urine (82%) and faeces (4%)

TREPROSTINIL (REMODULIN)

INDICATIONS
Approved: A continuous subcutaneous infusion for the treatment of pulmonary arterial hypertension in patients with NYHA class II-IV symptoms to diminish symptoms associated with exercise.

DOSE & DRUG ADMINISTRATION
Initial Dose: 1.25 ng/kg/min initial infusion rate, if not tolerated, reduce to 0.625 ng/kg/min. *Dose Increments:* Dose should be escalated slowly trying to ameliorate symptoms and have the fewest side effects possible. Dose increases are very individual, with increases of no more than 1.25 ng/kg/min per week for the first 4 weeks then no more than 2.5 ng/kg/min per week for the remaining duration of infusion. When a dose is reached which achieves a balance of symptomatic improvement and minimal side-effects dose increments are generally stopped. *Maintenance Dose:* Most infusion rates are < 40 ng/kg/min. *Infusion Rate (mL/hr)* = Dose (ng/kg/min) x Weight (kg) x [0.00006/Remodulin dosage strength concentration (mg/mL)];
Supplied: 20 mL Vials of 1, 2.5, 5, & 10 mg/mL

DOSE ADJUSTMENT

Hepatic Failure: Use with caution, maximum initial dose 0.625 ng/kg/min in mild to moderate hepatic impairment. No data on use in severe hepatic impairment.
Renal Failure: No specific dosage adjustment is recommended

ONSET OF ACTION

Initial Response: Studies have shown improvement in 6 minute walk testing (p=ns) and the Borg dyspnea scale at 12 weeks (p<0.05).

MONITORING

Patients require very close follow-up titrating the dose of treprostinil to maximize the benefits while monitoring for adverse events.

CONTRAINDICATIONS & PRECAUTIONS

(a) Known hypersensitivity to treprostinil; (b) Hepatic dysfunction

TOXICITY

Reversible: (a) Gen: Flushing, dizziness; *(b) CNS:* Headache; *(c) CVS:* Hypotension, edema; *(d) GI:* Nausea, diarrhea; *(e) Respiratory:* Dyspnea; *(f) MSK:* Jaw pain; *(g) Mucocut:* Rash, pruritis; *(h) Local infusion site pain and reaction:* Can be mild to severe and lead to discontinuation of the medication. May improve with time and with less frequent rotation of the infusion site (q3days vs q1day).
Potentially Serious: (a) Infection: Treprostinil is given by continuous subcutaneous infusion and thus requires an indwelling subcutaneous catheter which may be a portal of entry for infection; *(b) Withdrawal:* Abrupt withdrawal or sudden large reductions in dosage may result in symptoms associated with rebound pulmonary hypertension, including dyspnea and dizziness.

PREGNANCY & LACTATION

Pregnancy: NO EVIDENCE OF RISK IN HUMANS. (CATEGORY B)
Lactation: Unknown whether treprostinil is excreted in breast milk.

DRUG INTERACTIONS

Drugs which may ↑ toxicity of treprostinil: Anti hypertensives (may exacerbate hypotension), anti-platelet agents (bleeding); *Treprostinil may ↑ toxicity of:* Anti-platelet agents (bleeding), warfarin (bleeding)

MECHANISM OF ACTION

Treprostinil is a synthetic, stable form of prostacyclin. Treprostinil has 2 primary mechanisms of action: Direct vasodilation of pulmonary and systemic arterial vascular beds & inhibition of platelet aggregation via activation of intracellular adenylate cyclase with the resulting increase in cyclic adenosine monophosphate concentration within the platelets.

PHARMACOKINETICS

Bioavail: 100%; *Steady State Plasma Concn:* 10 hours; *1/2 Life:* 2-4 hours; *Metab:* Hepatic; *Prot Bind:* 91%; *Excret:* Metabolites in the urine (64%) and faeces (13%)

SALIVARY STIMULANTS

CEVIMELINE (EVOXAC)

INDICATIONS
Approved: Treatment of xerostomia (dry mouth) from salivary gland hypofunction in primary and secondary Sjögren's syndrome. Not Approved in Canada

DOSE & DRUG ADMINISTRATION
Dose: 30 mg PO TID (can start with 30 mg qhs); ***Maximum Dose:*** 90 mg/day; ***Supplied:*** 30 mg capsules

DOSE ADJUSTMENT
Hepatic Failure: Unknown
Renal Failure: Unknown

ONSET OF ACTION
Initial Response: 1 - 2 hours

MONITORING
Baseline: Nothing specifically recommended; ***Yearly:*** Nothing specifically recommended

CONTRAINDICATIONS & PRECAUTIONS
(a) Known hypersensitivity to cevimeline; (b) Significant cardiovascular disease; (c) Severe reactive airway disease; (d) Controlled asthma, chronic bronchitis, COPD; (e) Known or suspected cholelithiasis or biliary tract disease; (f) Narrow angle glaucoma; (g) Acute iritis

TOXICITY
Reversible: (a) Gen: Chills, flushing, hot flashes, rhinitis; ***(b) CNS:*** Headache, dizziness, asthenia; ***(d) Exocrine Gland:*** Sweating, hypersalivation, hyperlacrimation, salivary gland enlargement; ***(e) GU:*** Increased urinary frequency; ***(f) GI:*** Nausea, vomiting, diarrhea, biliary spasm
Potentially Serious: (a) Ophtho: Blurring of vision; ***(b) Resp:*** Increase airway resistance (bronchospasm); ***(c) CVS:*** AV block, bradycardia, tachycardia, hypotension, hypertension, arrhythmias; ***(d) CNS:*** Mental confusion, tremor

PREGNANCY & LACTATION
Pregnancy: RISK CANNOT BE RULED OUT. (CATEGORY C)
Lactation: Not known whether cevimeline is excreted in breast milk. Therefore, lactation is not recommended

DRUG INTERACTIONS
Cevimeline may ↓ efficacy of: Anticholinergic medications (TCAs, phenothiazines, atropine). ***Drugs which may ↑ toxicity of cevimeline:*** Drugs which inhibit CYP2D6 (amiodarone, fluoxetine, paroxetine, quinidine, ritonavir) and inhibit CYP3A4 (diltiazem, erythromycin, ketoconazole, itraconazole, verapamil); There is a possibility of conduction disturbances when given with beta adrenergic agonists

MECHANISM OF ACTION
Cevimeline is the active form of the medication. Cevimeline is a cholinergic parasympathomimetic agent exerting a broad spectrum of pharmacologic effects with predominant muscarinic action. Cevimeline, in appropriate dosage, can increase secretion by the exocrine glands.

PHARMACOKINETICS
Bioavail: Unknown; ***Max Plasma Concn:*** 1.5 - 2 hours; ***1/2 Life:*** 5 hours; ***Metab:*** Hepatic via CYP2D6 and CYP3A4; ***Prot Bind:*** < 20%; ***Excret:*** Urine as metabolites and unchanged drug

PILOCARPINE (SALAGEN)

INDICATIONS
Approved: Treatment of xerostomia (dry mouth) and xerophthalmia (dry eyes) from salivary gland hypofunction in primary and secondary Sjögren's syndrome

DOSE & DRUG ADMINISTRATION
Dose: 5 mg PO TID (can start with 5mg qhs); *Maximum Dose:* 30 mg/day;
Supplied: 5mg tablets

DOSE ADJUSTMENT
Hepatic Failure: Do not use in patients with severe hepatic impairment. Maximum dose of 5 mg BID in mild to moderate hepatic failure.
Renal Failure: Unknown

ONSET OF ACTION
Initial Response: 1 - 2 hours

MONITORING
Baseline: Nothing specifically recommended; *Yearly:* Nothing specifically recommended

CONTRAINDICATIONS & PRECAUTIONS
(a) Known hypersensitivity to pilocarpine; (b) Significant cardiovascular disease; (c) Severe reactive airway disease; (d) Controlled asthma, chronic bronchitis, COPD; (e) Known or suspected cholelithiasis or biliary tract disease; (f) Narrow angle glaucoma; (g) Acute iritis

TOXICITY
Reversible: (a) Gen: Chills, flushing, hot flashes; *(b) CNS:* Headache, dizziness, asthenia; *(c) Exocrine Gland:* Sweating, hypersalivation, hyperlacrimation; *(d) GU:* Increased urinary frequency; *(e) GI:* Nausea, vomiting, diarrhea
Potentially Serious: (a) Ocular: Blurring of vision; *(b) Resp:* Increase airway resistance; *(c) CVS:* AV block, bradycardia, tachycardia, hypotension, hypertension, arrhythmias; *(d) CNS:* Mental confusion, tremor

PREGNANCY & LACTATION
Pregnancy: RISK CANNOT BE RULED OUT. (CATEGORY C)
Lactation: Not known whether this drug is excreted in breast milk. Therefore, lactation is a relative contraindication unless the potential benefit of the medication justifies the potential risks to the baby.

DRUG INTERACTIONS
Pilocarpine may ↓ efficacy of: ACE-inhibitors & angiotensin receptor blockers, anticholinergic medications (antagonize effects); There is a possibility of conduction disturbances when given with beta adrenergic agonists

MECHANISM OF ACTION
Pilocarpine is the active form of the medication. Pilocarpine is a cholinergic parasympathomimetic agent exerting a broad spectrum of pharmacologic effects with predominant muscarinic action. Pilocarpine, in appropriate dosage, can increase secretion by the exocrine glands.

PHARMACOKINETICS
Bioavail: Unknown; *Max Plasma Concn:* 0.85 - 1.25 hours; *1/2 Life:* 0.76 - 1.35 hours; *Metab:* Unknown – thought to occur at neuronal synapses; *Prot Bind:* Unknown; *Excret:* Urine

VISCOSUPPLEMENTATION
HYLAN G-F 20 (Synvisc) & SODIUM HYALURONATE
(♣Neovisc, ♣Orthovisc, Hyalgan, Supartz, Durolane)

INDICATIONS
Synvisc®, Neovisc®, Orthovisc®, Hyalgan®, & Durolane® are indicated for the treatment of osteoarthritis (OA) of the knee in patients who have failed to respond adequately to conservative nonpharmacologic therapy and simple analgesics, e.g. acetaminophen.

DOSE & DRUG ADMINISTRATION
Dose: Administered by intra-articular injection of 16 mg (2 mL) hylan G-F 20 (Synvisc®), 16mg (2mL) Neovisc®, 30 mg (2 mL) Orthovisc®, or 20 mg (2mL) Hyalgan® once weekly for a total of three weeks. May repeat series of injections if inadequate response. Durolane® is given as a single injection of 60 mg (3 mL) of Non-Animal Stabilized Hyaluronic Acid (NASHA). *Max Dose:* Unknown;
Supplied: Synvisc: 2 mL glass syringes containing **8 mg/mL** of hylan G-F 20;
Hyalgan: 2 mL glass syringes containing **10 mg/mL** of sodium hyaluronate;
Supartz: 2.5 mL glass syringes containing **10 mg/mL** of sodium hyaluronate;
Durolane: 3 mL glass syringe containing 20 mg/mL of Non-Animal Stabilized Hyaluronic Acid (NASHA); ♣*Neovisc:* 2 mL glass syringes containing **8 mg/mL** of sodium hyaluronate; ♣*Orthovisc:* 2 mL glass syringes containing **15 mg/mL** of sodium hyaluronate;

DOSE ADJUSTMENT
Hepatic Failure: No dosage adjustment necessary
Renal Failure: No dosage adjustment necessary

ONSET OF ACTION
Initial Response: Variable

MONITORING
Nothing specifically recommended

CONTRAINDICATIONS & PRECAUTIONS
(a) Acute septic arthritis or overlying cellulitis; (b) Known hypersensitivity to hylan G-F 20 or hyaluronic acid; (c) Do not use disinfectants containing quaternary ammonium salts as they can precipitate; (d) Evidence of lymphatic or venous stasis in the leg; (e) Poultry allergy (all except Neovisc® & Durolane®)

TOXICITY
Reversible: (a) Local Reactions: Pain, swelling, and/or effusion in the injected knee. Reactions generally abate within a few days (~ 1 – 4% risk with injection); *(b) Gen:* Rash, hives, pruritis, fever, chills, malaise; *(c) MSK:* Muscle cramps, paresthesias, peripheral edema
Potentially Serious: (a) MSK: Septic arthritis

PREGNANCY & LACTATION
Pregnancy: The safety and effectiveness has not been established.
Lactation: The safety and effectiveness has not been established.

DRUG INTERACTIONS
None known

MECHANISM OF ACTION
The active ingredient in these devices is hyaluronic acid. The main source of hyaluronic acid is rooster combs, which contain the polymer at a higher concentration compared to other animal tissues. Neovisc is a biologically cultured product;

therefore, it can be used in patients with poultry allergies. Hylan G-F 20 (Synvisc) is a cross-linked polymer of hyaluronan (sodium hyaluronate), resulting in a higher molecular weight than the other available products. Durolane is a Non-Animal Stabilized Hyaluronic Acid designed to improve the half-life of the product within the articular space.

Pathologic changes in the synovium in osteoarthritic joints include disruption of hyaluronans. A lower concentration of these molecules is found, as well as a reduction in molecular weight as a result of both physical and chemical stresses.

The exact mechanism of viscosupplementation is unclear; current theories include: (a) Restoration of the elastoviscous properties of synovial fluid seems to be the most logical explanation, although, other mechanisms must exist due to the limited half life of exogenous hyaluronan within the synovial fluid; (b) Possible anti-inflammatory and anti-nociceptive properties; (c) Stimulation of de novo hyaluronic acid synthesis by the exogenously injected hyaluronic acid; (d) The actual period that the injected hyaluronic acid product stays within the joint space is on the order of hours to days, but the time of clinical efficacy is often on the order of months.

PHARMACOKINETICS

Not known

STRUCTURE OF ARTICULAR CARTILAGE

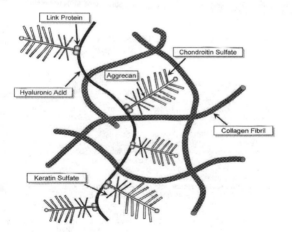

THE RHEUMATOLOGY LABORATORY

ANTI-DOUBLE STRANDED DNA (ANTI-dsDNA)

Antibodies directed against double-stranded DNA occur in approximately 60-83% of patients with SLE; when present in high titers they are highly specific (>90%) for SLE. In some SLE patients, the titer of anti-dsDNA may give an indication of disease activity. Anti-dsDNA may be detected using ELISA, indirect immunofluorescence (Crithidia luciliae) or radioimmunoassay (Farr assay) techniques. Antibodies to single-strand DNA are not specific for SLE and their measurement is generally not useful clinically.

ANTI-NEUTROPHIL CYTOPLASMIC ANTIBODIES (ANCA)

Antibodies directed against components of granules present in the cytoplasm of neutrophils occur frequently in certain vasculitides. Screening for ANCA is typically performed using an indirect immunofluorescence technique. Three patterns of immunofluorescence are recognized: cytoplasmic (cANCA), perinuclear (pANCA), and atypical perinuclear (xANCA). The cANCA pattern is usually associated with anti-proteinase 3 (PR3) antibodies and the pANCA pattern with anti-myeloperoxidase (MPO) antibodies. The xANCA pattern is most commonly associated with ulcerative colitis. If an immunofluorescent pattern is identified then additional testing for anti-MPO and/or anti-PR3 is performed using an ELISA technique.

Wegener's Granulomatosis: cANCA (PR3): 75-80%; pANCA (MPO):10-15%; Negative: 5-10%

Microscopic Polyangiitis: cANCA (PR3): 25-35%; pANCA (MPO):50-60%; Negative: 5-10%

Churg-Strauss Syndrome: cANCA (PR3): 1-5%; pANCA (MPO):70%; Negative: 20-30%

ANTI-NUCLEAR ANTIBODIES (ANA)

Antibodies directed against nuclear antigens occur frequently in various autoimmune diseases. Screening for ANA is performed using an indirect immunofluorescent technique typically using hep-2 cells as the substrate. A number of different patterns of immunofluorescence are recognized. If a significant immunofluorescent pattern is identified additional information may be obtained by testing for anti-dsDNA & ENAs

Conditions Associated with a Positive ANA: Rheumatic Diseases: (a) Drug-Induced Lupus (DILE) - 100%; (b) Chronic Active Hepatitis - 100%; (c) Systemic Lupus Erythematosus - 99%; (d) Systemic Sclerosis - 95%; (e) Mixed Connective Tissue Disease - 95-99%; (f) Polymyositis/Dermatomyositis - 90%; (g) Sjogren's Syndrome - 80%; (h) Rheumatoid Arthritis - 60%; *Non-Rheumatic Diseases:* (a) Thyroid; (b) Primary biliary cirrhosis; (c) Primary sclerosing cholangitis; (d) Viral hepatitis; (e) Primary pulmonary hypertension; (f) HIV; (g) Lymphoma; (h) Tuberculosis; (i) Myasthenia Gravis - 50%; *Normal:* 5-30%

Non-specific Disease Associations with ANA Patterns: (a) Homogenous Pattern - SLE, DILE, PM-SSc-SLE Overlap; (b) Speckled Pattern - SLE, SSc, SCLE; (c) Rim Pattern - SLE; (d) Nucleolar Pattern - SSc, PM-SSc overlap; (e) Centromere Pattern - SSc; (f) Cytoplasmic Pattern - SLE, PM/DM; **SCLE** = Subacute Cutaneous Lupus Erythematosus, **DILE** = Drug Induced Lupus Erythematosus, **NLE** = Neonatal Lupus Erythematosus, **SLE** = Systemic Lupus Erythematosus, **MCTD** = Mixed Connective Tissue Disease, **SSc** = Systemic Sclerosis, **PM** = Polymyositis, **DM** = Dermatomyositis

ANTI-PHOSPHOLIPID ANTIBODIES (APLA)

Antibodies directed against various phospholipids and phospholipid binding proteins occur in a variety of clinical settings. Antiphospholipid antibody syndrome is the association of certain clinical features (thrombosis, pregnancy morbidity) and the presence of antiphospholipid antibodies in serum. The two best characterized groups of APA are anticardiolipin antibodies and the lupus anticoagulant.

Associations with Increased Anti-Phospholipid Antibody Production: (a) Medications; (b) Autoimmune (SLE); (c) Infectious Disease (HIV); (d) Neoplastic Disease

ANTI-CARDIOLIPIN ANTIBODIES (aCL)

Antibodies directed against cardiolipin (a phospholipid) occur in the anti-phospholipid syndrome (APS), various infections, and autoimmune diseases. In APS the aCL are directed against the phospholipid binding protein beta-2 glycoprotein-I. Anti-cardiolipin antibodies occur in 80 to 90% of APS. They may be detected by the ELISA technique. Moderate to high titers of aCL are associated with thrombophilia with IgG more closely correlated than IgM.

ANTI-CYCLIC CITRULLINATED PEPTIDE (anti-CCP)

Filaggrin is a protein found in the epidermal matrix. Studies have found antibodies in rheumatoid arthritis (RA) which bind to filaggrin that has undergone post-translational modification by converting the amino acid arginine to citrulline. The present understanding is citrullinated peptides on filaggrin and possibly other proteins are recognized by antibodies in the serum of patients with RA. It is speculated that the target antigen in RA is actually citrullinated fibrin.

In early RA, symptoms may be milder and non-specific causing uncertainty about the diagnosis. Therefore, the detection of a disease specific antibody (like anti-CCP) could be of great diagnostic and therapeutic value. ELISA assays for anti-CCP are currently available and yield a diagnostic sensitivity of up to 80% and a specificity of 95-98%.

LUPUS ANTICOAGULANT (LA)

Lupus anticoagulants (LA) are antibodies directed against plasma proteins (usually prothrombin, occasionally beta-2 glycoprotein-I) bound to phospholipid. LA occur in the anti-phospholipid antibody syndrome, various infections, and autoimmune diseases. LA prolong phospholipid dependant clotting assays by interfering with initiation of clotting by the phospholipid. Lupus anticoagulant is actually a misnomer since LA usually have a pro-thrombotic effect in vivo; only in rare cases where there are specific antibodies directed against clotting factor II is there a possible bleeding diathesis. In unselected patients, LA are implicated as a cause in approximately 5-20% of recurrent fetal loss and 5-10% of recurrent thromboses. LA may be detected by various phospholipid dependent clotting tests (aPTT, DRVVT, KCT). No single test identifies all LA and therefore several tests and testing algorithms are used to establish the presence of LA.

Requirements for a Lupus Anticoagulant: (a) Prolongation of a phospholipid-dependent coagulation assay – aPTT; (b) Prolongation is due to inhibitor not a factor deficiency: No reversal on 1:1 mix of patient's plasma with normal platelet-free plasma; (c) Inhibitor is phospholipid dependent: Prolongation reversed or corrected by addition of excess phospholipid; (d) Prolongation is not due to inhibition of only one clotting factor

EXTRACTABLE NUCLEAR ANTIGEN ANTIBODIES (ENA)

Antibodies directed against particular nuclear antigens occur in various autoimmune diseases. The specificity of the antibodies helps identify the particular autoimmune disease. ENA in serum may be detected by the ELISA technique; commonly a panel of six antigens are used to identify the most common antibodies.

Disease Associations with ENA: (a) Anti-Ro/Anti-SSa: SS, SCLE, NLE, SLE; (b) Anti-La/anti-SSb: SS, SCLE, NLE, SLE; (c) Anti-Sm: SLE; (d) Anti-RNP: MCTD, SLE; (e) Anti-Scl 70: SSc; (f) Anti-Jo1: PM/DM; **SS** = Sjogren's Syndrome, **SCLE** = Subacute Cutaneous Lupus Erythematosus, **NLE** = Neonatal Lupus Erythematosus, **SLE** = Systemic Lupus Erythematosus, **MCTD** = Mixed Connective Tissue Disease, **SSc** = Systemic Sclerosis, **PM** = Polymyositis, **DM** = Dermatomyositis

ERYTHROCYTE SEDIMENTATION RATE (ESR)

The erythrocyte sedimentation rate (ESR) was first employed as a marker of pregnancy. Today it is used as a non-specific marker of inflammation. A 200 mm x 2.5 mm diameter vertically aligned anticoagulated tube of blood is left to stand for 1 hour. The distance the column of blood falls in one hour is the erythrocyte sedimentation rate.

Normal ESR (Rule of Thumb): (a) Men: Age/2; (b) Women: (Age+10)/2

Factors which may increase the ESR: (a) Inflammatory disease; (b) Hypoalbuminemia; (c) Hypergammaglobulinemia; (d) Tissue necrosis (MI, trauma); (e) Pregnancy; (f) Anemia; (g) Age; (h) Heparinized blood

Factors which may decrease the ESR: (a) Increased plasma viscosity; (b) Increased number of RBC; (c) Change in shape of RBC; (d) Decreased plasma proteins

C-REACTIVE PROTEIN (CRP)

C-reactive protein (CRP), a member of the pentraxin family of proteins, is a non-specific opsonin for bacteria named for its ability to precipitate the C-substance polysaccharide of streptococci. It is an acute phase reactant produced by the liver under the influence of IL-1 & IL-6. CRP is a very useful marker of acute inflammation since it increases within 6 hours of the onset of an inflammatory stimulus, peaks very quickly (<50 hrs), and falls rapidly once the inflammatory stimulus is removed (T1/2 = 8 hrs). It provides an immediate picture of inflammation. Since it is made in the liver, hepatocellular impairment interferes with a normal CRP response

Conditions Associated with Major CRP Elevation: (a) Infections; (b) *Hypersensitivity complications of infection:* Rheumatic fever, Erythema nodosum, Leprosum; *(c) Inflammatory Diseases:* Rheumatoid arthritis, Juvenile chronic arthritis, Ankylosing spondylitis, Psoriatic arthritis, Systemic vasculitis, Polymyalgia rheumatica, Reactive arthritis, Crohn's disease, Familial Mediterranean fever; *(d) Malignancy:* Lymphoma & Sarcoma; *(e) Necrosis:* Myocardial infarction, Tumor embolization, Acute pancreatitis; *(f) Trauma:* Burns & Fractures

Conditions Associated with Minor CRP Elevation: (a) Systemic Lupus Erythematosus; (b) Systemic Sclerosis; (c) Dermatomyositis; (d) Ulcerative Colitis; (e) Leukemia; (f) Graft Versus Host Disease

COMPLEMENT: THE SYSTEM

The complement system is a group of over 20 biologically active proteins and inhibitors produced in the liver. It was named for its ability to "complement" antibody in the killing of bacteria. It serves an important role in host defence; however, uncontrolled activation causes tissue injury in many autoimmune diseases. The complement system can be activated in one of two ways: *(see diagram)*

Classic Pathway: Initiated by an antigen-antibody complex; C1 is a large calcium dependant complex composed of C1q and the tetramer C1s-C1r-C1r-C1s; C1q (part of C1 complex) binds to the Fc portion of antibody; C1r cleaves itself from the complex and in turn cleaves C1s; C1s then cleaves C4 & C2; Cleaved components of C4 & C2 (C4b & C2a) come together to form C3-convertase (C4b2a); C3-convertase rapidly generates many activated C3 molecules (C3b); C3b then does the following: C3b deposits on targets and serves as an opsonin; C3b also binds to the C4b2a complex to form C5-convertase known as C5-convertase; C5-convertase generates active forms of C5 (C5b); Generation of C5b leads to the formation of the MAC (C5b+C6+C7+C8+multiple C9) – MAC ultimately forms a pore in the cell membrane which, through calcium flux and cellular activation, can result in cell lysis.

Alternate Pathway: A small amount of auto-activated C3 (C3b) is always present in the system; C3b attaches to foreign particles and then binds factor B; Factor B is cleaved by factor D to produce the fragments Ba & Bb; C3b binds to Bb to form the alternative pathway C3-convertase – C3bBb; This C3-convertase produces more C3b which: Deposits on targets and serves as an opsonin; Can activate MAC by the alternative pathway C5-convertase C3bBbC3b

Complement Components and their Functions: (a) C3a: Anaphylatoxin: vasodilatation & chemotaxis; (b) C3b: Opsonization & initiation of alternative pathway; (c) C4a: Mediates inflammation; (d) C5a: Anaphylatoxin: vasodilatation & chemotaxis; (e) C5b: Initiates assembly of Membrane Attack Complex (MAC); (f) C6,C7,C8,C9: Form the MAC with C5

COMPLEMENT: ROLE IN AUTOIMMUNE DISEASE

Hypocomplimentemia may occur in some autoimmune diseases for 2 reasons: (1) Diseases with immune complex formation (SLE, Glomerulonephritis, cryoglobulinemia, vasculitis, & serum sickness) may result in complement fixation and hypocomplimentemia (C3 & C4). (2) Hereditary deficiency of certain complement components (C1 or C2) is associated with some autoimmune diseases such as SLE.

COMPLEMENT: TOTAL HEMOLYTIC ASSAY (CH50)

The total hemolytic complement assay (CH50) is the best screening test for the integrity of the classical pathway of the complement system; it is used to investigate a suspected functional deficiency of complement. It measures the ability of the patient's serum to lyse 50% of a standard suspension of sheep erythrocytes coated with rabbit antibody. A low CH50 suggests a functional problem with the classical pathway which could stem from either consumption or a deficiency of complement.

COMPLEMENT: C1Q BINDING ASSAY

The C1q binding assay is a test for circulating immune complexes in the serum of a patient that bind to C1q. C1q (a component of C1) binds to the Fc portion of IgG or IgM initiating the classical pathway of the complement system. Normally, C1q has a weak affinity for the Fc regions of monomeric IgG and IgM. However, when IgG and IgM are part of an immune complex the Fc portion undergoes a conformational change which results in C1q having a much higher affinity for the complexed immunoglobulin. C1q binding may be assessed using the ELISA technique. This test can be used with a Raji cell preparation *(see below)*.

COMPLEMENT CASCADE

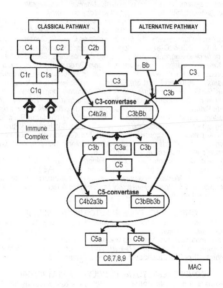

RAJI CELL

The Raji cell assay is a test for circulating immune complexes. Raji cells are a human lymphoblastoid cell line derived from a patient with Burkitt's lymphoma. Unique features of Raji cells include: (a) Surface receptors for complement components C1q, C3b, C3bi, C3d; (b) Lack of surface immunoglobulin; (c) Surface Fc IgG receptors which are low in avidity or low in number. Immune complexes containing complement bind to the complement surface receptors on Raji cells. This can then be used to help detect immune complexes capable of binding complement. This test can be used with a C1q binding assay *(see above)*. Warm reactive anti-lymphocyte antibodies and anti-dsDNA in the sera may cause false-positive results (i.e. SLE).

PROTEIN ELECTROPHORESIS (SPEP, UPEP)

Protein electrophoresis is used to separate and quantify proteins present in serum and/or urine. A patient's serum or urine sample is placed on an electrophoretic gel. An electric current is passed through the gel which causes the proteins (which are negatively charged or anions) to migrate towards the anode (+). Different proteins separate into distinct bands based on their different charges. The pattern on the gel is then read by a densitometer and the relative concn of each protein is determined.

Typical Electrophoretic Patterns

Acute phase reaction pattern: ↓ albumin & ↑ alpha-2-globulin
Chronic inflammatory pattern: ↓ albumin, ↑ alpha-2-globulin, & ↑ gammaglobulin
Nephrotic syndrome: ↓↓ albumin & ↑↑ alpha-2-globulin
Advanced cirrhosis: ↓ albumin, ↑ gammaglobulin, with beta-beta bridging
Polyclonal gammopathy (inflammatory conditions): Diffuse ↑ gammaglobulin
Hypogammaglobulinemia (e.g. light chain variant myeloma with urinary Bence-Jones protein loss): Diffuse ↓ gammaglobulin
Thin spike in the gammaglobulin region: Monoclonal gammopathy (multiple myeloma)

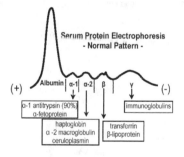

Serum Protein Electrophoresis
- Normal Pattern -

RHEUMATOID FACTOR (RF)

Rheumatoid factors are auto-antibodies directed against antigenic determinants on the Fc fragment of the immunoglobulin G (IgG) molecule. They can be of any isotype; however, IgM is only routinely tested for. They may be detected using latex agglutination or by nephelometry and are present in 70-85% of cases of established rheumatoid arthritis.

Rheumatic Conditions Associated with a Rheumatoid Factor: (a) Rheumatoid Arthritis; (b) Sjogren's Syndrome; (c) Systemic Lupus Erythematosus; (d) Mixed Connective Tissue Disease; (e) Myositis; (f) Cryoglobulinemia

Non-Rheumatic Conditions Associated with a Rheumatoid Factor: (a) Normal Aging; (b) Hepatitis B & C; (c) Human Immunodeficiency Virus (HIV); (d) Subacute Bacterial Endocarditis; (e) Tuberculosis; (f) Sarcoidosis; (g) Idiopathic Pulmonary Fibrosis

SYNOVIAL FLUID ANALYSIS (SF)

Synovial fluid aspirated from an inflamed joint may provide clues to the etiology of the arthropathy.

Characteristics of Normal Synovial Fluid: Appearance: Clear; < 200 WBC's/mm3; <25% PMNs; 95-100% of serum glucose level; No Crystals

Characteristics of Non-inflammatory Synovial Fluid: Appearance: Clear / Yellow; < 2000 WBC's/mm3; <25% PMNs; 95-100% of serum glucose level; No crystals

Characteristics of the Synovial Fluid in Acute Gout: Appearance: Turbid; 2000 – 100,000 WBC's/mm3; 80-100% of serum glucose level; Negative birefringent needle-like Crystals

Characteristics of the Synovial Fluid of Pseudogout: Appearance: Turbid; 2000 – 100,000 WBC's/mm3; >75% PMNs; 80-100% of serum glucose level; Positive birefringent rhomboid Crystals

Characteristics of the Synovial Fluid of Septic Arthritis: Appearance: Yellow / White; > 100,000 WBC's/mm3; >75% PMNs; < 50% of serum glucose level; No Crystals

Characteristics of Inflammatory Synovial Fluid: Appearance: Yellow / White; 2000 – 100,000 WBC's/mm3; 50-75% PMNs; ~ 75% of serum glucose level; No Crystals

CLASSIFICATION CRITERIA OF THE RHEUMATIC DISEASES

ANKYLOSING SPONDYLITIS: 1961 Rome Criteria

Clinical Criteria: (a) Low back pain and stiffness for more than 3 months not relieved by rest; (b) Pain and stiffness of the thoracic region; (c) Limited motion in the lumbar spine; (d) Limited chest expansion; (e) Evidence or history of iritis or its sequelae;

Requirements: Positive radiographs (bilateral SI) and one or more clinical criteria OR Four out of five clinical criteria

Adapted from: Kellgren JH, Jeffrey MR, Ball J Eds. The epidemiology of chronic rheumatism, Vol 1. Oxford:Blackwell, 1963:326.

ANKYLOSING SPONDYLITIS: 1966 New York Criteria

Clinical Criteria: (a) Presence of history of pain at dorso-lumbar junction or in lumbar spine; (b) Limitation of motion in anterior flexion, lateral flexion, and extension; (c) Limitation of chest expansion to 1 inch (2.5 cm) or less at the fourth intercostals space;

Requirements: Positive radiographs (grade 3-4 bilateral sacroiliac) and one or more clinical criteria OR Grade 3-4 unilateral or grade 2 bilateral SI with clinical criteria 2 or clinical criteria 1 & 3

Adapted from: Bennett PH, Wood PHN, eds. Population studies of the rheumatic diseases. Amsterdam: Excerpta Medica, 1900:166-7

ANTIPHOSPHOLIPID ANTIBODY SYNDRONE: International Consensus Statement on Preliminary Criteria for the Classification of the Antiphospholipid Syndrome

CLINICAL CRITERIA

Vascular Thrombosis: One or more clinical episodes of arterial, venous, or small-vessel thrombosis, occurring within any tissue or organ

Complications of Pregnancy: (a) One or more unexplained deaths of morphologically normal fetuses at or after the 10th week of gestation; (b) One or more premature births of morphologically normal neonates at or before the 34th week of gestation; (c) Three or more unexplained consecutive spontaneous abortions before the 10th week of gestation

LABORATORY CRITERIA

Anticardiolipin Antibodies: Anticardiolipin IgG or IgM antibodies present at moderate or high levels in the blood on two or more occasions at least six weeks apart

Lupus Anticoagulant Antibodies: Lupus anticoagulant antibodies detected in the blood on two or more occasions at least six weeks apart, according to the guidelines of the International Society on Thrombosis and Hemostasis

Requirements: A diagnosis of definite antiphospholipid syndrome requires the presence of at least one of the clinical criteria and at least one of the laboratory criteria. No limits are placed on the interval between the clinical event and the positive laboratory findings.

Adapted from: Wilson WA, Gharavi AE, Koike T, et al. International consensus statement on preliminary classification criteria for definite antiphospholipid syndrome. Report of an International Workshop. Arthritis Rheum 1999;42:1309-11

BEHCET'S DISEASE

Recurrent oral ulceration: Minor aphthous, major aphthous, or herpetiform ulceration observed by physician or patient, which recurred at least three times in one 12-month period

plus two (2) of:

Recurrent genital ulceration: Aphthous ulceration or scarring, observed by physician or patient;

Eye lesions: Anterior uveitis, posterior uveitis, or cells in vitreous on slit-lamp examination; or retinal vasculitis observed by ophthalmologist;

Skin lesions: Erythema nodosum observed by physician or patient, pseudofolliculitis, or papulopustular lesions; or acneiform nodules observed by physician in post-adolescent patients not on corticosteroid treatment;

Positive pathergy test: Read by physician at 24-48 hrs;

Adapted from: International Study Group for Behcet's Disease, Criteria for diagnosis of Behcet's Disease. Lancet 1990;335:1078-1080

CHURG-STRAUSS SYNDROME

Asthma: History of wheezing or diffuse high pitched rales on expiration;

Eosinophilia: Eosinophilia > 10% on white blood cell differential count;

History of allergy: History of seasonal allergy (e.g. allergic rhinitis) or other documented allergies, including food, contactants, and other, except drug allergy;

Mononeuropathy or Polyneuropathy: Development of mononeuropathy, multiple mononeuropathies, or polyneuropathy (i.e. glove/stocking distribution), attributable to a systemic vasculitis;

Pulmonary infiltrates, non-fixed: Migratory or transitory pulmonary infiltrates on radiographs (not including fixed infiltrates), attributable to a systemic vasculitis;

Paranasal sinus abnormality: History of acute or chronic paranasal sinus pain or tenderness or radiographic opacification of the paranasal sinuses;

Extravascular eosinophils: Biopsy including artery, arteriole, or venule, showing accumulations of eosinophils in extravascular areas

Adapted from: Masi AT, Hunder GG, Lie JT, Michel BA, Bloch DA, Arend WP, et al. The American College of Rheumatology 1990 criteria for the classification of Churg-Strauss syndrome (allergic granulomatosis and angiitis). Arthritis Rheum 1990;33:1094 – 100.

FIBROMYALGIA

History of Widespread Pain: Pain is considered widespread when all of the following are present: pain in the left side of the body, pain in the right side of the body, pain above the waist, and pain below the waist. In addition, axial skeletal pain (cervical spine or anterior chest or thoracic spine or low back) must be present. In this definition, shoulder and buttock pain is considered as pain for each involved. 'Low back' pain is considered lower segment pain.

Pain in 11 of 18 Tender Points on Digital Palpation: Pain, on digital palpation, must be present in at least 11 of the following 18 tender point sites: *(1) Occiput:* Bilateral, at the suboccipital muscle insertions; *(2) Low cervical:* Bilateral, at the anterior aspects of the intertransverse spaces at C5-C7; *(3) Trapezius:* Bilateral, at the midpoint of the upper border; *(4) Supraspinatus:* Bilateral, at origins, above the scapular spine near the medial border; *(5) Second rib:* Bilateral, at the second costochondral junctions, just lateral to the junctions on upper surfaces; *(6) Lateral epicondyle:* Bilateral, 2 cm distal to the epicondyles; *(7) Gluteal:* Bilateral, in upper outer quadrants of buttocks in anterior fold of muscle; *(8) Greater trochanter:* Bilateral, posterior to the trochanteric prominence; *(9) Knee:* Bilateral, at the medial fat pad proximal to the joint line; Digital palpation should be performed with an approximate force of 4 kg; For a tender point to be considered 'positive' the subject must state that the palpation was painful. 'Tender' is not to be considered 'painful'.

Requirements: For classification purposes, patients will be said to have fibromyalgia if: Widespread pain must have been present for at least 3 months AND Pain in 11 of 18 tender point sites on digital palpation. The presence of a second clinical disorder does not exclude the diagnosis of fibromyalgia.

Adapted from: Wolfe F, Smythe HA, Yunus MB, Bennett RM, Bombardier C, Goldenberg DL, et al. The American College of Rheumatology 1990 criteria for the classification of fibromyalgia: report of the multicenter criteria committee. Arthritis Rheum 1990;33:160 – 72.

GIANT CELL ARTERITIS: The 1990 Classification Criteria

Age at disease onset > 50 yr: Development of symptoms or findings beginning at age 50 yr or older;

New headache: New onset of or new type of localized pain in the head;

Temporal artery abnormality: Temporal artery tenderness to palpation or decreased pulsation, unrelated to arteriosclerosis of cervical arteries;

Elevated erythrocyte sedimentation rate: Erythrocyte sedimentation rate 50 mm/hr by the Westergren method;

Abnormal artery biopsy: Biopsy specimen with artery showing vasculitis characterized by a predominance of mononuclear cell infiltration or granulomatous inflammation, usually with multinucleated giant cells.

Requirements: A patient shall be said to have giant cell arteritis if at least three of five criteria are present. The presence of any three or more criteria yields a sensitivity of 93.5% and a specificity of 91.2%.

Adapted from: Hunder GG, Bloch DA, Michel BA, Stevens MB, Arend WP, Calabrese LH, et al. The American College of Rheumatology 1990 criteria for the classification of giant cell arteritis. Arthritis Rheum 1990;33:1122 – 8.

GOUT

The presence of characteristic urate crystals in the joint fluid *and/or* A tophus proved to contain urate crystals by chemical or polarized light microscopic means *and/or* The presence of six of the 12 clinical, laboratory, and radiographic phenomena listed below: Maximum inflammation in 1 day; More than one attack; Monoarticular arthritis; Redness; First metatarsophalangeal joint pain or swelling; Unilateral first MTP; Unilateral tarsal; Suspected tophus; Hyperuricemia; Asymmetric swelling; Sub-cortical cysts, no erosions; Negative organisms on culture

Adapted from: Wallace SL, Robinson H, Masi At et al. Preliminary criteria for the classification of the acute arthritis of primary gout. Arthritis Rheum 1977;20:895-900

HENOCH-SCHONLEIN PURPURA: 1990 Classification Criteria

Palpable purpura: Slightly raised, 'palpable' hemorrhagic skin lesions, not related to thrombocytopenia;

Age < 20 yr at disease onset: Patient 20 yr or younger at onset of first symptoms;

Bowel angina: Diffuse abdominal pain, worse after meals or the diagnosis of bowel ischemia, usually including bloody diarrhea;

Wall granulocytes on biopsy: Histologic changes showing granulocytes in the walls of arterioles or venules.

Requirements: A patient shall be said to have Henoch-Schonlein purpura if at least two of these four criteria are present. The presence of any two or more criteria yields a sensitivity of 87.1% and a specificity of 87.7%.

Adapted from: Mills JA, Michel BA, Bloch DA, Calabrese LH, Hunder GG, Arend WP, et al. The American College of Rheumatology 1990 criteria for the classification of Henoch-Schönlein purpura. Arthritis Rheum 1990;33:1114 - 21.

HYPERSENSITIVITY VASCULITIS: 1990 Classification Criteria

Age at disease onset >16 yr: Development of symptoms after age 16 yr;

Medication at disease onset: Medication was taken at the onset of symptoms that may have been a precipitating factor;

Palpable purpura: Slightly elevated purpuric rash over one or more areas of the skin; does not blanch with pressure and is not related to thrombocytopenia;

Maculopapular rash: Flat and raised lesions of various sizes over one or more areas of the skin;

Biopsy including arteriole and venule: Histological changes showing granulocytes in a perivascular or extravascular location.

Requirements: A patient shall be said to have hypersensitivity vasculitis if at least three of these five criteria are present. The presence of any three or more yields a sensitivity of 71.0% and a specificity of 83.9%.

Adapted from: Calabrese LH, Michel BA, Bloch DA, Arend WP, Edworthy SM, Fauci AS, et al. The American College of Rheumatology 1990 criteria for the classification of hypersensitivity vasculitis. Arthritis Rheum 1990;33:1108 – 13.

INFLAMMATORY MYOPATHIES: Diagnostic Criteria

Symmetrical weakness: Weakness of limb-girdle muscles and anterior neck flexors, progressing over weeks to months with or without dysphagia or respiratory muscle involvement;

Muscle biopsy evidence: Evidence of necrosis of type I and II fibers, phagocytosis, regeneration with basophilia, large vesicular sarcolemmal nuclei and prominent nucleoli, atrophy in a perifascicular distribution, variation in fiber size, and an inflammatory exudate, often perivascular;

Elevation of muscle enzymes: Elevation in serum of skeletal muscle enzymes, particularly creatine phosphokinase and often aldolase, serum glutamate oxaloacetate, pyruvate transaminases, and lactate dehydrogenase;

Electromyographic evidence: Electromyographic triad of short, small polyphasic motor units, fibrillations, positive sharp waves, insertional irritability, and bizarre, high frequency repetitive discharges;

Dermatologic features: A lilac discoloration of the eyelids (heliotrope) with periorbital edema, a scaly, erythematous dermatitis over the dorsum of the hands (especially the MCP and PIP joints, Gottron's sign), and involvement of the knees, elbows, and medial malleoli, as well as the face, neck, and upper torso

Requirements for Dermatomyositis: Definite diagnosis: Three of four criteria plus the rash must be present; Probable diagnosis: Two of four criteria plus the rash must be present; Possible diagnosis: One of four criteria plus the rash must be present;

Requirements for Polymyositis: Definite diagnosis: Four of four criteria without the rash must be present; Probable diagnosis: Three of four criteria without the rash must be present; Possible diagnosis: Two of four criteria without the rash must be present

Adapted from: Bohan A, Peter JB. Polymyositis and dermatomyositis (first of two parts). N Engl J Med 1975;292:344-347.

KAWASAKI SYNDROME

PRINCIPAL SYMPTOMS

Fever: Fever lasting from 1 to 2 weeks and not responding to antibiotics;

Bilateral congestion of ocular conjunctivae;

Changes in lips and oral cavity: dryness, redness and fissuring of lips; protuberance of tongue papillae (strawberry tongue); diffuse reddening of oral and pharyngeal mucosa.

Changes in peripheral extremities: reddening of palms and soles (initial stage); indurative edema (initial stage); membranous desquamation from fingertips (convalescent stage);

Polymorphous exanthema of body trunk without vesicles or crusts: Acute non-purulent swelling of cervical lymph nodes of 1.5 cm or more in diameter;

OTHER SIGNIFICANT SYMPTOMS OR FINDINGS

Carditis, especially myocarditis and pericarditis; Diarrhea; Arthralgia or arthritis; Proteinuria and increase of leukocytes in urine sediment;

Changes in blood tests: Leukocytosis with shift to the left; Slight decrease in erythrocyte and hemoglobin levels; Increased erythrocyte sedimentation rate; Positive C-reactive protein; Increased alpha 2-globulin; Negative anti streptolysin-O titer;

Changes occasionally observed: Aseptic meningitis; Mild jaundice or slight increase in serum transaminase

Adapted from: Kawasaki T, Kosaki T, Oksawa S et al. A new infantile acute febrile mucocutaneous lymph node syndrome (MLNS) prevailing in Japan. Pediatrics 1974;54:271-6.

OSTEOARTHRITIS OF THE HAND: Classification Criteria

Pain, aching, stiffness *and* three or four of the following features: (a) Hard tissue enlargement of two or more of 10 selected joints; (b) Hard tissue enlargement of two or more distal interphalangeal joints; (c) Fewer than three swollen metacarpophalangeal (MCP) joints; (d) Deformity of at least one of 10 selected joints. *Requirements:* The 10 selected joints are the second and third distal interphalangeal, the second and third proximal interphalangeal, and the first carpometacarpal joints of both hands. This classification method yields a sensitivity of 94% and a specificity of 87%.

Adapted from: Altman R, Alarcón G, Appelrouth D, Bloch D, Borenstein D, Brandt K, et al. The American College of Rheumatology criteria for the classification and reporting of osteoarthritis of the hand. Arthritis Rheum 1990;33:1601---10.

OSTEOARTHRITIS OF THE HIP: Clinical and Radiographic Classification Criteria

Hip pain *and* at least two of the following three features: (a) Erythrocyte sedimentation rate < 20 mm/hr; (b) Radiographic femoral or acetabular osteophytes; (c) Radiographic joint space narrowing (superior, axial, and/or medial). *Requirements:* This classification method yields a sensitivity of 89% and a specificity of 91%

Adapted from: Altman R, Alarcon G, Appelrouth D, et al. The American College of Rheumatology criteria for the classification and reporting of osteoarthritis of the hip. Arthritis Rheum 1991;34:505-514

OSTEOARTHRITIS OF THE KNEE: Classification Criteria

Clinical & Laboratory: Knee Pain AND at least 5 of 9: (a) Age > 50; (b) Stiffness < 30 min; (c) Crepitus; (d) Bony tenderness; (e) Bony enlargement; (f) No palpable warmth; (g) ESR < 40 mm/hr; (h) RF <1:40; (i) SF OA. Sensitivity: 92%, Specificity: 75%

Clinical & Radiographic: Knee Pain AND at least 1 of 3: (a) Age > 50 yr; (b) Stiffness < 30 min; (c) Crepitus & osteophytes. Sensitivity: 91%, Specificity: 86%

Clinical: Knee Pain; AND at least 3 of 6: (a) Age > 50 yr; (b) Stiffness < 30 min; (c) Crepitus; (d) Bony tenderness; (e) Bony enlargement; (f) No palpable warmth. Sensitivity: 95%, Specificity: 69%. *ESR* = Erythrocyte Sedimentation Rate; *RF* = Rheumatoid Factor; *SF OA* = Synovial Fluid Signs of Osteoarthritis (clear, viscous, or WBC < 2000/mm3)

Adapted from: Altman R, Alarcon G, Appelrouth D, et al. The American College of Rheumatology criteria for the classification and reporting of osteoarthritis of the hip. Arthritis Rheum 1991;34:505-514

OSTEOPOROSIS: World Health Organization Criteria

Normal: BMD not more than 1 standard deviation below peak adult bone mass (T-Score > -1.0)

Osteopenia: BMD that lies between 1 and 2.5 standard deviations below peak adult bone mass (T-Score between –1.0 and –2.5);

Osteoporosis: BMD more than 2.5 standard deviations below peak adult bone mass (T-Score -2.5;

Severe Osteoporosis: BMD more than 2.5 standard deviations below peak adult bone mass and the presence of one or more fragility fractures (T-Score -2.5 plus fragility fracture)

Adapted from: Assessment of fracture risk and its application to screening for postmenopausal osteoporosis. Report of a WHO study group. World Health Organ Techn Rep Ser 1994;843:1-129

POLYARTERITIS NODOSA: 1990 Classification Criteria

Weight loss > 4 kg: Loss of 4 kg or more of body weight since illness began, not due to dieting or other factors;

Livedo Reticularis: Mottled reticular pattern over the skin of portions of the extremities or torso;

Testicular pain or tenderness: Pain or tenderness of the testicles, not due to infections, trauma, or other causes;

Myalgias, weakness, or leg tenderness: Diffuse myalgias (excluding shoulder and hip girdle) or weakness of muscles or tenderness of leg muscles;

Mononeuropathy or polyneuropathy: Development of mononeuropathy, multiple mononeuropathies, or polyneuropathies;

Diastolic blood pressure > 90 mm Hg: Development of hypertension with diastolic blood pressure higher than 90 mm HG;

Elevated BUN or creatinine: Elevated BUN > 40 mg/dl or creatinine > 1.5mg/dl, not due to dehydration, or obstruction;

Hepatitis B virus: Presence of hepatitis B surface antigen or antibody in serum;

Arteriographic abnormality: Arteriogram showing aneurysms or occlusions of the visceral arteries, not due to arteriosclerosis, fibromuscular dysplasia, or other non-inflammatory causes;

Biopsy of small or medium-sized artery containing PMN: Histological changes showing the presence of granulocytes or granulocytes and mononuclear leukocytes in the artery wall.

Requirements: A patient shall be said to have polyarteritis nodosa if at least three of these 10 criteria are present. The presence of any three or more criteria yields a sensitivity of 82.2% and a specificity of 86.6%.

Adapted from: Lightfoot RW Jr, Michel BA, Bloch DA, Hunder GG, Zvaifler NJ, McShane DJ, et al. The American College of Rheumatology 1990 criteria for the classification of polyarteritis nodosa. Arthritis Rheum 1990;33:1088---93.

POLYMYALGIA RHEUMATICA

Characteristics: (a) Shoulder pain and/or stiffness bilaterally; (b) Onset of illness < 2 weeks' duration (refers to time taken for symptoms to reach their full-blown picture); (c) Initial erythrocyte sedimentation rate 40 mm/hr; (d) Morning stiffness duration > 1 hour; (e) Age > 65; (f) depression and/or loss of weight; (g) Upper arm tenderness bilaterally

Adapted from: Bird HA, Esselincks W, Dixon AJ et al. An evaluation of criteria for polymyalgia rheumatica. Ann Rheum Dis 1979;38;434-9

RHEUMATIC FEVER: Guidelines for the Diagnosis of an Initial Attack of Rheumatic Fever (Jones Criteria, 1992 Update)

Major Manifestations: (a) Carditis; (b) Polyarthritis; (c) Chorea; (d) Erythema marginatum; (e) Subcutaneous nodules;

Minor Manifestations: Clinical Findings: (a) Arthralgia; (b) Fever; *Laboratory Findings:* (a) Elevated acute-phase reactants: Erythrocyte sedimentation rate, C-reactive protein; (b) Prolonged PR interval; (c) Supporting evidence of antecedent group A streptococcal infection: Positive throat culture or rapid streptococcal antigen test, Elevated or rising streptococcal antibody titer.

Requirements: If supported by evidence of preceding group A streptococcal infection, the presence of two major manifestations or of one major and two minor manifestations indicates a high probability of acute rheumatic fever.

Adapted from: Special Writing Group of the Committee on Rheumatic Fever, Endocarditis and Kawasaki Disease of the Council on Cardiovascular Disease in the You of the American Heart Association. Guidelines for the diagnosis of rheumatic fever: Jones criteria, updated 1992. J Am Med Assoc 1992;268:2069-73. (Copyright 1992, American Medical Association).

RHEUMATOID ARTHRITIS: 1987 Revised Classification Criteria

Morning Stiffness: Morning stiffness in and around the joints, lasting at least 1 hour before maximal improvement;

Arthritis of 3 or more joint areas: At least three joint areas simultaneously have had soft tissue swelling or fluid (not bony overgrowth alone) observed by a physician. The 14 possible areas are right or left proximal interphalangeal (PIP), MCP, wrist, elbow, knee, ankle, and MTP joints.

Arthritis of the hand joints: At least one area swollen (as defined above) in a wrist, MCP, or PIP joint.

Symmetric arthritis: Simultaneous involvement of the same joint areas [as defined in (2)] on both sides of the body (bilateral involvement of PIPs, MCPs, or MTPs is acceptable without absolute symmetry).

Rheumatoid nodules: Subcutaneous nodules, over bony prominences, or extensor surfaces, or in juxta-articular regions, observed by a physician.

Serum rheumatoid factor: Demonstration of abnormal amounts of serum rheumatoid factor by any method for which the result has been positive in <5% of normal subjects.

Radiographic changes: Radiographic changes typical of rheumatoid arthritis on posteroanterior hand and wrist radiographs, which must include erosions or unequivocal bony decalcification localized in or most marked adjacent to the involved joints (osteoarthritis changes alone do not qualify).

Requirements: A patient shall be said to have rheumatoid arthritis if he/she has satisfied at least four of these seven criteria. Criteria (1)-(4) must have been present for at least 6 weeks. Patients with two clinical diagnoses are not excluded. Designation as classic, definite, or probable rheumatoid arthritis is not to be made.

Adapted from: Arnett FC, Edworthy SM, Bloch DA, McShane DJ, Fries JF, Cooper NS, et al. The American Rheumatism Association 1987 revised criteria for the classification of rheumatoid arthritis. Arthritis Rheum 1988;31:315-324

RHEUMATOID ARTHRITIS: Classes Based on Severity

Mild: At least 3 simultaneously inflamed joints; Arthralgias; Absence of extra-articular disease; Elevations of ESR or CRP; Negative rheumatoid factor; No evidence of erosions or cartilage loss

Moderate: Between 6 - 20 inflamed joints; Absence of extra-articular disease; Elevated ESR and CRP; Positive rheumatoid factor; Evidence of inflammation on plain radiography; Periarticular osteopenia & swelling; usually no erosions.

Severe: More than 20 persistently inflamed joints; A rapidly declining functional capacity; Elevated ESR or CRP; Anemia of chronic disease; Hypoalbuminemia; Positive rheumatoid factor (often high titer); Extra-articular disease (rheumatoid nodules, eye or lung inflammation, vasculitis, neuropathy)

RHEUMATOID ARTHRITIS: Assessment of Disease Activity

History: Degree and involvement of joints; Duration of morning stiffness; Duration of fatigue; Limitation of function.

Physical: Actively inflamed joints (joint count); Mechanical joint problems: loss of range of motion, crepitus, instability, malalignment and/or deformities; Extra-articular manifestations.

Laboratory: ESR and/or CRP; Rheumatoid factor; CBC, electrolytes, BUN, Cr, AST, ALT, ALP, albumin, bilirubin; Urinalysis; Synovial fluid analysis – if necessary.

Other: Functional status or quality of life assessment using standardized questionnaires; Physician's global assessment of disease activity; Patient's global assessment of disease activity;

Radiography: Radiographs of selected joints

RHEUMATOID ARTHRITIS: Classification of Functional Status

Class I: Completely able to perform usual activities of daily living (self-care, vocational, and avocational);

Class II: Able to perform usual self-care and vocational activities, but limited in avocational activities;

Class III: Able to perform usual self-care activities, but limited in vocational and avocational activities;

Class IV: Limited in ability to perform usual self-care, vocational, and avocational activities

Adapted from: Hochberg MC, Chang RW, Dwosh I et al. The American College of Rheumatology 1991 revised criteria for the classification of global functional status in rheumatoid arthritis. Arthritis Rheum 1992; 35:498-502

RHEUMATOID ARTHRITIS: Criteria for Clinical Remission

(a) Duration of morning stiffness not exceeding 15 minutes; (b) No fatigue; (c) No joint pain; (d) No joint tenderness or pain on motion; (e) No soft tissue swelling in joints or tendon sheaths; (f) ESR less than 30 mm/hr for a female or 20 mm/hr for a male

Adapted from: Pinals RS, Masi AT, Larsen RA, et al. Preliminary criteria for clinical remission in rheumatoid arthritis. Arthritis Rheum 1981; 24:1308-1315

RHEUMATOID ARTHRITIS: Classification of Progression

Stage I (Early): No destructive changes on radiographic examination; Radiographic evidence of osteoporosis may be present.

Stage II (Moderate): Radiographic evidence of osteoporosis, with or without slight subchondral bone destruction; slight cartilage destruction may be present; No joint deformities, although limitation of joint mobility may be present; Adjacent muscle atrophy; Extra-articular soft tissue lesions, such as nodules and tenosynovitis may be present.

Stage III (Severe): Radiographic evidence of cartilage and bone destruction in addition to osteoporosis. Joint deformity, such as subluxation, ulnar deviation, or hyperextension, without fibrosis or bony ankylosis; Extensive muscle atrophy; Extra-articular soft tissue lesions, such as nodules and tenosynovitis may be present.

Stage IV (Terminal): Fibrous or bony ankylosis; Criteria of stage III

Adapted from: Steinbrocker O, Traeger CH, Batterman RC. Therapeutic criteria in rheumatoid arthritis. JAMA 1949;140:659-662. (Copyright 1949, American Medical Association)

SJÖGREN'S SYNDROME: Preliminary Classification Criteria

Ocular Symptoms: Definition: a positive response to at least one of the following three questions: (a) Have you had daily, persistent, troublesome dry eyes for more than 3 months? (b) Do you have recurrent sensation of sand or gravel in the eyes? (c) Do you use tear substitutes more than three times a day?

Oral symptoms: Definition: a positive response to at least one of the following three questions: (a) Have you had a daily feeling of dry mouth for more than 3 months? (b) Have you had recurrent or persistently swollen salivary glands as an adult? (c) Do you frequently drink liquids to aid in swallowing dry foods?

Ocular Signs: Definition: Objective evidence of ocular involvement, determined on the basis of a positive result on at least one of the following two tests: (a) Schirmer-1 test (5 mm in 5 min); (b) Rose Bengal score (4, according to the van Bijsterveld scoring system).

Histopathological features: Definition: focus score 1 on minor salivary gland biopsy (focus defined as an agglomeration of at least 50 mononuclear cells; focus score defined as the number of foci in 4 mm2 of glandular tissue).

Salivary gland involvement: Definition: Objective evidence of salivary gland involvement, determined on the basis of a positive result on at least one of the following three tests: (a) Salivary scintigraphy; (b) Parotid sialography; (c) Unstimulated salivary flow (1.5 ml in 15 min)

Autoantibodies: Definition: Presence of at least one of the following serum autoantibodies: (a) Antibodies to Ro/SS-A or La/SS-B antigens; (b) Antinuclear antibodies; (c) Rheumatoid factor

Exclusion criteria: Pre-existing lymphoma, acquired immunodeficiency syndrome, sarcoidosis, or graft-vs-host disease

Adapted from: Vitali C, Bombardieri S, Moutsopoulos HM et al. Preliminary criteria for the classification of Sjogren's syndrome. Arthritis Rheum 1993; 36:340-347

SPONDYLOARTHROPATHIES: European Spondyloarthropathy Study Group Classification for spondyloarthropathy

Inflammatory spinal pain: History or present symptoms of spinal pain in back, dorsal, or cervical region, with at least four of the following: (a) onset before age 45, (b) insidious onset, (c) improved by exercise, (d) associated with morning stiffness, (e) at least 3 months' duration

OR

Synovitis (asymmetric or predominantly in the lower limbs): Past or present asymmetric arthritis or arthritis predominantly of the lower limbs.

AND, One or more of the following

Positive family history: Presence in first-degree or second-degree relatives of any of the following: (a) ankylosing spondylitis, (b) psoriasis, (c) acute uveitis, (d) reactive arthritis, (d) inflamm bowel disease;

Psoriasis: Past or present psoriasis diagnosed by a physician;

Inflammatory bowel disease: Past or present Crohn's disease or ulcerative colitis diagnosed by a physician and confirmed by radiographic examination or endoscopy;

Urethritis, cervicitis, or acute diarrhea within 1 month before arthritis: Episode of diarrhea occurring within one month before arthritis, Nongonococcal urethritis or cervicitis occurring within one month before arthritis;

Buttock pain alternating between right and left gluteal areas: Past or present alternating pain between the right and left gluteal regions;

Enthesopathy: Past or present spontaneous pain or tenderness at examination of the site of the insertion of the Achilles tendon or plantar fascia;

Sacroiliitis: Bilateral grade 2-4 or unilateral grade 3-4, according to the following radiographic grading system: 0=normal, 1=possible, 2=minimal, 3=moderate, and 4=ankylosis. This classification system yields a sensitivity of 78.4% and a specificity of 89.6%. When radiographic evidence of sacroiliitis was included, the sensitivity improved to 87.0% with a minor decrease in specificity to 86.7%.

Adapted from: Dougados M, Van Der Linden S, Juhlin R, et al. The European Spondyloarthropathy Study Group preliminary criteria for the classification of Spondyloarthropathy. Arthritis Rheum 1991; 34:1218-1227

SYSTEMIC LUPUS ERYTHEMATOSUS: The 1982 Revised Criteria for the Classification of Systemic Lupus Erythematosus

Malar rash: Fixed erythema, flat or raised, over the malar eminences, tending to spare the nasolabial folds;

Discoid rash: Erythematous raised patches with adherent keratotic scaling and follicular plugging; atrophic scarring may occur in older lesions;

Photosensitivity: Skin rash as a result of unusual reaction to sunlight, by patient history or physician observation;

Oral ulcers: Oral or nasopharyngeal ulceration, usually painless, observed by physician;

Arthritis: Non-erosive arthritis involving two or more peripheral joints, characterized by tenderness, swelling, or effusion;

Serositis: (a) Pleuritis: convincing history of pleuritic pain or rub heard by a physician or evidence of pleural effusion; or (b) Pericarditis: documented by ECG or rub or evidence of a pericardial effusion;

Renal disorder: (a) Persistent Proteinuria greater than 0.5 g/day or greater than 3+ if quantitation not performed; or (b) Cellular casts: may be red cell, hemoglobin, granular, tubular, or mixed;

Neurological disorder: (a) Seizures: in the absence of offending drugs or known metabolic derangements, e.g. uremia, ketoacidosis, or electrolyte imbalance; or (b) Psychosis: in the absence of offending drugs or known metabolic derangements, e.g. uremia, ketoacidosis, or electrolyte imbalance;

Hematological disorder: (a) Hemolytic anemia with reticulocytosis; or (b) Leukopenia: less than 4.00/mm3 total on two or more occasions; or (c) Lymphopenia: less than 1.55/mm3 on two or more occasions; or (d) Thrombocytopenia: less than 100 000/mm3 in the absence of offending drugs;

Immunological disorder (modified 1997): (a) Anti-DNA: antibody to native DNA in abnormal titer; or (b) Anti-Sm: presence of antibody to Sm nuclear antigen; or (c) Positive finding of antiphospholipid antibodies based on: (1) an abnormal serum level of IgG or IgM anticardiolipin antibodies; (2) a positive test result for lupus anticoagulant using a standard method; or (3) a false-positive serological test for syphilis known to be positive for at least 6 months and confirmed by Treponema pallidum immobilization or fluorescent treponemal antibody absorption test;

Antinuclear antibody: An abnormal titer of antinuclear antibody by immunofluorescence or an equivalent assay at any point in time and in the absence of drugs known to be associated with 'drug-induced lupus' syndrome.

Requirements: A patient shall be said to have systemic lupus erythematosus if any four or more of the 11 criteria are present, serially or simultaneously, during any interval of observation.

Adapted from: Tan EM, Cohen AS, Fries JF, Masi AT, McShane DJ, Rothfield NF, et al. The 1982 revised criteria for the classification of systemic lupus erythematosus. Arthritis Rheum 1982; 25:1271-7.

SYSTEMIC SCLEROSIS: Classification Criteria

Major Criteria: Proximal Scleroderma: Symmetrical thickening, tightening, and induration of the skin of the fingers and the skin proximal to the metacarpophalangeal or metatarsophalangeal joints. These changes may affect the entire extremity, face, neck, and trunk (thorax and abdomen).

Minor Criteria: (a) Sclerodactyly: Above-indicated skin changes limited to the fingers. (b) Digital pitting scars or loss of substance from the finger pad. Depressed areas at tips of fingers or loss of digital pad tissue as a result of ischemia. (c) Bibasilar pulmonary fibrosis: Bilateral reticular pattern of linear or lineonodular densities most pronounced in basilar portions of the lungs on standard chest radiograph; may assume appearance of diffuse mottling or "honeycomb lung". These changes should not be attributable to primary lung disease.

Requirements: A person shall be said to have systemic sclerosis (scleroderma) if one major and two or more minor criteria are present. Localized forms of scleroderma, eosinophilic fasciitis, and the various forms of pseudoscleroderma are excluded from these criteria.

Adapted from: Subcommittee for Scleroderma Criteria of the American Rheumatism Association Diagnostic and Therapeutic Criteria Committee. Preliminary criteria for the classification of systemic sclerosis (scleroderma). Arthritis Rheum 1980; 23:581-90.

TAKAYASU'S ARTERITIS: 1990 Classification Criteria

Age at disease onset < 40 yr: Development of symptoms or findings related to Takayasu's arteritis at age < 40 yr;

Claudication of extremities: Development and worsening of fatigue and discomfort in muscles of one or more extremity while in use, especially the upper extremities;

Decreased brachial artery pulse: Decreased pulsation of one or both brachial arteries;

Blood pressure difference > 10 mmHg: Difference of > 10 mmHg in systolic blood pressure between arms;

Bruit over subclavian arteries or aorta: Bruit audible on auscultation over one or both subclavian arteries or abdominal aorta;

Arteriogram abnormality: Arteriographic narrowing or occlusion of the entire aorta, its primary branches, or large arteries in the proximal upper or lower extremities, not due to arteriosclerosis, fibromuscular dysplasia, or similar causes: changes usually focal or segmental.

Requirements: A patient shall be said to have Takayasu's arteritis if at least three of these six criteria are present. The presence of any three or more criteria yields a sensitivity of 90.5% and a specificity of 97.8%.

Adapted from: Arend WP, Michael BA, Bloich DA et al. The American College of Rheumatology 1990 criteria for the classification of Takayasu's arteritis. Arthritis Rheum 1990; 33:1129-1132

WEGENER'S GRANULOMATOSIS:1990 Classification Criteria

Nasal or oral inflammation: Development of painful or painless oral ulcers or purulent or bloody nasal discharge;

Abnormal chest radiograph: Chest radiograph showing the presence of nodules, fixed infiltrates, or cavities;

Urinary sediment: Microhematuria (>5 red blood cells per high power field) or red cell casts in urine sediment;

Granulomatous inflammation on biopsy: Histological changes showing granulomatous inflammation in the wall of an artery or in the perivascular or extravascular area (artery or arteriole).

Requirements: A patient shall be said to have Wegener's granulomatosis if at least two of these four criteria are present. The presence of any two or more criteria yields a sensitivity of 88.2% and a specificity of 92.0%.

Adapted from: Leavitt RY, Fauci AS, Bloch DA, Michel BA, Hunder GG, Arend WP, et al. The American College of Rheumatology 1990 criteria for the classification of Wegener's granulomatosis. Arthritis Rheum 1990; 33:1101 – 7.

INDEX

A

Abenol 138
Acetaminophen 138
Acetylsalicylic Acid 197
Aciphex 188
Actiq 144
Actonel 220
Adalimumab 149
Adult Still's Disease (ASD) 6
Advil 201
Albert-Tiafen 209
Alendronate 211
Aleve 206
Allopurinol 190
Alora 214
Amigesic 208
Amitriptyline 138
ANA 232
Anakinra 150
Anaprox 206
ANCA 232
Ankylosing Spondylitis 8
    1961 Rome Criteria 239
    1966 New York Criteria 239
    Anterior uveitis 8
    Chest Expansion 10
    Modified Schober test 10
    Poor Prognosticators 11
    Sacroiliitis 10
    Syndesmophytes 11
Ansaid 200
Anterior 104
Anti-Cardiolipin Antibodies 233
Anti-Double Stranded DNA 232
Anti-dsDNA 232
Anti-Neutrophil Cytoplasmic Antibodies 232
Anti-Nuclear Antibodies 232
Anti-Phospholipid Antibodies 233
Antiphospholipid Antibody Syndrome (APLAS) 12

APLA 233
Aralon 165
Arava 178
Aredia 218
Aristospan 159
Arthrotec 198
ASA 197
Aspirin 197
Atasol 138
Aurolate 174
Avinza 145
Azasan 163
Azathioprine 163
Azulfidine 183
Azulfidine-EN 183

B

Bacterial Arthritis
    Gonococcal 39
    Non Gonococcal 15
Behcet's Disease (BD) 17
    Criteria 240
Betamethasone Sodium Phosphate 159
Boniva 217
Bosentan 224

C

C1Q Binding Assay 235
Calciferol 214
Calcimar 212
Calcitonin 212
Calcitriol 214
Calcium Pyrophosphate Deposition (CPPD) 20
Calcium Supplements 213
Cataflam 197
Celebrex 161
Celecoxib 161
Celestone 159
Cellcept 182
Cenestin 214
Ces 214
Cevimeline 228
CH50 235
Chlorambucil 164

Chloroquine Phosphate 165
Churg-Strauss Syndrome (CSS) 23
    Criteria 240
Climara 214
Clinoril 208
Codeine 143
Codeine-Contin 143
Colchicine 192
Complement
    Complement Components and their
    Functions 235
    Role of Complement in Autoimmune
    Disease 235
    The Complement System 235
    Total Hemolytic Complement Assay
    235
Complex Regional Pain Syndrome
(CRPS) 26
Corticosteroids
    Dexamethasone Sodium Phosphate
    157
    Hydrocortisone Sodium Succinate 157
    Intra-Articular Corticosteroids 159
    Methylprednisolone Sodium Succinate
    158
    Prednisone 158
C-Reactive Protein 234
Criteria for the Classification of the
Rheumatic Diseases 239
CRP 234
Cryoglobulinemia 130
Cuprimine 172
Cutaneous Vasculitis 29
Cyclobenzaprine 140
Cyclophosphamide - Intravenous 166
Cyclophosphamide - Oral 168
Cyclosporine 170
Cytotec 188
Cytoxan 166, 168

D

Dactylitis 4
Dapsone 172
Darvon 147

Darvon-N 147
Daypro 207
Decadron 157
Demerol 145
Depen 172
Depo-Medrol 159
Dermatomyositis 45
Diclofenac 197, 198
Didrocal 216
Didronel 216
Diffuse Idiopathic Skeletal Hyperostosis
(DISH) 32
Diflunisal 199
Dilaudid 144
Dilaudid-5 144
Disalcid 208
Dolobid 199
D-Penicillamine 172
Drug-Induced Myositis 46
Duragesic 144
Durolane 230

E

EC-Naprosyn 206
Elavil 138
Empracet 143
Emtec 143
ENA 234
Enbrel 151
Epoprostenol 225
Erythema Nodosum (EN) 34
Erythrocyte Sedimentation Rate 234
Esclim 214
Esomeprazole 188
ESR 234
Estrace 214
Estraderm 214
Estradiol 214
Estradot 214
Estrogen
    Conjugated Estrogen 214
    Estradiol 214
    Estrogen/Progesterone 214
    Estropipate 214

Transdermal Estrogen 214
Etanercept 151
Etidronate 216
Etodolac 199
Evista 219
Evoxac 228
Extractable Nuclear Antigen Antibodies 234

F

Famotidine 187
Feldene 207
FemPatch 214
Fenoprofen 200
Fentanyl 144
Fibromyalgia (FM) 36
    Criteria 240
Fioricet with Codeine 143
Fiorinal C1/2 143
Fiorinal C1/4 143
Fiorinal with Codeine 143
FK506 184
Flexeril 140
Flolan 225
Flurbiprofen 200
Forteo 221
Fosamax 211
Froben 200
Froben-SR 200
Frosst 143
Frosst 222 AF 138
Frosst 292 143

G

Gabapentin 141
Gastroprotection 187
Gengraf 170
Giant Cell Arteritis (GCA) 80
    1990 Classification Criteria 241
Gold Sodium Thiomalate 174
Gonococcal Arthritis 39
Gout 41
    Criteria 241
Gynodiol 214

H

Humira 149
Hyalgan 230
Hyaluronate 230
Hydromorph-Contin 144
Hydromorphone 144
Hydroxychloroquine 175
Hylan G-F 20 230
Hypersensitivity Vasculitis 29
    1990 Criteria for the Classification of
    Hypersensitivity Vasculitis 242

I

Ibandronate 217
Ibuprofen 201
Imuran 163
Inclusion body myositis 46
Indocid 202
Indocid-SR 202
Indomethacin 202
Inflammatory Myositis 45
    Criteria for the Diagnosis of
    Polymyositis and Dermatomyositis
    242
Infliximab 153
Intra-Articular Corticosteroids 159
Intravenous Immunoglobulin 176
IVIG 176

J

Juvenile Idiopathic Arthritis
    Pauciarticular 48
    Polyarticular 52
    Systemic 57

K

Kadian 145
Kawasaki Syndrome 243
Kenalog 159
Ketoprofen 202
Ketorolac 203
Kineret 150

L

Lansoprazole 188

Leflunomide 178
Lenoltec 143
Leukeran 164
Leukocytoclastic Vasculitis 29
Lodine 199
Lodine-XL 199
Losec 188
Lupus Anticoagulant 233
Lyme Disease 62

M

M.O.S. 145
Meclofenamate 203
Meclomen 203
Medications Used for the Treatment of
Gout & Hyperuricemia 190
Mefenamic Acid 204
Meloxicam 205
Meperidine 145
M-Eslon 145
Methotrexate 179
Methylprednisolone Acetate 159
Miacalcin 212
Microscopic Polyangiitis (MPA) 64
Minocin 181
Minocycline 181
Misoprostol 188, 198
Mixed Connective Tissue Disease
(MCTD) 67
Mobic 205
Mobicox 205
Mobiflex 209
Morphine Sulfate 145
Motrin 201
MS-Contin 145
Mycophenolate Mofetil 182
Myochrisine 174

N

Nabumetone 205
Nalfon 200
Naprelan 206
Naprosyn 206
Naproxen 206
Neoral 170

Neovisc 230
Neurontin 141
Neuropathic Arthropathy 70
Nexium 188
Non-Steroidal Anti-Inflammatory Drugs
(NSAIDs) 195

O

Oesclim 214
Ogen 214
Omeprazole 188
Opioid Analgesics 142
Oramorph-SR 145
Orthovisc 230
Orudis 202
Oruvail 202
Osteoarthritis (OA) 72
    Criteria for the Classification of
    Idiopathic Osteoarthritis of the Hip 243
    Criteria for the Classification of
    Idiopathic Osteoarthritis of the Knee
    244
Osteoporosis (OP) 75, 211
Oxaprozin 207
Oxycocet 146
Oxycodan 146
Oxycodone 146
OxyContin 146
OxyFAST 146
OxyIR 146

P

Paget's Disease 83
Pamidronate 218
Panadol 138
Pantoloc 188
Pantoprazole 188
Pariet 188
Pentazocine 147
Pepcid 187
Percocet 146
Percocet-Demi 146
Percodan 146
Percodan-Demi 146
Percolone 146

Pethidine 145
Pilocarpine 229
Piroxicam 207
Plaquenil 175
Polyarteritis Nodosa (PAN) 85
    1990 Criteria for the Classification of
    Polyarteritis Nodosa 244
Polymyalgia Rheumatica (PMR) 80
    Criteria 245
Polymyositis 45
Ponstan 204
Ponstel 204
Prednisone 158
Premarin 214
Premplus 214
Prempro 214
Prevacid 188
Prilosec 188
Probonocid 193
Progesterone 215
Prograf 184
Propoxyphene 147
Protein Electrophoresis 237
Proton Pump Inhibitors 188
Protonix 188
Provera 215
Psoriatic Arthritis (PsA) 88
Pulmonary-Renal Syndrome 65

R

Rabeprazole 188
Raji Cell 236
Raloxifene 219
Raynaud's Phenomenon (RP) 91
Reactive Arthritis (ReA) 94
Relafen 205
Relapsing Polychondritis (RP) 97
Remicade 153
Remodulin 226
RF 237
Rheumatic Fever
    Guidelines for the Diagnosis of an
    Initial Attack of Rheumatic Fever
    (Jones Criteria, 1992 Update) 245

Rheumatoid Arthritis (RA) 99
    1087 Revised Classification Criteria
    245
    Assessment of Disease Activity 246
    Classification of Functional Status 246
    Classification of Progression 247
    Clinical Classes of Rheumatoid
    Arthritis Based on Severity 246
    Criteria for Clinical Remission 247
Rheumatoid Factor 237
Rheumatology Laboratory 232
Rheumatrex 179
Rhodis 202
Rhovail 202
Risedronate 220
Rocaltrol 214
Roxicet 146
Roxicodone 146

S

Salagen 229
Salazopyrin 183
Salazopyrin-EN 183
Salflex 208
Salivary Stimulants 228
Salsalate 208
Sandimmune 170
Sarcoidosis 103
Sjogren's Syndrome (SS) 108
    Preliminary Criteria for the
    Classification of Sjogren's syndrome
    247
Solu-Cortef 157
Solu-Medrol 158
Soluspan 159
SPEP 237
Spondyloarthropathies
    European Spondyloarthropathy Study
    Group Classification for
    Spondyloarthropathy 248
Statex 145
Sulfasalazine 183
Sulfinpyrazone 194
Sulindac 208

Supartz 230
Supeudol 146
Surgam 209
Synovial Fluid Analysis 238
Synvisc 230
Systemic Lupus Erythematosus
  1982 Revised Criteria for the
  Classification of Systemic Lupus
  Erythematosus 248
  Acute Lupus Pneumonitis 113
  Alopecia 112
  Anemia 113
  Cardiac Involvement 114
  Chilblains 112
  Discoid Lupus 112
  Gastrointestinal Involvement 116
  Hematologic Involvement 113
  Leukopenia 113
  Lupus nephritis 112
  Lupus Pernio 112
  Malar Rash 112
  Mucocutaneous Involvement 112
  Neuro-Psychiatric Involvement 114
  Pulmonary Involvement 113
  Renal Involvement 112
  Subacute Cutaneous Lupus 112
  Thrombocytopenia 113
Systemic Sclerosis (SSc) 123
  Classification Criteria 249

T

Tacrolimus 184
Takayasu Arteritis (TA) 127
  Classification Criteria 250
Talwin 147
Talwin-NX 147
Tempra 138
Tenoxicam 209
Teriparatide 221
Tiaprofenic Acid 209
Tolectin 210
Tolmetin 210
Toradol 203
Tracleer 224

Tramacet 148
Tramadol 148
Trendelenburg Test 10
Treprostinil 226
Trexall 179
Triamcinolone Acetonide 159
Triamcinolone Hexacetonide 159
Tylenol 138
Tylenol 2, 3, 4 143
Tylox 146

U

Ultracet 148
Ultradol 199
Ultram 148
UPEP 237

V

Vanatrip 138
Viral Arthritis
  Hepatitis B 130
  Hepatitis C 130
  HIV 130
  Parvovirus B19 130
  Rubella 130
Viscosupplementation 230
Vitamin D 214
Vivelle 214
Vivelle-Dot 214
Voltaren 197
Voltaren-SR 197
Voltaren-XR 197

W

Wegener's Granulomatosis (WG) 134
  1990 Criteria for the Classification of
  Wegener's Granulomatosis 250

Z

Zoledronic Acid 222
Zometa 222
Zyloprim 190